The Clinical Utility of Food Addiction and Eating Addiction

The Clinical Utility of Food Addiction and Eating Addiction

Editors

Stephanie Cassin
Sanjeev Sockalingam

MDPI • Basel • Beijing • Wuhan • Barcelona • Belgrade • Manchester • Tokyo • Cluj • Tianjin

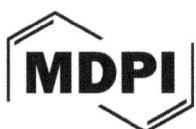

Editors
Stephanie Cassin
Ryerson University
Canada

Sanjeev Sockalingam
Centre for Addiction and Mental Health
Canada

Editorial Office
MDPI
St. Alban-Anlage 66
4052 Basel, Switzerland

This is a reprint of articles from the Special Issue published online in the open access journal *Nutrients* (ISSN 2072-6643) (available at: https://www.mdpi.com/journal/nutrients/special_issues/clinical_food_eating_addiction).

For citation purposes, cite each article independently as indicated on the article page online and as indicated below:

LastName, A.A.; LastName, B.B.; LastName, C.C. Article Title. *Journal Name* **Year**, *Volume Number*, Page Range.

ISBN 978-3-0365-1108-5 (Hbk)
ISBN 978-3-0365-1109-2 (PDF)

© 2021 by the authors. Articles in this book are Open Access and distributed under the Creative Commons Attribution (CC BY) license, which allows users to download, copy and build upon published articles, as long as the author and publisher are properly credited, which ensures maximum dissemination and a wider impact of our publications.

The book as a whole is distributed by MDPI under the terms and conditions of the Creative Commons license CC BY-NC-ND.

Contents

About the Editors vii

Stephanie E. Cassin and Sanjeev Sockalingam
Advances and Future Directions in the Clinical Utility of Food Addiction
Reprinted from: *Nutrients* **2021**, *13*, 708, doi:10.3390/nu13020708 1

Edgar Oliveira, Hyoun S. Kim, Emilie Lacroix, Mária de Fátima Vasques, Cristiane Ruiz Durante, Daniela Pereira, Janice Rico Cabral, Paula Sanches Bernstein, Ximena Garcia, Emma V. Ritchie and Hermano Tavares
The Clinical Utility of Food Addiction: Characteristics and Psychosocial Impairments in a Treatment-Seeking Sample
Reprinted from: *Nutrients* **2020**, *12*, 3388, doi:10.3390/nu12113388 5

Tracy Burrows, Antonio Verdejo-Garcia, Adrian Carter, Robyn M. Brown, Zane B. Andrews, Chris V. Dayas, Charlotte A. Hardman, Natalie Loxton, Priya Sumithran and Megan Whatnall
Health Professionals' and Health Professional Trainees' Views on Addictive Eating Behaviours: A Cross-Sectional Survey
Reprinted from: *Nutrients* **2020**, *12*, 2860, doi:10.3390/nu12092860 15

David Wiss and Timothy Brewerton
Separating the Signal from the Noise: How Psychiatric Diagnoses Can Help Discern Food Addiction from Dietary Restraint
Reprinted from: *Nutrients* **2020**, *12*, 2937, doi:10.3390/nu12102937 31

Stephanie Cassin, Samantha Leung, Raed Hawa, Susan Wnuk, Timothy Jackson and Sanjeev Sockalingam
Food Addiction Is Associated with Binge Eating and Psychiatric Distress among Post-Operative Bariatric Surgery Patients and May Improve in Response to Cognitive Behavioural Therapy
Reprinted from: *Nutrients* **2020**, *12*, 2905, doi:10.3390/nu12102905 61

Ashley A. Wiedemann, Valentina Ivezaj, Ralitza Gueorguieva, Marc N. Potenza and Carlos M. Grilo
Examining Self-Weighing Behaviors and Associated Features and Treatment Outcomes in Patients with Binge-Eating Disorder and Obesity with and without Food Addiction
Reprinted from: *Nutrients* **2020**, *13*, 29, doi:10.3390/nu13010029 73

Eliza L. Gordon, Lisa J. Merlo, Patricia E. Durning and Michael G. Perri
Longitudinal Changes in Food Addiction Symptoms and Body Weight among Adults in a Behavioral Weight-Loss Program
Reprinted from: *Nutrients* **2020**, *12*, 3687, doi:10.3390/nu12123687 85

Robert H. Lustig
Ultraprocessed Food: Addictive, Toxic, and Ready for Regulation
Reprinted from: *Nutrients* **2020**, *12*, 3401, doi:10.3390/nu12113401 103

David A. Wiss, Nicole Avena and Mark Gold
Food Addiction and Psychosocial Adversity: Biological Embedding, Contextual Factors, and Public Health Implications
Reprinted from: *Nutrients* **2020**, *12*, 3521, doi:10.3390/nu12113521 129

Laurie Zawertailo, Sophia Attwells, Wayne K. deRuiter, Thao Lan Le, Danielle Dawson and Peter Selby
Food Addiction and Tobacco Use Disorder: Common Liability and Shared Mechanisms
Reprinted from: *Nutrients* **2020**, *12*, 3834, doi:10.3390/nu12123834 . . . . **155**

Nicolette Stogios, Emily Smith, Roshanak Asgariroozbehani, Laurie Hamel, Alexander Gdanski, Peter Selby, Sanjeev Sockalingam, Ariel Graff-Guerrero, Valerie H. Taylor, Sri Mahavir Agarwal and Margaret K. Hahn
Exploring Patterns of Disturbed Eating in Psychosis: A Scoping Review
Reprinted from: *Nutrients* **2020**, *12*, 3883, doi:10.3390/nu12123883 . . . . **177**

Marzena Jezewska-Zychowicz, Aleksandra Małachowska and Marta Plichta
Does Eating Addiction Favor a More Varied Diet or Contribute to Obesity?—The Case of Polish Adults
Reprinted from: *Nutrients* **2020**, *12*, 1304, doi:10.3390/nu12051304 . . . . **217**

About the Editors

Stephanie Cassin is an Associate Professor of Psychology and Director of the Healthy Eating and Lifestyle (HEAL) Lab at Ryerson University. She also holds a faculty appointment in the Department of Psychiatry at the University of Toronto. Prior to working in academia, she was a staff clinical psychologist in the Bariatric Surgery Program at Toronto Western Hospital. She has expertise in psychosocial interventions for binge eating and obesity. Her research focuses primarily on psychosocial predictors of bariatric (weight loss) surgery outcomes, and psychosocial interventions with the potential to improve outcomes, including cognitive behavioural therapy and motivational interviewing. She also investigates health care innovations that increase treatment accessibility, such as virtual interventions. Dr. Cassin has developed treatment manuals for a number of clinical trials and has published her research widely in peer-reviewed scholarly journals. She is the co-editor of the book *Psychological Care in Severe Obesity: A Practical and Integrated Approach* and regularly trains health care professionals in evidence-based psychosocial interventions for disordered eating and obesity.

Sanjeev Sockalingam is a Professor of Psychiatry at the University of Toronto and the Director of the Bariatric Surgery Psychosocial Program at the Toronto Western Hospital, University Health Network. He is a Clinician Scientist and Vice President of Education at the Centre for Addiction and Mental Health. He is Vice-Chair, Education for Psychiatry at the University of Toronto. He is also the Co-Chair of ECHO Ontario Mental Health, which is a provincial hub-and-spoke knowledge network. Dr. Sockalingam has >190 peer-reviewed publications and is co-editor of the book *Psychiatric Care in Severe Obesity*, a comprehensive summary of an integrated approach to the assessment and managing psychosocial care in severe obesity, and a newly released book by Cambridge University Press, *Psychological Care in Severe Obesity: A Practical Approach*. He has funding from CIHR and other peer-reviewed agencies examining psychosocial outcomes related to obesity care, psychological treatments for obesity, and exploring the construct of food addiction. He is the co-principal investigator on a large multi-site CIHR funded study to evaluate the long-term outcomes of telephone-based cognitive behavioural therapy after bariatric surgery. Dr. Sockalingam is a co-author on the 2020 Canadian Obesity Guidelines.

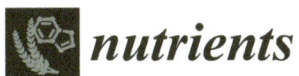

Editorial

Advances and Future Directions in the Clinical Utility of Food Addiction

Stephanie E. Cassin [1,2,3,*] **and Sanjeev Sockalingam** [2,3,4,5,*]

1. Department of Psychology, Ryerson University, 350 Victoria St, Toronto, ON M5B 2K3, Canada
2. Department of Psychiatry, University of Toronto, Toronto, ON M5T 1R8, Canada
3. Centre for Mental Health, University Health Network, Toronto, ON M5G 2C4, Canada
4. Bariatric Surgery Program, University Health Network, Toronto, ON M5T 2S8, Canada
5. Centre for Addiction and Mental Health, 1025 Queen Street West, B1 2nd Floor, Room 2300, Toronto, ON M6J 1H4, Canada
* Correspondence: stephanie.cassin@ryerson.ca (S.E.C.); sanjeev.sockalingam@camh.ca (S.S.)

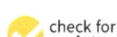

Citation: Cassin, S.E.; Sockalingam, S. Advances and Future Directions in the Clinical Utility of Food Addiction. *Nutrients* **2021**, *13*, 708. https://doi.org/10.3390/nu13020708

Received: 9 February 2021
Accepted: 19 February 2021
Published: 23 February 2021

Publisher's Note: MDPI stays neutral with regard to jurisdictional claims in published maps and institutional affiliations.

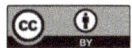

Copyright: © 2021 by the authors. Licensee MDPI, Basel, Switzerland. This article is an open access article distributed under the terms and conditions of the Creative Commons Attribution (CC BY) license (https://creativecommons.org/licenses/by/4.0/).

The body of research examining the validity of food addiction and eating addiction far exceeds the research examining their clinical utility. Although neither food addiction nor eating addiction are officially recognized diagnoses, many individuals self-identify as "food addicts" and/or exceed the cut-offs on measures of addictive-like eating. To be clinically useful, a diagnosis should inform the treatment plan and predict clinical outcomes. This special issue presents a collection of articles, contributed by renowned experts, researchers, and clinicians spanning different disciplines, that adds to the knowledge on the clinical utility of food addiction and eating addiction. The articles in this collection include reviews [1–5] as well as original research utilizing a variety of methodologies and study designs such as clinical trials [6–8], cross-sectional studies [9,10], and surveys [11].

Oliveria et al. [10] examined the characteristics of individuals seeking treatment for food addiction and found that they were very likely to present with comorbid diagnoses (83% of patients). On average, patients presented with 2 to 3 comorbid conditions, with anxiety and mood disorders being the most common. They also reported impairment in psychological, physical, and social functioning, and food addiction was a significant predictor of social impairment even when controlling for binge eating, depression, and anxiety severity.

In their international survey of health care professionals who potentially work with patients presenting with addictive eating behaviour (e.g., dietitians, psychologists), Burrows et al. [11] reported that the majority of respondents had been asked about addictive eating before (72%) and were interested or very interested in receiving training regarding addictive eating. They specifically reported a need for training in assessment/diagnosis (77%) and evidence-based treatments (81%). Therefore, knowledge translation of and training in food addiction assessment and treatment is needed to build capacity amongst healthcare providers.

Wiss & Brewerton [3] contributed a helpful guide to this special issue that can assist with the assessment of food addiction and differential diagnosis. Specifically, they described a comprehensive approach for assessing food addiction that takes into consideration factors such as dietary restraint and comorbid psychiatric disorders. By helping to distinguish food addiction from other forms of eating pathology, this approach aims to guide case formulation and treatment planning. Importantly, the authors concluded that "one size will not fit all in food addiction treatment" (p. 17).

A number of authors contributed papers to this special issue that emphasize the need for individual-level and societal-level interventions for food addiction. In a sample of post-operative bariatric surgery patients, Cassin et al. [6] found that those with food addiction reported greater binge eating characteristics and psychiatric distress relative to those without, and there was preliminary evidence that a brief telephone-based cognitive behavioural therapy intervention may lead to short-term improvement in food addiction symptoms. Two other studies examined food addiction in the context of behavioural weight loss programs. In a sample of individuals with obesity and binge eating disorder participating in a behavioural weight loss program, Wiedemann et al. [7] found that those with food addiction reported a stronger negative reaction to weekly weighing and less acceptance of their weight and shape throughout treatment, and the authors recommended that body image concerns be targeted in treatment given that both of these factors prospectively predicted greater eating disorder psychopathology. Gordon et al. [8] found that food addiction symptoms improved during a behavioural weight loss program; however, more severe food addiction symptomatology was associated with less weight loss. Interestingly, reduced intake of hyperpalatable foods during the program was associated with short-term improvements in food addiction symptoms but not with long-term improvements in food addiction symptoms or weight, suggesting that the association among hyperpalatable foods, food addiction, and weight is a complex one.

In his review and commentary, Lustig [1] provides a compelling argument that "personal intervention must be balanced with societal intervention" (p. 17) and presents evidence that added sugar, and by extension the category of ultraprocessed foods, meets the criteria deemed necessary and sufficient for public health regulatory policy. He then proposes a number of societal interventions, including public education, taxation, subsidies, and restricted access, that have been found effective in reducing the risk and impact of other public health issues. Wiss, Avena, & Gold [4] present a conceptual biopsychosocial model showing how early adversity, trauma, and stress may become biologically embedded and interact with psychological, social, and environmental factors to increase the risk of addiction, including food addiction. Following this model, they recommend a multilevel approach for reducing the risk and impact of food addiction that includes both individual and public health interventions.

Other authors examined the similarities between food addiction and other forms of addiction, or the presence of addictive-like eating in other clinical populations. Zawertailo et al. [5] conducted a narrative scoping review to examine commonalities between food addiction and tobacco use disorder and identified some shared biopsychosocial vulnerability factors (e.g., childhood adversity, attachment insecurity, dopaminergic neurocircuitry) and underlying mechanisms that may help to inform treatment options. They also included the results of a small pilot study examining food addiction among individuals seeking treatment for tobacco use disorder. The research conducted to date has primarily examined food addiction among individuals with other forms of addictions or eating disorders given their overlap, and Stogios et al. [2] extended this line of research into a new clinical population in their scoping review of eating behaviours among individuals with psychosis.

Collectively, the articles included in this special issue suggest that individuals with food addiction, and particularly those presenting for treatment of food addiction, often have comorbid psychiatric diagnoses, body image concerns, and impaired quality of life, and that many health care professionals who potentially work with such patients feel that they need additional knowledge of, and training in, assessment and evidence-based treatments for food addiction. Similar to other addictions such as tobacco use disorder, a multicomponent approach including both individual and societal intervention is warranted to reduce the personal and public health impact of food addiction.

As research attention shifts from examining the validity to the clinical utility of food and eating addiction, many questions remain to be answered. What factors predict treatment seeking among individuals with food or eating addiction? What are the treatment preferences of individuals with food or eating addiction? Are existing evidence-based treatments for eating disorders or substance-related and addictive disorders effective among individuals with food or eating addiction? What can be done to improve the durability of treatment effects of those interventions that have already been examined and found to improve only short-term outcomes? What is the evidence for abstinence-based versus moderation approaches? How do patients experience each of these interventions?

What do they find helpful and unhelpful, and what do they attribute any changes to? Recognizing that "one size will not fit all", how can we move to personalized approaches to food addiction treatment (i.e., what treatment for whom)? We hope that the articles included in this special issue will provide the impetus to explore these important questions and generate knowledge to inform clinical practice guidelines.

Author Contributions: Both authors conceptualized and contributed to writing this editorial. All authors have read and agreed to the published version of the manuscript.

Funding: This research received no external funding.

Conflicts of Interest: The authors declare no conflict of interest.

References

1. Lustig, R.H. Ultraprocessed Food: Addictive, Toxic, and Ready for Regulation. *Nutrients* **2020**, *12*, 3401. [CrossRef] [PubMed]
2. Stogios, N.; Smith, E.; Asgariroozbehani, R.; Hamel, L.; Gdanski, A.; Selby, P.; Sockalingam, S.; Graff-Guerrero, A.; Taylor, V.H.; Agarwal, S.M.; et al. Exploring Patterns of Disturbed Eating in Psychosis: A Scoping Review. *Nutrients* **2020**, *12*, 3883. [CrossRef] [PubMed]
3. Wiss, D.; Brewerton, T. Separating the Signal from the Noise: How Psychiatric Diagnoses Can Help Discern Food Addiction from Dietary Restraint. *Nutrients* **2020**, *12*, 2937. [CrossRef] [PubMed]
4. Wiss, D.A.; Avena, N.; Gold, M. Food Addiction and Psychosocial Adversity: Biological Embedding, Contextual Factors, and Public Health Implications. *Nutrients* **2020**, *12*, 3521. [CrossRef] [PubMed]
5. Zawertailo, L.; Attwells, S.; deRuiter, W.K.; Le, T.L.; Dawson, D.; Selby, P. Food Addiction and Tobacco Use Disorder: Common Liability and Shared Mechanisms. *Nutrients* **2020**, *12*, 3834. [CrossRef] [PubMed]
6. Cassin, S.; Leung, S.; Hawa, R.; Wnuk, S.; Jackson, T.; Sockalingam, S. Food Addiction Is Associated with Binge Eating and Psychiatric Distress among Post-Operative Bariatric Surgery Patients and May Improve in Response to Cognitive Behavioural Therapy. *Nutrients* **2020**, *12*, 2905. [CrossRef] [PubMed]
7. Wiedemann, A.A.; Ivezaj, V.; Gueorguieva, R.; Potenza, M.N.; Grilo, C.M. Examining Self-Weighing Behaviors and Associated Features and Treatment Outcomes in Patients with Binge-Eating Disorder and Obesity with and without Food Addiction. *Nutrients* **2021**, *13*, 29. [CrossRef] [PubMed]
8. Gordon, E.L.; Merlo, L.J.; Durning, P.E.; Perri, M.G. Longitudinal Changes in Food Addiction Symptoms and Body Weight among Adults in A Behavioral Weight-Loss Program. *Nutrients* **2020**, *12*, 3687. [CrossRef] [PubMed]
9. Jezewska-Zychowicz, M.; Małachowska, A.; Plichta, M. Does Eating Addiction Favor A More Varied Diet or Contribute to Obesity?—The Case of Polish Adults. *Nutrients* **2020**, *12*, 1304. [CrossRef] [PubMed]
10. Oliveira, E.; Kim, H.S.; Lacroix, E.; de Fátima Vasques, M.; Durante, C.R.; Pereira, D.; Cabral, J.R.; Bernstein, P.S.; Garcia, X.; Ritchie, E.V.; et al. The Clinical Utility of Food Addiction: Characteristics and Psychosocial Impairments in A Treatment-Seeking Sample. *Nutrients* **2020**, *12*, 3388. [CrossRef] [PubMed]
11. Burrows, T.; Verdejo-Garcia, A.; Carter, A.; Brown, R.M.; Andrews, Z.B.; Dayas, C.V.; Hardman, C.A.; Loxton, N.; Sumithran, P.; Whatnall, M. Health Professionals' and Health Professional Trainees' Views on Addictive Eating Behaviours: A Cross-Sectional Survey. *Nutrients* **2020**, *12*, 2860. [CrossRef] [PubMed]

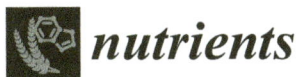

Article

The Clinical Utility of Food Addiction: Characteristics and Psychosocial Impairments in a Treatment-Seeking Sample

Edgar Oliveira [1,*], Hyoun S. Kim [2,*], Emilie Lacroix [3], Mária de Fátima Vasques [1], Cristiane Ruiz Durante [1], Daniela Pereira [1], Janice Rico Cabral [1], Paula Sanches Bernstein [1], Ximena Garcia [3], Emma V. Ritchie [4] and Hermano Tavares [1]

1. Department of Psychiatry, University of São Paulo, Rua Artur de Azevedo, 145, Cerqueira Cesar, São Paulo CEP 05404-010, SP, Brasil; vasquesfatima10@gmail.com (M.d.F.V.); crisnutrition@hotmail.com (C.R.D.); dani.psico8@gmail.com (D.P.); janice.rcabral@gmail.com (J.R.C.); paulabernstein@ciencias.com.br (P.S.B.); hermanot@usp.br (H.T.)
2. Department of Psychology, Ryerson University, 350 Victoria Street, Toronto, ON M5B 2K3, Canada
3. Department of Psychology, University of Calgary, 2500 University Drive, NW, Calgary, AB T2N 1N4, Canada; emilie.lacroix@ucalgary.ca (E.L.); xgarcia@ucalgary.ca (X.G.)
4. Department of Psychology, York University, 4700 Keele St, Toronto, ON M3J 1P3, Canada; evritchi@yorku.ca
* Correspondence: dredgaroliveirapq@gmail.com (E.O.); andrewhs.kim@ryerson.ca (H.S.K.)

Received: 9 October 2020; Accepted: 2 November 2020; Published: 4 November 2020

Abstract: Little is known about the characteristics of individuals seeking treatment for food addiction (FA), and the clinical utility of FA has yet to be established. To address these gaps, we examined (i) the demographic, eating pathology, and psychiatric conditions associated with FA and (ii) whether FA is associated with psychosocial impairments when accounting for eating-related and other psychopathology. Forty-six patients seeking treatment for FA completed self-report questionnaires and semi-structured clinical interviews. The majority of the sample were women and self-identified as White, with a mean age of 43 years. Most participants (83.3%) presented with a comorbid psychiatric condition, most commonly anxiety and mood disorders, with a mean of 2.31 comorbid conditions. FA was associated with binge eating severity and anxiety symptoms, as well as psychological, physical, and social impairment. In regression analyses controlling for binge eating severity, food cravings, depression, and anxiety, FA remained a significant predictor only of social impairment. Taken together, the results suggest that individuals seeking treatment for FA are likely to present with significant comorbid conditions, in particular anxiety disorders. The results of the present research provide evidence for the clinical utility of FA, particularly in explaining social impairment.

Keywords: food addiction; clinical utility; psychosocial impairment; comorbidity; quality of life

1. Introduction

The food addiction (FA) hypothesis posits that foods that are highly processed and rich in salt, sugar, and fat have "addictive potential". In other words, certain foods may have the ability to provoke symptoms of substance use disorders [1]. Empirical research on the concept of food addiction is rapidly growing, and animal and human studies have demonstrated similarities between food and drugs that are abused, particularly with respect to their effects on reward pathways in the brain [2,3]. FA, assessed using the self-report Yale Food Addiction Scale [4], which applies substance use disorder criteria to food and eating has been found to be relatively common, ranging from 3% to 20% in non-clinical samples [4]. Rates of FA are higher in eating disorder samples, with some studies finding rates as high as 95% among women with bulimia nervosa [4]. FA is also relatively common in Brazil, with Nunes-Neto and colleagues (2018) reporting a prevalence rate of 4.3% in a large web-based sample [5].

The concept of FA is heavily debated, with some arguing that it pathologizes everyday eating behaviors [6] or does not hold incremental clinical utility beyond existing eating disorder diagnoses [7]. According to the 5th edition of the Diagnostic and Statistical Manual of Mental Disorders, "The diagnosis of a mental disorder should have clinical utility: it should help clinicians to determine prognosis, treatment plans, and potential outcomes for their patients" (p. 20) [8]. However, the clinical utility of FA constitutes an important gap in the field. A systematic review examining the correlates of FA reported a relationship with body mass index, binge eating, and mixed results with other psychopathology including depression [9]. Since the review, studies have also revealed an association between FA and demographic characteristics [10], lower quality of life [11], psychological distress [12,13], problematic eating behaviors [13–15], and impulsivity [5,14]. Regarding psychosocial impairments, FA has been shown to have moderate to strong associations that remain significant when other forms of eating pathology are controlled for [16]. Within a Brazilian context, Nunes-Neto and colleagues also found associations between FA and psychopathology and lower quality of life in psychological, physical, social, and environment domains [5]. Thus, there is evidence to suggest that FA may be associated with unique characteristics and psychosocial impairments, providing preliminary support for its clinical utility.

Although these studies are informative, a major limitation is that they have all consisted of non-clinical samples or people experiencing difficulties with weight and eating disorders. Additionally, previous studies have not controlled for the impact of comorbid psychopathology on psychosocial impairments. As such, it is unclear whether the documented clinical characteristics and psychosocial impairments stem from FA or from other conditions, which provides a limited understanding of the clinical utility of FA. Furthermore, the incremental clinical utility of FA is not known, that is, whether it contributes useful information above and beyond what may be explained by the comorbid psychopathology. It is critical to examine the incremental utility of FA among individuals seeking treatment for this concern, given that there is already emerging literature recommending various treatment strategies for FA [17,18]. In this light, the aim of the present study was to address gaps in the understanding of the clinical utility of FA by examining clinical characteristics (demographics, eating disorders, cravings, psychiatric conditions) and psychosocial impairments (controlling for common psychopathology) in a clinical sample with the primary concern of FA.

2. Materials and Methods

2.1. Participants and Procedures

Participants were 46 patients seeking treatment for food addiction at a specialized university outpatient clinic associated with the University of São Paulo, Faculty of Medicine in São Paulo, Brazil. Patients were self-referred through the community or referred by other treatment programs affiliated with the University. At intake, patients were assessed by a registered psychiatrist to determine their suitability for treatment. The eligibility criteria for treatment were as follows: (i) meet criteria for moderate-to-severe FA as assessed by the Yale Food Addiction Scale 2.0 (YFAS 2.0) [19] and (ii) 18 years of age or over. Exclusion criteria included (i) an organic condition that may explain eating pathology (e.g., endocrine disturbances); (ii) acute psychosis, mania, or borderline personality disorder; (iii) cognitive impairments that may interfere with treatment; and (iv) being currently pregnant or breastfeeding. Current psychiatric conditions were assessed by psychiatrists using the Brazilian Portuguese version of the Mini International Neuropsychiatric Interview (MINI) [20] using the Diagnostic and Statistical Manual of Mental Disorders - IV criteria. The MINI is a brief, semi-structured clinical interview with strong psychometric properties and high inter-rater reliability compared to the Structured Clinical Interview for the DSM [20]. The treatment consisted of 15 weekly sessions of group schema therapy and six sessions of behavioral nutrition delivered by two psychologists and two nutritionists [21].

Ethics approval was obtained from the Faculty of Medicine, University of São Paulo (12820813.5.0000.0068). The research was conducted in accordance with the Declaration of Helsinki. All patients were informed that research participation was voluntary and would not impact their treatment. All participants provided their consent to participate in the study.

2.2. Measures

2.2.1. Demographic Information

Participants reported their age, gender, ethnicity, and marital and employment status.

2.2.2. Food Addiction Severity

The Yale Food Addiction Scale 2.0 (YFAS 2.0) [19] was used to assess FA severity. The YFAS 2.0 contains 35 items ($\alpha = 0.90$) assessing the 11 DSM-5 substance use disorder criteria applied to FA, including two items to assess distress and impairment. The items are anchored from 0 (never) to 7 (every day) with total scores ranging from 0 to 235. In addition to providing a total score, the YFAS 2.0 provides a total symptom count, as well as a categorical "diagnosis" of food addiction (None = ≤1 symptom and/or lack of distress or impairment; Mild = 2 to 3 symptoms plus distress and/or impairment; Moderate = 4 to 5 symptoms plus distress and/or impairment; Severe = ≥6 symptoms plus distress and/or impairment). The YFAS 2.0 was translated and back-translated to Brazilian Portuguese by the senior author (H.T.), a content expert who is fluent in both languages.

2.2.3. Binge Eating Severity

Binge eating severity was assessed using the Brazilian-Portuguese version of the Binge Eating Scale (BES) [22]. The BES consists of 16 items ($\alpha = 0.80$) assessing the behavioral, affective, and cognitive components associated with binge eating. The response options for BES range from 0 to 3, with two questions containing three response options. As such, the total scores on the BES range from 0 to 46, with higher scores indicating greater binge eating severity.

2.2.4. Food Craving (Trait)

The Brazilian-Portuguese validated version of the Food Cravings Questionnaire—Trait version (FCQ-T) [23] was used to assess the frequency and intensity of participants' food-related cravings. The FCQ-T contains 39 items ($\alpha = 0.94$) assessing a variety of dimensions related to food cravings. The items are anchored from 1 (never or not applicable) to 6 (always). Total scores (39–234) are calculated by summing the items with higher scores indicating greater food-related cravings.

2.2.5. Psychiatric Comorbidities

Symptoms of depression and anxiety were assessed using the Brazilian-Portuguese validated versions of the 21-item Beck Depression Inventory (BDI-II) [24] ($\alpha = 0.90$) and the 21-item Beck Anxiety Inventory (BAI) [25] ($\alpha = 0.87$), respectively. Both the BDI and BAI are anchored from 0 to 3 with total scores ranging from 0 to 63. The MINI provided diagnostic coverage of current psychiatric conditions, including mood, anxiety, substance use, and eating disorders.

2.2.6. Quality of Life

A Brazilian-Portuguese validated version of the WHOQOL-bref [26] was used to assess quality of life in four domains: psychological, physical, social, and environment. The WHOQOL-bref contains 26 items ($\alpha = 0.91$) with items ranging from 1 to 5. Mean scores were computed for each domain, with lower scores indicating worse quality of life in the domains.

2.3. Data Analytic Plan

First, descriptive statistics were used to examine demographic characteristics and current psychiatric conditions. Next, two-tailed bivariate correlation analyses were conducted to examine associations among YFAS 2.0 total scores, food cravings, binge eating severity, symptoms of depression/anxiety, and quality of life. Lastly, a multiple regression analysis was conducted with the psychological, physical, social, and environmental domains of the WHOQOL-bref as the criterion variable and binge eating severity, food craving, symptoms of depression, and anxiety as the predictor variables to examine whether FA predicted psychosocial impairments above and beyond common comorbidities associated with FA.

3. Results

3.1. Clinical Characteristics

The sample consisted of more women ($n = 37$; 80.4%) than men ($n = 9$; 19.6%). The mean age was 43.28 (*Standard Deviation [SD]* = 10.82) years. Regarding ethnicity, the majority of the sample self-identified as White ($n = 36$; 78.3%), five as mixed (10.9%), three as Black (6.5%), and one as Asian (2.2%). One participant did not disclose their ethnicity. Roughly half ($n = 24$; 52.2%) of the participants reported being in a relationship, and the majority ($n = 43$; 93.48%) reported being employed. The mean score on the YFAS 2.0 was 9.12 ($SD = 1.81$), which corresponds to severe symptoms of food addiction.

Of the 42 patients who completed the MINI, 35 (83.3%) met criteria for at least one current psychiatric condition, with a mean of 2.31 ($SD = 1.87$) comorbid conditions (Table 1). The most common current psychiatric condition was generalized anxiety disorder ($n = 26$; 61.9%), followed by major depressive episode ($n = 20$; 47.6%), suicidality ($n = 11$; 26.8%), agoraphobia ($n = 9$; 21.4%), and social anxiety ($n = 8$; 19.0%). Regarding eating disorders, seven (16.7%) participants met criteria for bulimia nervosa, and none met criteria for anorexia nervosa. Relatively few, if any, participants met current diagnostic criteria for post-traumatic stress disorder ($n = 1$; 2.4%) or alcohol or substance use/dependence ($n = 1$; 2.4%).

Table 1. Frequencies of current psychiatric conditions met by participants using the Mini International Neuropsychiatric Interview (MINI).

Psychiatric Diagnoses	Yes	No
Major Depressive Episode	20 (47.6%)	22 (52.4%)
Dysthymia	4 (9.5%)	38 (90.5%)
Suicidality	11 (26.8%)	30 (73.2%)
Panic Disorder	4 (9.5%)	38 (90.5%)
Agoraphobia	9 (21.4%)	33 (78.6%)
Social Anxiety	8 (19.0%)	34 (81.0%)
Generalized Anxiety	26 (61.9%)	15 (38.1%)
Obsessive Compulsive Disorder	6 (14.3%)	36 (85.7%)
Post-Traumatic Stress Disorder	1 (2.4%)	41 (97.6%)
Alcohol Abuse/Dependence	1 (2.4%)	41 (97.6%)
Substance Abuse/Dependence	0 (0.0%)	42 (100.0%)
Anorexia Nervosa	0 (0.0%)	42 (100.0%)
Anorexia Nervosa Binge/Purge Type	0 (0.0%)	42 (100.0%)
Bulimia Nervosa	7 (16.7%)	35 (83.3%)
Any Current Condition	35 (83.3%)	7 (16.7%)

3.2. Correlation Analyses

Means, standard deviations, and correlations among the variables of interest are presented in Table 2. Food addiction severity was positively correlated with binge eating severity and anxiety symptoms, and negatively correlated with the psychological, physical, and social domains of the WHOQOL-bref. Food addiction severity was not significantly correlated with food craving, depression symptoms, or the environment domain of the WHOQOL-bref, $p > 0.055$.

Table 2. Means, standard deviation, and correlations between our variables of interest.

	M	SD	1	2	3	4	5	6	7	8	9
1. YFAS2.0	142.45	34.89	-	0.42 **	0.26	0.28	0.50 ***	−0.37 *	−0.32 *	−0.44 **	−0.29
2. BES	30.46	7.60		-	0.63 ***	0.43 **	0.36 *	−0.54 **	−0.63 ***	−0.12	−0.22
3. FCQ-T	166.39	30.27			-	0.22	0.30 *	−0.35 *	−0.39 **	−0.09	−0.14
4. BDI	20.31	10.37				-	0.53 **	−0.86 ***	−0.73 ***	−0.43 **	−0.53 ***
5. BAI	16.66	10.42					-	−0.57 ***	−0.55 ***	−0.25	−0.42 **
6. WHO_Psyc	10.77	2.94						-	0.81 ***	0.52 ***	0.64 ***
7. WHO_Phys	12.07	2.74							-	0.42 **	0.51 ***
8. WHO_Soc	11.68	3.63								-	0.56 ***
9. WHO_Env	12.65	2.36									-

Note. YFAS 2.0 = Yale Food Addiction Scale 2.0; BES = Binge Eating Scale; FCQ-T = Food Craving Questionnaire—Trait; BDI = Beck Depression Inventory; BAI = Beck Anxiety Inventory; WHO = WHOQOL-bref; Psyc = psychological; Phys = physical; Soc = social; Env = environmental. * $p < 0.05$; ** $p < 0.01$; *** $p < 0.001$. M = Mean, SD = Standard deviation.

3.3. Multiple Regression

3.3.1. Psychological Impairment

The multiple regression model predicting psychological impairment was statistically significant $F(5,35) = 29.84$, $p < 0.001$, adj. $R^2 = 0.78$. In this model, only symptoms of depression significantly predicted psychological impairment. FA, binge eating, symptoms of anxiety, and food craving were not significant predictors (Table 3). A post hoc power analysis indicated a power of 1.0 based on our results.

Table 3. Multiple regression results predicting psychological impairments measured using the WHOQOL-bref.

Psychological Impairment	b	LL	UL	SE b	B	adj. R^2	R^2C
Model						0.78	0.81 ***
Constant	17.62 ***	14.92	20.33				
Food Addiction	−0.01	−0.02	0.01	0.01	−0.08		
Anxiety Symptoms	−0.01	−0.06	0.05	0.03	−0.03		
Depression Symptoms	−0.22 ***	−0.27	−0.17	0.03	−0.78 ***		
Binge Eating Symptoms	−0.07	−0.13	−0.01	0.04	−0.19		
Food Craving	0.003	−0.02	0.02	0.01	0.04		

Note. b = unstandardized beta, LL = Lower limit, UL = Upper limit, SE b = Standard error of unstandardized beta, B = standardized beta, adj.R^2 = adjusted R^2, R^2C = R^2 Change. *** $p < 0.001$.

3.3.2. Physical Impairment

The multiple regression model was statistically significant, $F(5,35) = 13.36$, $p < 0.001$, adj. $R^2 = 0.61$. Symptoms of depression and binge eating significantly predicted physical impairments. On the other hand, FA, symptoms of anxiety, and food craving were not significant predictors of physical impairments (Table 4). A post hoc power analysis indicated a power of 0.99 based on our results.

Table 4. Multiple regression results predicting physical impairments measured using WHOQOL-bref.

Physical Impairment	b	LL	UL	SE b	B	adj. R^2	R^2C
Model						0.61	0.66 ***
Constant	19.24 ***	15.68	22.79				
Food Addiction	0.01	−0.01	0.03	0.01	0.09		
Anxiety Symptoms	−0.05	−0.12	0.02	0.03	−0.17		
Depression Symptoms	−0.13 ***	−0.20	−0.06	0.03	−0.48 ***		

Table 4. *Cont.*

Physical Impairment	b	LL	UL	SE b	B	adj. R^2	R^2C
Binge Eating Symptoms	−0.14 **	−0.23	−0.04	0.05	−0.38 **		
Food Craving	−0.003	−0.03	0.02	0.01	−0.04		

Note. b = unstandardized beta, LL = Lower limit, UL = Upper limit, SE b = Standard error of unstandardized beta, B = standardized beta, adj.R^2 = adjusted R^2, R^2C = R^2 Change. ** $p < 0.01$, *** $p < 0.001$.

3.3.3. Social Impairment

The multiple regression model was statistically significant, $F(5,35) = 4.10$, $p = 0.005$, adj. $R^2 = 0.28$. FA and symptoms of depression were significant predictors of social impairments. Symptoms of anxiety, binge eating severity, and food craving were not significant predictors (Table 5). A post hoc power analysis indicated a power of 0.95 with the parameters of our observed results. FA symptoms remained a significant predictor of social impairment $b = -0.049$, $t = -3.20$, $p = 0.004$ when controlling for age, gender, marital status, ethnicity, and body mass index.

Table 5. Multiple regression results predicting social impairments measured using WHOQOL-bref.

Social Impairment	b	LL	UL	SE b	B	adj. R^2	R^2C
Model						0.28	0.37 **
Constant	16.57 ***	10.38	22.77				
Food Addiction	−0.05 **	−0.08	−0.02	0.02	−0.49 **		
Anxiety Symptoms	0.05	−0.08	0.17	0.06	0.13		
Depression Symptoms	−0.18 **	−0.29	−0.06	0.06	−0.50 **		
Binge Eating Symptoms	0.09	−0.08	0.26	0.09	0.19		
Food Craving	0.01	−0.03	0.05	0.02	0.09		

Note. b = unstandardized beta, LL = Lower limit, UL = Upper limit, SE b = Standard error of unstandardized beta, B = standardized beta, adj.R^2 = adjusted R^2, R^2C = R^2 Change. ** $p < 0.01$; *** $p < 0.001$.

3.3.4. Environmental

The multiple regression model predicting environmental impairment was statistically significant, $F(5,35) = 3.17$, $p = 0.018$, adj. $R^2 = 0.21$. In this model, only symptoms of depression were significant. FA, binge eating, symptoms of anxiety, and food craving were not significant predictors of environmental impairments (Table 6). A post hoc power analysis indicated a power of 0.88 based on our results.

Table 6. Multiple regression results predicting environmental impairments measured using WHOQOL-bref.

Environmental Impairment	b	LL	UL	SE b	B	adj. R^2	R^2C
Model						0.21	0.31 *
Constant	14.51 ***	10.28	18.74				
Food Addiction	−0.01	−0.03	0.01	0.01	−0.16		
Anxiety Symptoms	−0.02	−0.10	0.06	0.04	−0.09		
Depression Symptoms	−0.11 **	−0.19	−0.03	0.04	−0.48 **		
Binge Eating Symptoms	−0.001	−0.12	0.12	0.06	−0.004		
Food Craving	0.01	−0.02	0.04	0.02	0.15		

Note. b = unstandardized beta, LL = Lower limit, UL = Upper limit, SE b = Standard error of unstandardized beta, B = standardized beta, adj.R^2 = adjusted R^2, R^2C = R^2 Change. * $p < 0.05$; ** $p < 0.01$; *** $p < 0.001$.

4. Discussion

The present study is, to our knowledge, the first to examine the clinical characteristics and psychosocial impairments of individuals for whom FA is the primary concern and reason for seeking treatment. Regarding demographic characteristics, the sample consisted mainly of women, consistent with previous studies reporting a higher prevalence of FA among women [4]. A potential explanation for this gender difference is that the weight gain associated with or expected to occur as a consequence of food addiction may be more distressing to women given they are under greater sociocultural pressure to conform to a thin body ideal [27]. As a result, women may be more likely to be distressed by and seek treatment for FA. Nonetheless, in the current study, roughly one in five participants seeking treatment were men, providing further evidence for the clinical significance of FA among individuals of both these genders. Future studies investigating gender differences in the clinical characteristics of those seeking treatment for FA would be highly informative. Indeed, to increase the generalizability of characterizations of FA across the gender spectrum, it is important to avoid under-representation of men and individuals who identify as transgender or gender non-binary in studies of FA.

Regarding the relationship between FA and binge eating, the mean score of the participants on the BES was in the severe range, and FA was moderately ($r = 0.42$) associated with binge eating, consistent with previous research [15]. These findings suggest binge eating disorder may be a common comorbidity; however, given that the correlation between FA and BES scores was far from perfect, there does not appear to be a complete overlap between these two constructs. Regarding other eating disorders, no participants met the diagnostic criteria for anorexia nervosa including the binge/purge subtype, and less than 1 in 5 participants met diagnostic criteria for bulimia nervosa. These results may be partly attributable to the low base rates of anorexia nervosa and bulimia nervosa and are consistent with prior evidence that FA can occur outside the context of eating disorders [28,29].

The majority of participants reported a current psychiatric condition, with patients meeting criteria for two diagnoses on average. However, it should be noted that 16.7% of the participants did not meet criteria for any current psychiatric conditions. This result suggests that there likely exists a group of individuals with FA who may not meet criteria for a recognized eating disorder or other psychiatric condition, yet still experience psychosocial impairment severe enough to warrant seeking treatment. Addictive disorders were not very common in the sample, which is surprising given the conceptualization of FA as an addiction and given that addictive disorders tend to co-occur [30,31]. Additionally, FA was not related to cravings, which is also a hallmark symptom of addictive disorders. A potential reason for this finding may be due to the relatively small sample size as the association between FA and craving was approaching significance with close to a moderate effect size ($p = 0.087$, $r = 0.26$). Thus, future research with large samples is needed to further investigate the association of FA with other addictive behaviors, to examine whether they are likely to co-occur, and whether FA is associated with hallmark characteristics of addictive disorders such as heightened levels of impulsivity.

The most frequent comorbid conditions were anxiety and mood disorders. Interestingly, however, FA was not significantly correlated with severity of depression in contrast to previous findings but in line with others [9]. Given the mixed findings in the literature regarding the association between FA and depression, further research is warranted. On the other hand, FA was significantly associated with severity of anxiety. Furthermore, anxiety disorders were the most frequent disorders in patients seeking treatment for FA. Longitudinal studies would be highly valuable in determining the temporal relationships between FA and anxiety.

FA was significantly associated with physical, psychological, and social impairment in our univariate analyses. FA remained a significant predictor of social impairment when controlling for binge eating, craving, depression, and anxiety. These results provide some support for the incremental clinical utility of FA, specifically in regard to social impairment, and suggest that individuals seeking treatment for FA may experience significant impairments in their social and interpersonal lives. These results are consistent with qualitative research [32], wherein people with FA described significant interpersonal difficulties as a result of FA. They reported that the shame, secrecy, and judgment by others regarding their difficulties with FA led them to withdraw from social situations, resulting in social and interpersonal harm.

Taken together, the results of the present research hold some implications for the clinical utility (i.e., prognosis, treatment plans, potential outcomes) of FA. Given the cross-sectional nature of our data, it would be premature to draw definitive conclusions regarding the prognosis or treatment of FA. Nonetheless, our findings identified factors worthy of further study using longitudinal and experimental designs, to examine whether they play a causal role in the generation or maintenance of FA symptoms or in recovery from FA. For example, given the significant association between FA and anxiety, it is plausible that excessive food consumption may represent a maladaptive coping mechanism to manage symptoms of anxiety, as was described by participants in an earlier qualitative study conducted by our team [32]. Using addictive behaviors to regulate one's emotions is a hallmark characteristic of addictions. Previous reports have distinguished two types of emotion regulation goals that may motivate addictive behavior: reducing aversive emotional states such as anxiety (a form of negative reinforcement) or increasing positive affect via the introduction of a pleasurable stimulus (a form of positive reinforcement). Some addictive behaviors such as alcohol abuse may be more motivated by the former goal, whereas others, such as gambling, may be motivated by the latter [33,34]. Our findings suggest that, in FA, eating may be used primarily as a means of reducing aversive emotional states, rather than for increasing positive affect. This finding is consistent with a prior qualitative study where participants emphasized eating as a means of temporarily reducing aversive emotional states [32].

From a potential treatment perspective, if addictive-like eating represents a maladaptive response to anxiety, then clinicians may wish to employ an integrated treatment model to address difficulties with anxiety and FA simultaneously, by the same team of clinicians. Indeed, an integrative approach has been associated with improved outcomes compared to a sequential or parallel treatment approach when addressing multiple concerns [35]. Regarding social impairments, should social functioning be identified as a causal or perpetuating factor in the development and maintenance of FA symptoms, incorporating aspects of social skill training into the treatment plan may lead to improved prognosis, and social impairment may represent an outcome to track in progress monitoring. That said, more research is needed regarding the associations between FA and anxiety as well as social impairments before recommending potential treatment strategies for FA. Lastly, the results suggest that it may be helpful to monitor treatment outcomes not only for FA but also for related conditions given the high rates of psychiatric conditions, in particular anxiety disorders, and the strong associations between FA, binge eating, and depression.

Limitations

Several limitations are worth noting. First, the cross-sectional design does not allow for causal inferences between FA and our variables of interest. Second, given the relatively small sample size, future research with larger samples is needed to replicate the findings of the present research. Having said that, the sample in the present study is one of the largest clinical samples of FA, and to our knowledge, the only study investigating clinical characteristics of people seeking treatment whose primary concern is FA. Third, the version of the MINI used in the present research captured DSM-IV diagnoses and as such did not capture binge eating disorder. Rather, in the present research, the well-known and used Binge Eating Scale was used to examine the relationship between FA and binge eating disorder. However, the BES was developed prior to the inclusion of binge eating disorder in the DSM-5 and thus was not designed to diagnose binge eating disorder [27]. Importantly, FA predicted social impairments when controlling for binge eating symptoms, providing some support for the clinical utility of FA. Lastly, although FA predicted social impairment when controlling for demographic factors and Body mass index, it is possible that other variables may have influenced the results. As such, future research controlling for other confounding variables would provide further support for our results.

5. Conclusions

In the past decade, there has been an increased empirical interest in FA. Although our knowledge of FA has grown exponentially, less is known regarding the clinical utility of FA, which impedes progress in developing efficacious treatments for this relatively common concern. The current study suggests that people seeking treatment for FA are likely to present with co-occurring psychiatric conditions and experience impairments in social functioning, over and beyond other psychopathology. Taken together, the results suggest FA holds some clinical utility. The results of the present research, as well as future research investigating the clinical utility of FA, may help in providing knowledge on the potential treatment possibilities for people with FA.

Author Contributions: Conceptualization, E.O., H.S.K., M.d.F.V., C.R.D., and E.L.; methodology, E.O. and H.T.; formal analysis, H.S.K.; investigation, C.R.D., D.P., J.R.C., and P.S.B.; resources, H.T.; data curation X.G. and E.V.R.; supervision, M.d.F.V. and H.T.; writing—original draft preparation, E.O., H.S.K., and E.L.; writing—review and editing, X.G., E.V.R., and H.T. All authors have read and agreed to the published version of the manuscript.

Funding: This research received no external funding.

Conflicts of Interest: The authors declare no conflict of interest.

References

1. Ifland, J.R.; Preuss, H.G.; Marcus, M.T.; Rourke, K.M.; Taylor, W.C.; Burau, K.; Jacobs, W.S.; Kadish, W.; Manso, G. Refined food addiction: A classic substance use disorder. *Med. Hypotheses* **2009**, *72*, 518–526. [CrossRef]
2. Gearhardt, A.N.; Corbin, W.R.; Brownell, K. Food addiction: An examination of the diagnostic criteria for dependence. *J. Addict. Med.* **2009**, *3*, 1–7. [CrossRef] [PubMed]
3. Meule, A.; Gearhardt, A.N. Food addiction in the light of DSM-5. *Nutrients* **2014**, *6*, 3653–3671. [CrossRef]
4. Meule, A.; Gearhardt, A.N. Ten years of the Yale Food Addiction Scale: A review of Version 2.0. *Curr. Addict. Rep.* **2019**, *6*, 218–228. [CrossRef]
5. Nunes-Neto, P.R.; Köhler, C.A.; Schuch, F.B.; Solmi, M.; Quevedo, J.; Maes, M.; Murru, A.; Vieta, E.; McIntyre, R.S.; McElroy, S.L.; et al. Food addiction: Prevalence, psychopathological correlates and associations with quality of life in a large sample. *J. Psychiatr. Res.* **2018**, *96*, 145–152. [CrossRef] [PubMed]
6. Finlayson, G. Food addiction and obesity: Unnecessary medicalization of hedonic overeating. *Nat. Rev. Endocrinol.* **2017**, *13*, 493–498. [CrossRef] [PubMed]
7. Davis, C. Compulsive overeating as an addictive behavior: Overlap between food addiction and binge eating disorder. *Curr. Obes. Rep.* **2013**, *2*, 171–178. [CrossRef]
8. American Psychiatric Association. *Diagnostics and Statistical Manual of Mental Disorders*, 5th ed.; (DSM-5); American Psychiatric Publishing: Washington, DC, USA, 2013.
9. Long, C.G.; Blundell, J.E.; Finlayson, G. A systematic review of the application and correlates of YFAS-diagnosed "food addiction" in humans: Are eating-related "addictions" a cause for concern or empty concepts? *Obes. Facts* **2015**, *8*, 386–401. [CrossRef]
10. Schulte, E.M.; Gearhardt, A.N. Associations of food addiction in a sample recruited to be nationally representative of the United States. *Eur. Eat. Disord. Rev.* **2018**, *26*, 112–119. [CrossRef]
11. Wiedemann, A.A.; Lawson, J.L.; Cunningham, P.M.; Khalvati, K.M.; Lydecker, J.A.; Ivezaj, V.; Grilo, C.M. Food addiction among men and women in India. *Eur. Eat. Disord. Rev.* **2018**, *26*, 597–604. [CrossRef]
12. Raymond, K.L.; Lovell, G.P. Food addiction associations with psychological distress among people with type 2 diabetes. *J. Diabetes Complicat.* **2016**, *30*, 651–656. [CrossRef] [PubMed]
13. Koball, A.M.; Clark, M.M.; Collazo-Clavell, M.; Kellogg, T.; Ames, G.; Ebbert, J.; Grothe, K.B. The relationship among food addiction, negative mood, and eating-disordered behaviors in patients seeking to have bariatric surgery. *Surg. Obes. Relat. Dis.* **2016**, *12*, 165–170. [CrossRef] [PubMed]
14. Meadows, A.; Nolan, L.J.; Higgs, S. Self-perceived food addiction: Prevalence, predictors, and prognosis. *Appetite* **2017**, *114*, 282–298. [CrossRef]
15. Burrows, T.; Skinner, J.; McKenna, R.; Rollo, M. Food addiction, binge eating disorder, and obesity: Is there a relationship? *Behav. Sci.* **2017**, *7*, 54. [CrossRef]
16. Lacroix, E.; von Ranson, K. Prevalence of social, cognitive, and emotional impairment among individuals with food addiction. *Eat. Weight Disord.* **2020**. [CrossRef] [PubMed]
17. Cassin, S.E.; Sijercic, I.; Montemarano, V. Psychosocial interventions for food addiction: A systematic review. *Curr. Addict. Rep.* **2020**, *7*, 9–19. [CrossRef]

18. Vella, S.L.C.; Pai, N.B. A narrative review of potential treatment strategies for food addiction. *Eat. Weight Disord.* **2017**, *22*, 387–393. [CrossRef]
19. Gearhardt, A.N.; Corbin, W.R.; Brownell, K.D. Development of the Yale Food Addiction Scale Version 2.0. *Psychol. Addict. Behav.* **2016**, *30*, 113–121. [CrossRef]
20. Amorim, P. Mini International Neuropsychiatric Interview (MINI): Validação de entrevista breve para diagnóstico de transtornos mentais. *Rev. Braz. Psiquiatr.* **2000**, *22*, 106–115. [CrossRef]
21. Oliveira, E.; Lacroix, E.; Stravogiannis, A.; de Vasques, M.F.; Durante, C.R.; Duran, E.P.; Pereira, D.; Cabral, J.R.; Tavares, H. Treatment of food addiction: Preliminary results. *Arch. Clin. Psychiatry* **2020**, *47*, 163–164.
22. Freitas, S.R.; Lopes, C.S.; Appolinario, J.C.; Coutinho, W. The assessment of binge eating disorder in obese women: A comparison of the binge eating scale with the structured clinical interview for the DSM-IV. *Eat. Behav.* **2006**, *7*, 282–289. [CrossRef] [PubMed]
23. Queiroz de Medeiros, A.C.; Campos Pedrosa, L.F.; Hutz, C.S.; Yamamoto, M.E. Brazilian version of food cravings questionnaires: Psychometric properties and sex differences. *Appetite* **2016**, *105*, 328–333. [CrossRef]
24. Gomes-Oliveira, M.H.; Gorenstein, C.; Neto, F.L.; Andrade, L.H.; Wang, Y.P. Validação da versão Brasileira em Português do Inventário de Depressão de Beck-II numa amostra da comunidade. *Rev. Bras. Psiquiatr.* **2012**, *34*, 389–394. [CrossRef]
25. Quintão, S.; Delgado, A.R.; Prieto, G. Validity study of the beck anxiety inventory (Portuguese version) by the rasch rating scale model. *Psicol. Reflex. Crit.* **2013**, *26*, 305–310. [CrossRef]
26. Fleck, M.; Louzada, S.; Xavier, M.; Chachamovich, E.; Vieira, G.; Santos, L.; Pinzon, V. Application of the Portuguese version of the abbreviated instrument of quality life WHOQOL-bref. *Rev. Saude Publica* **2000**, *34*, 178–183. [CrossRef]
27. Polivy, J.; Herman, C.P. Sociocultural idealization of thin female body shapes: An introduction to the special issue on body image and eating disorders. *J. Soc. Clin. Psychol.* **2004**, *23*, 1–6. [CrossRef]
28. Gearhardt, A.N.; White, M.A.; Masheb, R.M.; Morgan, P.T.; Crosby, R.D.; Grilo, C.M. An examination of the food addiction construct in obese patients with binge eating disorder. *Int. J. Eat. Disord.* **2012**, *45*, 657–663. [CrossRef]
29. Avena, N.M.; Gearhardt, A.N.; Gold, M.S.; Wang, G.J.; Potenza, M.N. Tossing the baby out with the bathwater after a brief rinse? The potential downside of dismissing food addiction based on limited data. *Nat. Rev. Neurosci.* **2012**, *13*, 514. [CrossRef]
30. Konkolÿ Thege, B.; Hodgins, D.C.; Wild, T.C. Co-occurring substance-related and behavioral addiction problems: A person-centered, lay epidemiology approach. *J. Behav. Addict.* **2016**, *5*, 614–622. [CrossRef] [PubMed]
31. Kim, H.S.; Hodgins, D.C.; Kim, B.; Wild, T.C. Transdiagnostic or disorder specific? Indicators of substance and behavioral addictions nominated by people with lived experience. *J. Clin. Med.* **2020**, *9*, 334. [CrossRef]
32. Lacroix, E.; Oliveira, E.; Saldanha de Castro, J.; Cabral, J.R.; Tavares, H.; von Ranson, K.M. "There is no way to avoid the first bite": A qualitative investigation of addictive-like eating in treatment-seeking Brazilian women and men. *Appetite* **2019**, *137*, 35–46. [CrossRef]
33. De Castro, V.; Fong, T.; Rosenthal, R.J.; Tavares, H. A comparison of craving and emotional states between pathological gamblers and alcoholics. *Addict. Behav.* **2007**, *32*, 1555–1564. [CrossRef]
34. Tavares, H.; Zilberman, M.L.; Hodgins, D.C.; El-Guebaly, N. Comparison of craving between pathological gamblers and alcoholics. *Alcohol. Clin. Exp. Res.* **2005**, *29*, 1427–1431. [CrossRef] [PubMed]
35. Karapareddy, V. A review of integrated care for concurrent disorders: Cost effectiveness and clinical outcomes. *J. Dual Diagn.* **2019**, *15*, 56–66. [CrossRef]

Publisher's Note: MDPI stays neutral with regard to jurisdictional claims in published maps and institutional affiliations.

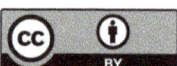

© 2020 by the authors. Licensee MDPI, Basel, Switzerland. This article is an open access article distributed under the terms and conditions of the Creative Commons Attribution (CC BY) license (http://creativecommons.org/licenses/by/4.0/).

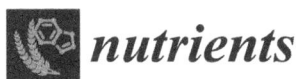

Article

Health Professionals' and Health Professional Trainees' Views on Addictive Eating Behaviours: A Cross-Sectional Survey

Tracy Burrows [1,2,*], Antonio Verdejo-Garcia [3], Adrian Carter [3], Robyn M. Brown [4], Zane B. Andrews [4,5], Chris V. Dayas [6,7], Charlotte A. Hardman [8], Natalie Loxton [9,10], Priya Sumithran [11,12] and Megan Whatnall [1,2]

1. Priority Research Centre for Physical Activity and Nutrition, University of Newcastle, Callaghan, NSW 2308, Australia; megan.whatnall@newcastle.edu.au
2. School of Health Sciences, Faculty of Health and Medicine, University of Newcastle, Callaghan, NSW 2308, Australia
3. Turner Institute for Brain and Mental Health, Monash University, Clayton, VIC 3800, Australia; antonio.verdejo@monash.edu (A.V.-G.); adrian.carter@monash.edu (A.C.)
4. Florey Institute of Neuroscience and Mental Health, University of Melbourne, Parkville, VIC 3052, Australia; robyn.brown@florey.edu.au (R.M.B.); zane.andrews@monash.edu (Z.B.A.)
5. Monash Biomedicine Discovery Institute and Department of Physiology, Monash University, Clayton, VIC 3800, Australia
6. School of Biomedical Sciences & Pharmacy, Faculty of Health and Medicine, University of Newcastle, Callaghan, NSW 2308, Australia; christopher.dayas@newcastle.edu.au
7. Hunter Medical Research Institute (HMRI), New Lambton Heights, NSW 2305, Australia
8. Department of Psychology, Institute of Population Health, University of Liverpool, Liverpool L69 7ZA, UK; cah@liverpool.ac.uk
9. School of Applied Psychology, Griffith University, Brisbane, QLD 4122, Australia; n.loxton@griffith.edu.au
10. Centre for Youth Substance Abuse Research, University of Queensland, Brisbane, QLD 4072, Australia
11. Department of Medicine (Austin), University of Melbourne, Heidelberg, VIC 3084, Australia; priyas@unimelb.edu.au
12. Department of Endocrinology, Austin Health, Heidelberg Heights, VIC 3081, Australia
* Correspondence: tracy.burrows@newcastle.edu.au

Received: 13 August 2020; Accepted: 17 September 2020; Published: 18 September 2020

Abstract: Despite increasing research on the concept of addictive eating, there is currently no published evidence on the views of health professionals who potentially consult with patients presenting with addictive eating behaviours, or of students training to become health professionals. This study aimed to explore the views and understanding of addictive eating behaviours among health professionals and health professionals in training and to identify potential gaps in professional development training. An international online cross-sectional survey was conducted in February–April 2020. The survey (70 questions, 6 key areas) assessed participants' opinions and clinical experience of addictive eating; opinions on control, responsibility, and stigma relating to addictive eating; and knowledge of addictive eating and opinions on professional development training. In total, 142 health professionals and 33 health professionals in training completed the survey (mean age 38.1 ± 12.5 years, 65% from Australia/16% from the U.K.) Of the health professionals, 47% were dietitians and 16% were psychologists. Most participants ($n = 126$, 72%) reported that they have been asked by individuals about addictive eating. Half of the participants reported that they consider the term food addiction to be stigmatising for individuals ($n = 88$). Sixty percent ($n = 105$) reported that they were interested/very interested in receiving addictive eating training, with the top two preferred formats being online and self-paced, and face-to-face. These results demonstrate that addictive eating is supported by health professionals as they consult with patients presenting with this behaviour, which supports the views of the general community and demonstrates a need for health professional training.

Keywords: addictive eating; food addiction; health professional; clinician

1. Introduction

Addictive eating (i.e., an abnormal, recurrent pattern of excessive food consumption despite negative consequences) [1], often referred to as food addiction, is not currently recognised in the Diagnostic and Statistical Manual of Mental Disorders as a distinct diagnosis from other eating and substance use disorders. There exists an ongoing scientific debate in this regard, which centres around whether the symptoms of addictive eating are covered appropriately under other recognised disorders, such as binge eating disorder [2,3]. If addictive eating is a distinct disorder, the debate is also around whether it should be considered a substance (i.e., food) addiction or a behavioural (i.e., eating) addiction, or on a spectrum of overeating [2,3]. Further, there is the question of what the addictive substance/s are or whether it relates to the level of food processing [2,3]. Regardless of whether addictive eating should be recognised, 15–20% of the population report experiencing symptoms that align with addictive eating as determined by self-reported tools [4]. This is higher among certain groups, including females, those with binge eating disorder and other mental health conditions, and those with overweight and obesity [4]. Further, rates of self-perceived addictive eating among community samples range from 27% to 50% [5]. There is also widespread support from community samples that the concept of addictive eating exists [5,6]. For example, a survey of over 600 American and Australian adults reported that 86% believed certain foods may be addictive, and 72% believed addictive eating is linked with an increased risk of obesity [6].

Unhealthy lifestyle behaviours such as poorer dietary intake, physical inactivity, greater time spent sitting, and poor sleep quality are associated with addictive eating [7,8]. This association extends to conditions such as depression, anxiety, and overweight and obesity [9,10]. In terms of clinical management of addictive eating, the published evidence is scarce [11,12]. A recent systematic review conducted by Cassin et al. to assess psychosocial interventions for addictive eating identified only eight studies [12]. Of these, only two studies included individuals with addictive eating and interventions that specifically targeted addictive eating symptoms. The two interventions were abstinence-based (i.e., abstaining from overeating, snacking, and/or from identified problem foods), while the remaining studies included an outcome measure of addictive eating in intervention studies targeting either bulimia nervosa or overweight and obesity. Additionally, all of the included studies were deemed to exhibit poor or fair methodological quality, and most were pilot or feasibility studies. Importantly, the review was limited to psychosocial interventions and did not consider alternate options such as dietary advice alone. Overall, the review's authors concluded that no effective psychosocial interventions currently exist for the treatment of addictive eating. There is however a high volume of self-help support groups for individuals with addictive eating [13]. A recent review of websites identified 13 online support groups for addictive eating; however only three of these involved credentialed health professionals [13]. Evidently, research exploring the clinical utility of recognising addictive eating as a diagnostic entity and evidence-based best practices for treatment are limited.

There is currently no published evidence on the views of health professionals who likely consult with patients who report addictive eating behaviours, or of those training to become health professionals. Research should examine clinicians' and future clinicians' understanding of addictive eating, their support for it as a diagnostic category, and whether professional development training is needed regarding understanding and treating addictive eating. This work is critical to advancing the field of addictive eating in terms of treatment and informing best practice. The aims of this study were to explore the opinions and understanding of addictive eating behaviours among health professionals with experience in weight management and students undertaking relevant health professional training. The study also aimed to explore the needs and preferences for professional development training in addictive eating.

2. Materials and Methods

2.1. Study Design

An international online cross-sectional survey was conducted. An online survey was used as a convenient method of completion for participants and to maximise the survey reach and response rate. The survey was hosted via Qualtrics (https://www.qualtrics.com/au/) and was open from 21 February to 27 April 2020. The survey took approximately 25 min to complete and was initially pilot tested among a sample of five health professionals and university students to assess for readability and comprehension. The survey consisted of 70 questions including demographic questions and questions across six key areas (opinions and clinical experience of addictive eating; opinions on control, responsibility, and stigma relating to addictive eating; knowledge of addictive eating and opinions on professional development training; opinions on weight gain; treatment of disordered eating and overweight/obesity; and agreement with statements regarding addictive eating symptoms). This paper reports on the questions relating to opinions and clinical experience of addictive eating; opinions on control, responsibility, and stigma relating to addictive eating; and knowledge of addictive eating and opinions on professional development training. Questions relating to the other key areas were outside the scope of the current paper (see File S1 and Table S1). The survey questions used were developed by the research team for the purpose of this study. The survey was set up to require a response to each question before participants could progress to the next question, with the exception of the qualitative questions, which were optional to complete. Survey logic was used so that only relevant questions were displayed to each participant, based on their previous responses. The use of survey logic also limits participants from being able to go back and change previous responses. The study conduct and reporting comply with the Strengthening the Reporting of Observational Studies in Epidemiology (STROBE) guidelines for cross-sectional studies [14]. All participants gave informed consent prior to completing the survey. Participation was voluntary, and no incentives were offered for participation. Ethical approval for the study was obtained from the University of Newcastle Human Research Ethics Committee (H-2019-0349).

2.2. Participants and Recruitment

Individuals were eligible to participate if they were a health professional with experience in the management or research of overweight or obesity or disordered eating, or were a student currently enrolled in health professional training at a university. Relevant disciplines included allied health professionals; medical professionals; psychologists; other health professionals; public health, nutrition, or other health researchers; or university students training in one of these professions. University students of relevant disciplines were also included as they represent the next generation of health professionals. Individuals from any country were eligible to participate; however, the survey was written in English. Health professionals and university students completed the same survey; however, some of the survey questions were worded differently by asking health professionals about their practical experience and university students about their opinions. Additionally, the questions regarding experience in treating clients were only asked of health professionals. Recruitment was via convenience sampling and used a range of strategies. Email invitations were sent from the members of the research team to their networks of health professionals and students and contained a link to the online survey. The survey was also advertised via posts from the research team on Twitter, a brief advertisement in the member e-newsletter of Dietitians Australia (professional body for Dietitians in Australia), and an advertisement to students was posted via the online learning management system at the University of Newcastle, Australia. All advertisements used the same recruitment materials and information, which described the survey as a "cross-sectional survey to identify the current understanding of addictive eating behaviours and whether a need exists for professional development training."

2.3. Measures

2.3.1. Demographic Characteristics

Demographic data collected included age, gender, country of residence, and highest qualification completed. Health professionals were also asked their occupation, primary work setting (e.g., hospital, private practice, research), the population group/life stage they primarily work with (e.g., adolescents, adults), and whether they provide advice to individuals with disordered eating or overweight/obesity. University students were also asked the degree for which they were currently studying.

2.3.2. Opinions and Clinical Experience of Addictive Eating

The survey included 14 questions about opinions and clinical experiences regarding addictive eating. Participants were asked whether they had encountered patients/individuals asking or speaking about addictive eating, their thoughts around whether people can develop compulsive eating patterns that resemble an addictive disorder, and whether addictive eating exists (yes, no, or maybe). Of those who indicated that addictive eating does or may exist, participants were asked whether they think different populations may be more vulnerable. Of those who indicated that they provide advice to individuals with disordered eating or overweight/obesity, participants were asked what proportion of their clients may benefit from a specific treatment of addictive eating, if available. Participants were also asked to rate their level of interest in addictive eating becoming a diagnostic term and a referral pathway being introduced for the treatment/management of addictive eating (1/very interested to 5/not at all interested). In terms of treatment for addictive eating, participants were asked their opinion on which health professionals would be best placed to identify and treat people with addictive eating, and which services they would be more/less likely to refer individuals to, as well as whether any particular sub-groups of overweight and obese people would benefit more from a diagnosis of addictive eating. Two open-ended questions were also asked of those who indicated that addictive eating does or may exist, including what they thought were the strengths and weaknesses of using the addictive eating concept to explain eating and weight to individuals.

2.3.3. Opinions on Control, Responsibility, and Stigma Relating to Addictive Eating

Three questions were included relating to opinions on control and responsibility for eating and weight. Participants were asked to rate how much they think it is the responsibility of the individual with addictive eating to gain control over their eating and weight status (1/not responsible to 5/100% responsible) and how much control they think individuals have over their eating and weight (1/a great deal to 5/none at all). Three questions were included relating to their opinions around the different terminology used for addictive eating and stigma. Participants were asked how well they think the term food addiction relates to the experiences of people with weight issues, whether they think the term food addiction is stigmatising, and to indicate which term (if any) they think is most appropriate to describe food addiction/addictive eating.

2.3.4. Knowledge of Addictive Eating and Opinions on Professional Development Training

Three questions asked about participants' knowledge of addictive eating. Participants were asked what sources of information informed their understanding of addictive eating and to rate their current knowledge of addictive eating and their level of confidence in their knowledge. Six questions asked about participants' professional development training needs and preferences. Participants were asked about what kinds of professional development training on addictive eating assessment and treatment would be needed, who should receive this training, and their preferred method of training delivery. They were also asked to rate their level of interest in receiving addictive eating training delivered online, whether this would be of interest to colleagues/peers, and whether individuals/clients would be interested in training/management/treatment delivered online.

2.4. Analysis

Data were analysed using Stata statistical software version 14.2. In total, 274 individuals accessed the online survey, of these, 175 consented and completed all survey questions (i.e., 64% of those who accessed the survey). Of those that did not complete the survey (n = 99), 14 opened the link/viewed the first page but did not start the survey, one did not provide consent and exited the survey, 15 filled in some of the demographics questions only, and the remaining 69 completed the demographics questions and some but not all of the rest of the survey. Quantitative data are reported as number and percentage for categorical variables and mean and standard deviation for continuous variables. Open-response questions are described qualitatively. Qualitative data were analysed using a theoretical thematic analysis approach [15], including (1) identifying codes from the responses based on keywords/phrases, (2) grouping codes into themes, (3) reviewing themes in relation to the contributing codes, and (4) defining and naming themes. One researcher initially conducted the thematic analysis, and this was checked by a second researcher, with any discrepancies discussed and results amended. Themes are presented in the order of most to least frequent/recurrent. Results for health professional and health professional trainee participants were compared using chi-square tests for questions with mutually exclusive response options, to determine whether these were significantly different. There were differences between responses for nine of the questions; however, with further investigation these differences were driven by the large number of response options. As the pattern of the most common responses were similar between the two groups, and due to the small sample size of the health professionals in training, it was deemed appropriate to combine the responses for reporting (see Table S2 for responses by group).

3. Results

3.1. Sample Characteristics

Of the 175 participants, 81% (n = 142) were health professionals, and 19% (n = 33) were university students (Table 1). The mean ± SD age of participants was 38.1 ± 12.5 years, the majority were female (n = 150, 86%), and participants were from six different countries with most residing in Australia (n = 113, 65%) or the U.K. (n = 28, 16%). Among the health professional participants, the most common occupations were dietitian (n = 66, 47%) and psychologist (n = 23, 16%), with the highest proportion working in hospitals (n = 39, 28%) and private practice (n = 39, 28%), and working with population groups of adults 25–65 years (n = 109, 77%) and young adults 18–24 years (n = 52, 37%). Sixty-three percent of health professional participants (n = 90) reported that they provide advice to clients for disordered eating, while 70% (n = 100) provide advice to clients for overweight/obesity.

Table 1. Demographic characteristics of health professionals participating in a survey on addictive eating (n = 175).

Demographic Characteristic	n	%
Age (years) Mean ± SD	38.1 ± 12.5	
Gender		
Female	150	85.7
Male	22	12.6
Other	3	1.7
Country of residence		
Australia	113	64.6
U.K.	28	16.0
USA	23	13.1
Other	11	6.3

Table 1. *Cont.*

Demographic Characteristic	n	%
Highest qualification completed		
School certificate/Higher school certificate	21	12.0
Trade or diploma	2	1.1
Undergraduate university degree	50	28.6
Postgraduate university degree	71	40.6
Higher research degree	31	17.7
Occupation		
Dietitian	66	37.7
Tertiary health or medical student [a]	33	18.9
Psychologist	23	13.1
Other health practitioner	18	10.3
Health researcher	12	6.9
Tertiary academic/teacher	6	3.4
Medical specialist/registrar	4	1.7
General practitioner	3	1.7
Counsellor	3	1.7
Pharmacist	3	1.7
Psychotherapist	2	1.1
Social worker	2	1.1
Primary work situation [b]		
Hospital	39	27.5
Private practice	39	27.5
Research and teaching	29	20.4
Community/population/public health program	19	13.4
Primary care	7	4.9
Food service	1	0.7
Other	8	5.6
Population group worked with [b,c]		
Infants < 2 years	13	9.2
Children 2–12 years	20	14.1
Adolescents 13–17 years	39	23.2
Young adults 18–24 years	52	36.6
Adults 25–65 years	109	76.8
Adults > 65 years	41	28.9
Not applicable	4	2.8

[a] Of the tertiary health and medical students, n = 29 (88%) were studying a degree in Nutrition and Dietetics. [b] Responses are for health professionals only (n = 142). [c] Multiple response question i.e., percentages add to >100.

3.2. Description of Quantitative Results

3.2.1. Opinions and Clinical Experience of Addictive Eating

The majority of participants (n = 126, 72%) reported that they have been asked by individuals about addictive eating (Table 2). Sixty percent of participants (n = 105) indicated that they think addictive eating exists. The proportion of the sample who reported being interested/very interested in addictive eating being a diagnostic term was 48% (n = 83).

Table 2. Opinions and clinical experience of addictive eating among health professionals participating in a survey on addictive eating ($n = 175$).

Survey Item	n	%
Have you experienced individuals asking or speaking about addictive eating?		
Yes	126	72.0
Maybe	14	8.0
No	35	20.0
In your opinion, do you feel that people can develop compulsive patterns of eating that resemble an addictive disorder?		
Yes	120	68.6
Maybe	33	18.9
No	22	12.6
In your opinion, does addictive eating exist?		
Yes	105	60.0
Maybe	33	18.9
No	37	21.1
In your opinion, do you feel that there are population groups who may be more vulnerable to addictive eating? [a]		
Yes	75	54.3
Unsure	18	13.0
No	45	32.6
Estimated percentage of clients to benefit from a specific treatment of addictive eating (Mean SD) [b]	40.9 ± 27.9	
How interested would you be in addictive eating being a diagnostic term?		
Very interested	43	24.6
Interested	40	22.9
Somewhat interested	29	16.6
Not very interested	23	13.1
Not at all interested	40	22.9
How interested would you be if there was a referral pathway for the treatment/management of addictive eating?		
Very interested	72	41.1
Interested	41	23.4
Somewhat interested	20	11.4
Not very interested	6	3.4
Not at all interested	36	20.6
Who do you think would be best placed to identify people with behaviours suggestive of addictive eating? [c]		
Dietitians/nutritionists	99	56.6
Psychologists	93	53.1
Psychiatrists	51	29.1
Counsellor	49	28.0
General practitioner	48	27.4
Medical specialists	30	17.1
All of the above	75	42.9
Other	30	17.1
Who do you think is best placed to provide treatment for people with addictive eating? [c]		
Psychologists	114	65.1
Dietitians/nutritionists	107	61.1
Psychiatrists	52	29.7
Counsellor	49	28.0
General practitioner	16	9.1
Medical specialists	17	9.7
All of the above	34	19.4
Other	29	16.6
Are there any services you would be more likely to refer to or suggest to clients/individuals with addictive eating? [c]		
Psychologist	124	70.9
Counselling	77	44.0
Addiction specialist	75	42.9
General practitioner	19	10.9
Pharmacological	8	4.6
All of the above	96	54.9
Other	14	8.0
None	34	19.4

Table 2. *Cont.*

Survey Item	n	%
Are there any services you would be less likely to refer to or suggest to clients/individuals with addictive eating? [c]		
Pharmacological	86	49.1
General practitioner	76	43.4
Addiction specialist	33	18.9
Counselling	6	3.4
Psychologist	2	1.1
All of the above	7	4.0
Other	3	1.7
None	46	26.3
Are there any particular sub-groups of overweight and obese people you feel would benefit more from a diagnosis of addictive eating? [c]		
Individuals with binge eating disorder	80	45.7
Overeaters	79	45.1
Individuals with a mental health condition	60	34.3
Individuals with other mental illnesses	44	25.1
Individuals with substance disorders	36	20.6
Individuals with low motivation to engage with treatment	30	17.1
Children	14	8.0
Other	17	9.7
No	58	33.1

[a] n = 138 responses (i.e., those that believe addictive eating exists). [b] n = 80 responses from health professionals (i.e., those that believe addictive eating exists and provide treatment for overweight/obesity and/or disordered eating). [c] Multiple response questions, i.e., percentages add to >100.

3.2.2. Opinions on Control, Responsibility, and Stigma Relating to Addictive Eating

The largest proportion of participants reported that they think individuals with addictive eating have "a little" control over their eating habits (n = 89, 51%) and weight (n = 77, 44%) (Table 3). However, the majority reported that individuals with addictive eating are very/moderately responsible for gaining control over their eating and weight (n = 118, 67%). Half of the participants reported that they think food addiction is a stigmatising term for individuals (n = 88). Participants' preferences regarding the terminology used to describe addictive eating/food addiction were varied. From the proposed list of terms, the largest proportion of participants selected compulsive overeating (n = 41, 23%), followed by addictive eating (n = 34, 19%), and other (n = 29, 17%). Of those that selected other, some indicated that eating disorder terminology should be used, some indicated that more than one term is needed as the most appropriate term may differ for different clients/individuals, while other suggested terms included disordered eating, eating addiction, highly processed food addiction, refined food addiction, and restriction–rebound overeating.

Table 3. Opinions on control, responsibility, and stigma relating to addictive eating among health professionals participating in a survey on addictive eating (n = 175).

Survey Item	n	%
In your opinion, how much control does someone with addictive eating have over their eating habits?		
A great deal	5	2.9
A lot	9	5.1
A moderate amount	60	34.3
A little	89	50.9
None at all	12	6.9
In your opinion, how much control does someone with addictive eating have over their weight?		
A great deal	2	1.1
A lot	2	1.1
A moderate amount	44	25.1
A little	77	44.0
None at all	50	28.6

Table 3. Cont.

Survey Item	n	%
In your opinion, how much responsibility does someone with addictive eating have to gain control over their eating and weight?		
100% responsible	12	6.9
Very responsible	51	29.1
Moderately responsible	67	38.3
Not very responsible	20	11.4
Not responsible	25	14.3
Do you think that the term "food addiction" is stigmatising for individuals?		
Yes	88	50.3
Unsure	52	29.7
No	35	20.0
How well do you think the term food addiction relates to the experiences of people with weight issues?		
Extremely/very well	59	33.7
Neutral	35	20.0
Not well	81	46.3
Select which term you feel is most appropriate to describe food addiction/addictive eating?		
Compulsive overeating	41	23.4
Addictive eating	34	19.4
Compulsive overeating disorder	27	15.4
Food addiction	23	13.1
None, no term needed	21	12.0
Other	29	16.6

3.2.3. Knowledge of Addictive Eating and Opinions on Professional Development Training

The majority of participants rated their knowledge of addictive eating as average or poor (n = 106, 61%) (Table 4). The most common source of information that participants used to inform their understanding of addictive eating was colleagues (n = 123, 70%), followed by the scientific literature (n = 116, 66%). Sixty percent of participants (n = 105) reported that they were interested/very interested in receiving training on addictive eating delivered via technologies such as the internet and/or smartphones. When participants were asked who should be trained in addictive eating, the most common responses were dietitians (n = 87, 50%) and psychologists (n = 82, 47%). In terms of the types of professional development training that is needed, most commonly, participants indicated training in evidence-based treatment (n = 142, 81%), followed by understanding medical and non-medical treatments (n = 134, 77%) and assessment and diagnosis (n = 134, 77%).

Table 4. Knowledge of addictive eating and opinions on professional development training among health professionals participating in a survey on addictive eating (n = 175).

Survey Item	n	%
How confident do you feel in your knowledge on the latest evidence relating to addictive eating (i.e., assessment methodologies/treatment)?		
Extremely confident	26	14.9
Very confident	26	14.9
Neutral	41	23.4
Somewhat confident	34	19.4
Not at all confident	48	27.4
How would you rate your current knowledge about addictive eating?		
Excellent	30	17.1
Good	36	20.6
Average	57	32.6
Poor	49	28.0
Terrible	3	1.7

Table 4. *Cont.*

Survey Item	n	%
What sources of information have informed your understanding of addictive eating? [a]		
Colleagues	123	70.3
Scientific literature	116	66.3
Education	102	58.3
Conferences	68	38.9
Social media	36	20.6
Other reading	27	15.4
Traditional media	21	12.0
Have not heard of addictive eating	7	4.0
If training for addictive eating were available, how interested would you be in participating in training delivered using technologies such as the internet and/or smartphones?		
Very interested	75	42.9
Interested	30	17.1
Somewhat interested	24	13.7
Not very interested	10	5.7
Not at all interested	36	20.6
In your opinion, who should be trained in addictive eating assessment and treatment? [a]		
Dietitians	87	49.7
Psychologists	82	46.9
Psychiatrists	55	31.4
General practitioners	52	29.7
Undergraduate students	38	21.7
Medical specialists	33	18.9
Practice nurses	25	14.3
All of the above	73	41.7
Other	38	21.7
If food addiction/addictive eating became a diagnostic term, what kinds of professional development training do you think would be needed (for yourself/other professions)? [a]		
Evidence-based treatment	142	81.1
Understanding treatment (medical and non-medical)	134	76.6
Assessment/diagnosis	134	76.6
Treatment approaches focusing on other behaviours as well as food, e.g., sleep, physical activity	129	73.7
Understanding addiction terminology	123	70.3
Neuroscience behind addictive eating	119	68.0
How to minimise stigma	114	65.1
Foods to avoid	59	33.7
Other	36	20.6
What would be your preferred method of delivery for professional development training? [b]		
Face to face	81	46.3
Online, self-paced	77	44.0
Professional development	65	37.1
Structured short course	63	36.0
Delivered by a credential source	51	29.1
Other	13	7.4
Do you think online training/management/treatment delivered by health professionals would be of interest to clients/individuals?		
Yes/Maybe	157	89.7
No	18	10.3
Do you think online training would be of interest to your co-workers/colleagues/peers?		
Yes/Maybe	154	88.0
No	21	12.0

[a] Multiple response questions i.e., percentages add to >100. [b] Reported as the n(%) who ranked responses as 1 or 2.

3.2.4. Description of Qualitative Results

Thematic analysis results are presented in Table 5. Sixty-three percent ($n = 111$) of the participants responded to the question "What are some strengths/benefits to using the addictive eating approach to explain eating and weight to clients/individuals?" Five themes were identified, including from most to least frequent: (1) provides an explanation/assists understanding; (2) relieves guilt/stigma; (3) provides acknowledgement/validation; (4) provides a framework/pathway for future treatment;

and (5) encourages hope for overcoming addictive eating. Fifty-nine percent ($n = 103$) of participants responded to the question "What are some of the downsides/weaknesses to using the addictive eating approach to explain eating and weight to clients/individuals?" Six themes were identified, including from most to least frequent: (1) reason/barrier not to change; (2) negative response from clients/individuals; (3) stigma; (4) lack of evidence/recognition; (5) implications for treatment; and (6) clinician training/time.

Table 5. Qualitative findings among health professionals participating in a survey on addictive eating ($n = 175$).

	Question: What are some strengths/benefits to using the addictive eating approach to explain eating and weight to clients/individuals?
Themes and quotes	(1) Provides an explanation/assists understanding "Help clients realise the link between behaviours, thoughts, and food … " "Help people understand the role of psychology in food choice"
	(2) Relieves guilt/stigma "May help to reduce stigma and some of the extreme negative thoughts people have in relation to their eating." "Clients may feel less guilty about weight/weight gain."
	(3) Provides acknowledgement/validation "Legitimises their problem" "'Giving it a name' may help people externalise and tackle the issue better."
	(4) Provides a framework/pathway for future treatment "Current knowledge about addiction medicine would provide potential avenues for treatment."
	(5) Encourages hope for overcoming addictive eating "When they [clients] feel understanding and empowered it is easier to facilitate health promoting changes and more effective strategies."
	Question: What are some of the downsides/weaknesses to using the addictive eating approach to explain eating and weight to clients/individuals?
Themes and quotes	(1) Reason/barrier not to change "Some people may like another label as a reason not to try to change." "Dissolves some responsibility for lifestyle decisions that are outside of addictive behaviours."
	(2) Negative response from clients/individuals "[It] may induce a sense of helplessness." "Some people may get offended when using the word addictive, may bring up deep rooted emotional issues associated with why they overeat."
	(3) Stigma "It can become a stigmatised label of being an 'addict', which may impact on their recovery journey."
	(4) Lack of evidence/recognition "I do not see this [food addiction] at the moment as true addiction." "The fact that scientific literature and other health care professionals don't support this."
	(5) Implications for treatment "The abstinence model may have the potential to increase binge eating if it is too restrictive regarding food rules." "Limited psychological support to help manage the condition"
	(6) Clinician training/time "Clinicians need to be trained to identify and safely address addictive eating … Identifying the eating behaviour without appropriate treatment may be detrimental."

Questions were only asked of those participants who responded yes or maybe to the question, "do you believe addictive eating exists?"

4. Discussion

This study aimed to explore the opinions and understanding of addictive eating in an international sample of practising health professionals and health professionals in training. The needs and preferences for professional development training in addictive eating were also explored. The majority of the survey sample reported that they support that addictive eating exists, have experienced individuals/patients asking about addictive eating, and expressed interest in receiving training about addictive eating. Overall, the study findings provide important insight into the perspective of currently practicing health professionals and health professionals in training (i.e., future health professionals) on addictive eating.

This adds to and provides a point of comparison for the larger evidence base of opinions among the general population.

Sixty percent of the health professionals and health professionals in training surveyed supported that addictive eating exists, while a higher proportion (69%) expressed the view that people can develop compulsive patterns of eating resembling an addictive disorder. These results are substantially lower than in community samples such as the survey by Lee et al. where 86% of adults believed that certain foods may be addictive [6]. Results show that over 70% of health professionals reported that individuals had enquired about addictive eating. Moreover, participants expressed interest in addictive eating being officially recognised as a formal diagnosis and in the use of a specific referral pathway. However, self-rating of knowledge of addictive eating was rated below average in the majority of participants and confidence in knowledge of the evidence base was low. Thus, it is potentially not surprising that our data revealed a definite interest for training and education in this specific topic. Two-thirds of health professionals were interested or very interested in receiving addictive eating training, with almost half reporting that they would prefer training to be online and self-paced and almost half preferring face-to-face training. The most common types of professional development training that were reportedly needed included training in evidence-based treatment, understanding medical and non-medical treatments, and training in assessment and diagnosis. Participants identified dietitians and psychologists as the two major professions who should receive training, followed by psychiatrists and general practitioners, while the majority reported that training in addictive eating would also be useful for individuals or clients. This is not surprising given the pertinent roles that these health professionals have in other recognised forms of disordered eating. These findings indicate that this is a significant issue faced by clients and health professionals.

Overall, there was a mixed response in terms of the preferred terminology to be used to describe this compulsive form of eating. Compulsive overeating was the most preferred term, indicated by 23% of participants, followed by addictive eating (19%). However, a large proportion of participants indicated other responses including that more than one term may be needed as the most appropriate term may differ between clients/individuals. This difference may suggest that a multidimensional or domain-based approach is needed rather than a categorical diagnosis. This also shows that reaching a consensus on a common term may not be achievable. Despite there being a lack of consensus in existing research over the preferred terminology [16,17], the term "food addiction" was the least preferred. This illustrates the recognition amongst those surveyed of the highly stigmatising nature of this descriptor. Indeed, the majority of participants expressed a belief that the term food addiction is stigmatising, which supports consumer research [18]. Many existing research reports discuss the terminology, and it may be time to move beyond the terminology to focus on greater understanding and possible management options, given that many health professionals in the current study have patients seeking help for this behaviour. The qualitative findings from the current study also provide further insight into the discussion of stigma, as this was a recurrent theme when health professionals were asked to explain the benefits and downsides of using the addictive eating approach to explain eating and weight to individuals. Views were divided, in that, some health professionals commented that it may reduce stigma, while others explained that it may introduce the stigma that is associated with addictions and other mental health conditions in general. This may be linked with the number of views expressed about the terminology. Further exploration of the views of health professionals regarding addictive eating and stigma is warranted [19].

The survey identified mixed opinions regarding the relationship between addictive eating behaviours and weight. Over two-thirds of the participants reported that individuals with addictive eating have little to no control over their eating habits and weight. This highlights acceptance of the lack of control experienced by those with addictive eating; yet, approximately half of the participants reported that addictive eating does not relate well to the experiences of people with weight issues. These findings could relate to the fact that individuals may not have been directed to the appropriate services for the management of their addictive eating, i.e., the lack of control relates to numerous unsuccessful attempts at treatment/management by the individual with addictive eating. Comparatively, the study by Lee et al. found that among the community sample of >600 adults, almost three-quarters supported that addictive eating causes obesity, while views were divided close to 50:50 in terms of individuals having control over their weight and eating [6]. These are important findings, as the way that health professionals view these factors would have implications for the treatment that they may provide or refer individuals on to. Further, if these views differ from those of the general population and/or their patients, this may also influence the efficacy of treatment. There has been increasing research of the overlap of disordered eating and obesity [20]. Given that addictive eating often overlaps with binge eating and presents with obesity, this offers an interesting opportunity for further exploration.

The major strength of this study is that it is the first to explore opinions on addictive eating in a sample of health professionals and health professionals in training. Further, a moderate sample size was obtained, which is a strength given the challenges of engaging health professionals in research (e.g., due to busy workloads). The sample was an international sample with health professionals from a range of backgrounds, which is a strength for this exploratory study as it provides a broad range of perspectives; however, the fact that different countries have different professional standards and structures is also a potential limitation. In terms of limitations, health professionals who have an interest in or have been asked about addictive eating may have been motivated to participate in the current study, while a large proportion were dietitians or psychologists. Therefore, the representativeness of the sample is a limitation, and the views presented may not represent the generalised community of health professionals and students. Further, females were over-represented in the study population. However, this can be explained by the higher percentage of women among the health professions surveyed [21] and by the fact that females are more likely to participate in online survey studies than males [22]. The use of convenience sampling is also a limitation in terms of the representativeness of the sample, for example, this likely contributed to the high percentage of dietitians and participants residing in Australia. The survey included a large number and scope of questions as it is the first to explore this topic among health professionals and the intention was to obtain a broad overview of opinions. However, this may have contributed to some participants not completing the survey. Additionally, the survey is based on self-report and, while some qualitative data were collected, the survey included primarily quantitative questions, which may limit the scope of opinions. Many of the participants surveyed also rated their knowledge of addictive eating as below average and their confidence in their knowledge of the latest evidence as low, which could be a limitation to their views on the topic.

The implications of the study findings for research and practice include that practitioners are being asked about addictive eating and there is a need for practitioners to understand addictive eating and the related comorbidities with weight and other mental health conditions such as depression. This would ensure that individuals are provided or directed to the most appropriate service rather than just standard dietary, weight management or psychology advice. One avenue for this could be achieved through professional development training. The focus of professional development training will need to consider the needs of different health professions based on their role in the referral or treatment pathway, for example, focusing on awareness of addictive eating and appropriate services to refer individuals to, compared with evidence-based treatment approaches for those delivering/managing treatment. Despite the lack of consistent terminology, addictive eating may be a means of people seeking help for a mental illness evidenced through having an unhealthy relationship with food. Therefore, there is a need for greater understanding of addictive eating behaviour and possible management options regardless of the terminology that is used to describe it. Future studies should aim to include a varied representation of health professions who may have a role in the care of individuals presenting with addictive eating. For example, GPs who may be the first point of contact for individuals and psychologists, dietitians, or other health professionals who may provide ongoing treatment. As addictive eating is an emerging field of research, health professionals' views on the topic may change over time, and research into this should be updated accordingly.

5. Conclusions

Overall, this survey of an international sample of practising health professionals and health professionals in training identified support for the concept of addictive eating and interest in professional development training. Additional exploration of health professionals' views on addictive eating is warranted, as this information is critical to advancing the field of addictive eating and informing best practice for assessment and treatment.

Supplementary Materials: The following are available online at http://www.mdpi.com/2072-6643/12/9/2860/s1, File S1: Health professionals' and health professional trainees' views on addictive eating behaviours: A cross sectional survey - Additional results, Table S1: Opinions on weight gain, and treatment of individuals with disordered eating or overweight/obesity among health professionals participating in a survey on addictive eating (n = 175), Table S2: Responses of participants in a survey on addictive eating, by health professionals and health professionals in training (n = 175).

Author Contributions: Conceptualisation, T.B., A.V.-G., A.C., R.M.B., Z.B.A., C.V.D., C.A.H., N.L., and P.S.; methodology, T.B., A.V.-G., A.C., R.M.B., Z.B.A., C.V.D., C.A.H., N.L., P.S., and M.W.; data curation, M.W. and T.B.; formal analysis, M.W. and T.B.; writing—original draft preparation, M.W. and T.B.; writing—review and editing, T.B., A.V.-G., A.C., R.M.B., Z.B.A., C.V.D., C.A.H., N.L., P.S., and M.W. All authors have read and agreed to the published version of the manuscript.

Funding: This research received no external funding. T.B. and P.S. are supported by Investigator Grant's from the National Health and Medical Research Council (NHMRC). A.C. is supported by an NHMRC Career Development Fellowship (ID: APP1123311). R.M.B. is supported by an Australian Research Council (ARC) Discovery Early Career Researcher Award (DECRA) Fellowship (DE190101244). A.V.G. is supported by a Medical Research Future Fund Next Generation of Clinical Researchers Fellowship (MRF1141214).

Conflicts of Interest: The authors declare no conflict of interest for this research. C.A.H. has received research funding from the American Beverage Association and speaker fees from the International Sweeteners Association for work outside of the submitted manuscript.

References

1. Gearhardt, A.N.; Corbin, W.R.; Brownell, K.D. Food Addiction: An Examination of the Diagnostic Criteria for Dependence. *J. Addict. Med.* **2009**, *3*, 1–7. [CrossRef]
2. Davis, C. From passive overeating to "food addiction": A spectrum of compulsion and severity. *ISRN Obes.* **2013**, *2013*, 435027. [CrossRef]
3. Fletcher, P.C.; Kenny, P.J. Food addiction: A valid concept? *Neuropsychopharmacology* **2018**, *43*, 2506–2513. [CrossRef] [PubMed]
4. Pursey, K.M.; Stanwell, P.; Gearhardt, A.N.; Collins, C.E.; Burrows, T.L. The prevalence of food addiction as assessed by the Yale Food Addiction Scale: A systematic review. *Nutrients* **2014**, *6*, 4552–4590. [CrossRef] [PubMed]
5. Ruddock, H.K.; Hardman, C.A. Food Addiction Beliefs Amongst the Lay Public: What Are the Consequences for Eating Behaviour? *Curr. Addict. Rep.* **2017**, *4*, 110–115. [CrossRef] [PubMed]
6. Lee, N.M.; Lucke, J.; Hall, W.D.; Meurk, C.; Boyle, F.M.; Carter, A. Public Views on Food Addiction and Obesity: Implications for Policy and Treatment. *PLoS ONE* **2013**, *8*, e74836. [CrossRef]
7. Li, J.T.E.; Pursey, K.M.; Duncan, M.J.; Burrows, T. Addictive Eating and Its Relation to Physical Activity and Sleep Behavior. *Nutrients* **2018**, *10*, 1428. [CrossRef]
8. Pursey, K.M.; Collins, C.E.; Stanwell, P.; Burrows, T.L. Foods and dietary profiles associated with 'food addiction' in young adults. *Addict. Behav. Rep.* **2015**, *2*, 41–48. [CrossRef]
9. Pedram, P.; Wadden, D.; Amini, P.; Gulliver, W.; Randell, E.; Cahill, F.; Vasdev, S.; Goodridge, A.; Carter, J.C.; Zhai, G.; et al. Food Addiction: Its Prevalence and Significant Association with Obesity in the General Population. *PLoS ONE* **2013**, *8*, e74832. [CrossRef]
10. Burrows, T.; Skinner, J.; McKenna, R.; Rollo, M. Food Addiction, Binge Eating Disorder, and Obesity: Is There a Relationship? *Behav. Sci.* **2017**, *7*, 54. [CrossRef]
11. Wiss, D.A.; Brewerton, T.D. Incorporating food addiction into disordered eating: The disordered eating food addiction nutrition guide (DEFANG). *Eat. Weight Disord. EWD* **2017**, *22*, 49–59. [CrossRef] [PubMed]
12. Cassin, S.E.; Sijercic, I.; Montemarano, V. Psychosocial Interventions for Food Addiction: A Systematic Review. *Curr. Addict. Rep.* **2020**. [CrossRef]

13. McKenna, R.A.; Rollo, M.E.; Skinner, J.A.; Burrows, T.L. Food Addiction Support: Website Content Analysis. *JMIR Cardio* **2018**, *2*, e10. [CrossRef] [PubMed]
14. Vandenbroucke, J.P.; von Elm, E.; Altman, D.G.; Gotzsche, P.C.; Mulrow, C.D.; Pocock, S.J.; Poole, C.; Schlesselman, J.J.; Egger, M. Strengthening the Reporting of Observational Studies in Epidemiology (STROBE): Explanation and elaboration. *Epidemiology* **2007**, *18*, 805–835. [CrossRef]
15. Braun, V.; Clarke, V. Using thematic analysis in psychology. *Qual. Res. Psychol.* **2006**, *3*, 77–101. [CrossRef]
16. Hebebrand, J.; Albayrak, Ö.; Adan, R.; Antel, J.; Diéguez, C.; De Jong, J.; Leng, G.; Menzies, J.; Mercer, J.G.; Murphy, M.; et al. "Eating addiction", rather than "food addiction", better captures addictive-like eating behavior. *Neurosci. Biobehav. Rev.* **2014**, *47*, 295–306. [CrossRef]
17. Ruddock, H.K.; Christiansen, P.; Halford, J.C.G.; Hardman, C.A. The development and validation of the Addiction-like Eating Behaviour Scale. *Int. J. Obes.* **2017**, *41*, 1710–1717. [CrossRef]
18. DePierre, J.A.; Puhl, R.M.; Luedicke, J. Public perceptions of food addiction: A comparison with alcohol and tobacco. *J. Subst. Use* **2014**, *19*, 1–6. [CrossRef]
19. Cassin, S.E.; Buchman, D.Z.; Leung, S.E.; Kantarovich, K.; Hawa, A.; Carter, A.; Sockalingam, S. Ethical, Stigma, and Policy Implications of Food Addiction: A Scoping Review. *Nutrients* **2019**, *11*, 710. [CrossRef]
20. da Luz, F.Q.; Hay, P.; Touyz, S.; Sainsbury, A. Obesity with Comorbid Eating Disorders: Associated Health Risks and Treatment Approaches. *Nutrients* **2018**, *10*, 829. [CrossRef]
21. Australian Institute of Health & Welfare. Health Workforce Snapshot. Available online: https://www.aihw.gov.au/reports/australias-health/health-workforce (accessed on 25 August 2020).
22. Cull, W.L.; O'Connor, K.G.; Sharp, S.; Tang, S.-F.S. Response rates and response bias for 50 surveys of pediatricians. *Health Serv. Res.* **2005**, *40*, 213–226. [CrossRef] [PubMed]

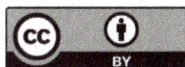

© 2020 by the authors. Licensee MDPI, Basel, Switzerland. This article is an open access article distributed under the terms and conditions of the Creative Commons Attribution (CC BY) license (http://creativecommons.org/licenses/by/4.0/).

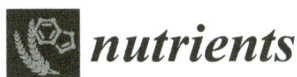

Review

Separating the Signal from the Noise: How Psychiatric Diagnoses Can Help Discern Food Addiction from Dietary Restraint

David Wiss [1],* and Timothy Brewerton [2]

[1] Department of Community Health Sciences, Fielding School of Public Health, University of California Los Angeles, Los Angeles, CA 90025, USA
[2] Department of Psychiatry and Behavioral Sciences, Medical University of South Carolina, Charleston, SC 29425, USA; drtimothybrewerton@gmail.com
* Correspondence: dwiss@ucla.edu; Tel.: +310-403-1874

Received: 30 August 2020; Accepted: 23 September 2020; Published: 25 September 2020

Abstract: Converging evidence from both animal and human studies have implicated hedonic eating as a driver of both binge eating and obesity. The construct of food addiction has been used to capture pathological eating across clinical and non-clinical populations. There is an ongoing debate regarding the value of a food addiction "diagnosis" among those with eating disorders such as anorexia nervosa binge/purge-type, bulimia nervosa, and binge eating disorder. Much of the food addiction research in eating disorder populations has failed to account for dietary restraint, which can increase addiction-like eating behaviors and may even lead to false positives. Some have argued that the concept of food addiction does more harm than good by encouraging restrictive approaches to eating. Others have shown that a better understanding of the food addiction model can reduce stigma associated with obesity. What is lacking in the literature is a description of a more comprehensive approach to the assessment of food addiction. This should include consideration of dietary restraint, and the presence of symptoms of other psychiatric disorders (substance use, posttraumatic stress, depressive, anxiety, attention deficit hyperactivity) to guide treatments including nutrition interventions. The purpose of this review is to help clinicians identify the symptoms of food addiction (true positives, or "the signal") from the more classic eating pathology (true negatives, or "restraint") that can potentially elevate food addiction scores (false positives, or "the noise"). Three clinical vignettes are presented, designed to aid with the assessment process, case conceptualization, and treatment strategies. The review summarizes logical steps that clinicians can take to contextualize elevated food addiction scores, even when the use of validated research instruments is not practical.

Keywords: food addiction; eating disorder; dietary restraint; substance use disorder; posttraumatic stress disorder; trauma; adverse childhood experience; early life adversity; psychiatric comorbidity; clinical vignette

1. Background

The Yale Food Addiction Scale (YFAS) was created in 2009 to match criteria for Substance Abuse in the Diagnostic and Statistical Manual of Mental Disorders (DSM-IV) and has been validated as a tool for identifying eating patterns which resemble alcohol and drug addictions [1]. The YFAS 2.0 (released 2016) reflects updated criteria in the DSM-5 [2]. Prevalence estimates of food addiction (FA) in a nationally representative US sample are approximately 15%, with higher rates in those who are obese [3]. A meta-analysis of 51 studies suggests the mean prevalence of FA worldwide is 16.2% [4]. Unlike obesity, rates of FA in the US are elevated among individuals with higher incomes [3]. In other studies of patients with obesity seeking weight loss, prevalence estimates range from 6.7–16.5% [5,6]

which closely mirror national prevalence rates for alcohol and substance use disorders (SUDs) [7]. Estimates are lower in adolescents [8], suggesting that FA develops over time. There has been a growing interest in early life psychosocial risk factors (e.g., trauma—defined as a deeply distressing or disturbing experience) in the development of both FA and obesity [9–12]. The current review employs a biopsychosocial perspective on FA, considering predisposing factors such as early life adversity which occurs in the first 18 years of life and can become biologically embedded, impacting reward function and eating behavior over the life course.

There has been considerable debate regarding the utility of an FA "diagnosis" without considering the contribution of dietary restraint in increasing FA symptoms [13–17]. While FA is not recognized by the DSM, the term diagnosis is used loosely throughout this manuscript. A common criticism of the YFAS in clinical applications is that the measure itself does not detect restrained eating (tendency to restrict food intake for weight control). The Disordered Eating and Food Addiction Nutrition Guide (DEFANG) attempted to conceptualize a role for FA into the common eating disorder (ED) paradigm which rejects the concept of food having addictive qualities by favoring an "all foods fit" ("no bad foods") approach [18]. However, the DEFANG did not incorporate restrained eating into the framework, nor did it consider the impact of trauma. The current review aims to help clinicians consider divergent nutritional strategies in patients with elevated YFAS scores, and to avoid misconceptions regarding treatment. Importantly, FA does not always necessitate rigid nutrition interventions. Arguments for and against the FA construct in the context of binge eating have recently been published [15]. Here, the position that FA can be relevant as a clinical entity is presented, and it is suggested that the presence of other psychiatric conditions such as ED, SUD, and posttraumatic stress disorder (PTSD) can be useful in determining if an individual requires targeted nutritional treatment (e.g., abstinence from specific foods). Alternatively, related psychopathology (e.g., chronic dieting based on body dissatisfaction) might indicate an opposite approach (e.g., inclusion of the foods persistently avoided). An understanding of different FA phenotypes may help guide intervention strategies.

1.1. Food Addiction Stigma

Alcohol use disorder (AUD) and SUDs were once viewed as individual choices but scientific progress and changing social norms have reduced this stigma. A survey study found that FA is more vulnerable to stigmatization than alcohol and may be perceived as a behavioral rather than substance addiction [19]. This position has favored the term "eating addiction" which has gained some traction and stimulated scholarly debate [20,21]. Meanwhile, FA is becoming increasingly accepted by the lay public, as evidenced by growing numbers of self-perceived food addicts [22,23]. Study participants express a desire to have their perceived condition formally recognized in order to receive more appropriate treatment [24]. While some research suggests that the FA label may increase stigmatizing attitudes [25], other studies show that the FA explanation reduces weight stigma [26,27]. It has also been suggested that while FA reduces externalized stigma, it may increase internalized stigma [28]. Furthermore, believing that certain food products can be addictive has been associated with support for policies intended to curb their use [29]. However, it remains unclear how a better understanding of FA neurobiology can reduce stigma in the context of ED treatment and recovery.

1.2. Food Addiction Controversy

Efforts to clear confusion around the FA construct have focused on semantics. For example, some authors have proposed the terms "refined food addiction" or "processed food addiction" to better capture FA as a substance-related disorder [30,31]. This approach targets specific foods which have been identified as addictive, such as chocolate, ice cream, French fries, pizza, cookies, chips, and cake [32]. More importantly, individuals would identify foods to avoid ("trigger foods") as part of their personal recovery program, which has been endorsed by some 12-Step groups (whereas other 12-Step groups have fixed food plans for all members). These approaches have come under scrutiny because success rates have not been well documented. Meanwhile, some authors posit that saying abstinence is ineffective because people binge when they finally eat sweets is like saying that abstinence from alcohol is ineffective because those with AUD binge after taking the first drink [31]. Another reason "abstinence-based" approaches are criticized is because they often place emphasis on weight loss, which current data suggests is not sustainable over the long term. A study based on a large prospective cohort from the UK suggests that over a 9-year period, the probability of going from obese to normal was 1 in 210 for men, and 1 in 124 for women [33]. Understandably, with such small chances of sustaining weight loss, classic ED treatment has favored targeting dietary restraint rather than weight loss, or the removal of specific foods.

1.3. Dietary Restraint

In 2003, Fairburn introduced a transdiagnostic theory of EDs proposing that diagnosis is not relevant to the treatment [34], when binge eating disorder (BED) was in the DSM-IV appendix and not yet an official diagnosis. A core assumption is that dieting precipitates bingeing; therefore, the pursuit of weight loss will be counterproductive with most ED presentations. However, among women with body image concerns (n = 1165), weight suppression correlated with future onset of EDs characterized by dietary restriction or compensatory weight control behaviors, but not with BED [35]. In one study of BED outpatients (n = 98), 65% reported an onset of dieting prior to their first binge and 35% reported that binge eating preceded their first diet [36]. Thus, dieting may not necessarily be a precursor to all forms of binge eating [37,38]. There is less consensus regarding the pursuit of weight loss in the presence of FA without an ED. Some advocates for reconceptualizing weight as a social justice issue believe that no person at all should engage in weight-loss behaviors. Rather, treatment professionals should target the problem of fat shame in society [39]. Others support the idea that new treatments are needed to address ED pathology and weight loss concurrently [40]. A recent systematic review and meta-analysis found that structured and professionally run obesity treatments are associated with reduced ED prevalence, risk, and symptoms in children [41]. However, because clinicians who work with patients with EDs often discover that the onset of disordered eating follows the first attempt to diet, many prefer a "do no harm" approach. Additionally, many professionals who work with these populations have abandoned weight loss [42] in some cases to avoid being targeted (shamed) by colleagues.

The current standard ED treatment is associated with high rates of relapse and poor long-term outcomes [43–45]. It has been suggested that contemporary ED models devote relatively little attention to biological factors driving binge eating, and that changes in the food environment interacting with individual vulnerability are key predisposing risk factors [46]. Newly proposed models suggest that clinicians go beyond a "no dieting" approach for all ED presentations and should incorporate addiction neuroscience [46,47]. Some authors recommend that researchers and clinicians distinguish between flexible and rigid restraint [14]. In some cases, restraint is related to a lower body weight, better weight regulation, and a better diet quality while in others, restraint predicts poor diet, overeating, and obesity [48]. While short-term deprivation increases cravings for avoided foods, long-term restriction results in reduction of food cravings that can facilitate extinction of conditioned responses [16]. Meule states that "the wide-held notion that dieting inevitably leads to food cravings is strongly oversimplified as the relationship between food restriction and food craving is more complex" [16]. This paper explores the nuances of different FA phenotypes, which have not been adequately described.

2. Eating Disorders

2.1. Bulimia Nervosa and Anorexia Nervosa

The highest prevalence rates of YFAS 2.0 diagnoses have been found in individuals with bulimia nervosa (BN) [49]. The relationship between FA and BMI has been described as non-linear: FA symptomatology can be higher in some underweight groups, in some cases related to compensatory behaviors that maintain lower BMIs [50]. In fact, some studies suggest that when separating anorexia nervosa restrictive type (AN-R) with the binge–purge type (AN-BP), FA prevalence is the highest in AN-BP [51]. Compensatory weight control behaviors in individuals with BN and AN-BP likely dampen the association between FA and BMI [52]. Several key reviews have summarized neurobiological overlaps with BN and SUDs, including dopamine (DA) D2 receptor-related vulnerabilities, structural and functional alterations in the frontal cortex, glutamatergic signaling, and the opioid system [53–55]. A recent systematic review of neuroimaging studies on BN and BED found diminished activity in frontostriatal circuits (associated with self-regulation) [56]. Treatment studies suggest that FA most likely improves when BN symptoms remit [57]. In an intervention study among women with BN ($n = 66$), those with higher FA severity at baseline were less likely to obtain abstinence from binge–purge episodes following treatment [58]. Taken together, there is preliminary support for the role of FA in the maintenance of BN via neuroadaptive changes in reward circuits. The challenge is discerning which came first (or would be considered "primary") in order to conceptualize an effective nutrition strategy. Here, it is suggested that consideration of the temporal sequence of disorder onset can be useful in discerning the truly positive FA "signal" from the falsely positive "noise," but that no rule can be applied to all cases.

2.2. Binge Eating Disorder

It has been suggested that subtyping BED based on psychiatric comorbidity may have important implications for treatment [59]. Researchers question whether the presence of BED vs. FA vs. BED + FA requires tailored treatment approaches [60]. One study suggested that when diagnostic subtypes are considered separately, FA is associated with a poor prognosis in the BED group [61]. It is possible that poor BED outcomes stem from the transdiagnostic assumption that BED patients do not need to emphasize the quality of their food ("it's not about the food"). Patient interest in weight loss may increase their risk of dropout from nonspecific ED treatment (not tailored to BED) [62]. Different phenotypes in BED are likely related to their dopaminergic response to highly palatable foods. For example, some individuals may develop particular eating expectancies in the face of poor emotion regulation and high anticipatory rewards [63]. The presence of FA may represent a more disturbed group of BED characterized by greater psychopathology [64]. To illustrate, in one study of 788 adults enrolled in BED treatment, shape/weight overvaluation differentiated BED severity more strongly than binge eating frequency [65]. Relatedly, those with heightened body image disturbance are more likely to engage in dietary restraint [66] which may contribute to bingeing as well as FA symptoms. Importantly, fear of being stigmatized predicts worsening FA status over time [67]. Stigma leads to maladaptive eating behaviors, stress, and weight gain [68]. Meanwhile, other findings do not support prevailing models that posit dietary or cognitive restraint as the predominant risk factor in BED [69]. Taken together, there appears a timely need to identify phenotypes of BED that require different treatment strategies, specifically those that would aim to reduce addiction-like eating versus those that would aim to reduce dietary restraint.

3. Substance Use Disorders

Given the neurobiological overlap between SUDs, EDs, and FA, considering an individual's relationship to alcohol, drugs, and other substances such as nicotine and caffeine may be helpful in separating the FA signal from the noise. For example, in a sample of Dutch adolescents ($n = 2653$), symptoms of FA were positively associated with alcohol use, cannabis use, smoking, and sugar intake [8]. Men with heroin use disorder ($n = 100$) had triple the odds of meeting criteria for BED or FA compared to controls [70]. Not surprisingly, FA diagnosis was associated with more severe craving. In a community-based sample of women ($n = 3756$), those with lifetime AUD or nicotine dependence were at higher risk for ED symptoms and diagnoses [71]. Based on the concept of reward dysfunction (reviewed below), it is likely that such ED symptoms represent those that overlap with FA. A recent systematic review and meta-analysis confirmed a higher prevalence of comorbid SUD in binge–purge ED presentations [72]. Among individuals with EDs, the pooled lifetime prevalence of comorbid SUD was 21.9% [72]. In an Italian sample of SUD patients ($n = 575$), the prevalence of FA was 20.2% [73], which is very close to the prevalence of ED estimated in meta-analysis. In a large longitudinal study from Australia, illicit substance users had significant risk of developing recurrent binge eating in addition to, or in place of, their substance use; however, the reverse was not found [74]. This suggests that individuals who engage in dysfunctional food-related behaviors prior to using drugs and alcohol may represent a different phenotype than those who develop addiction-like eating as a result of their drug use. In a study of women in SUD treatment ($n = 297$), a third reported starting drug use (in part) to lose weight and nearly half were concerned that gaining weight could trigger relapse [75]. In a non-treatment sample of drug-using women (college setting), 15.3% reported drug use for weight control purposes [76]. Patients with co-occurring SUD and ED are more sensitive to reward, have more difficulty engaging in goal-directed activity, are more impulsive, and have less access to emotion regulation skills [77]. The assessment of other addictions may prove helpful in determining the underpinnings of a high FA score, specifically as they relate to reward dysfunction and impulsivity. Meanwhile, genome wide association studies have found limited support for shared underpinnings for FA and SUD [78] whereas other lines of research have implicated DA-D2 receptors [79–83].

3.1. Reward Dysfunction

Convergence from neuroscience findings with case reports from the field have made clear that dysregulation of DA function is important for reward-related processes driving substance-seeking behavior [84]. Many authors have speculated that the bidirectional association between food and alcohol/drug dysfunction represents an "addiction transfer" [85] which has been supported by many studies of bariatric patients [86]. In a large twin study from the Netherlands, genetic factors explained 48% of the variation in high sugar consumption (52% explained by unique environmental factors), suggesting that neuronal circuits underlying the development of addiction and obesity are related, possibly due to DA receptor dysfunction that lead to difficulties resisting rewarding stimuli [87]. DA contributes to addiction and obesity through its differentiated role in reinforcement, motivation, and self-regulation [88]. In addition to deficiencies identified at striatal DA-D2 receptors [89,90], individuals with obesity and BED have widespread reduction in binding at mu-opioid receptors (MOR) [91]. The mesolimbic dopaminergic circuit is clearly affected by both highly palatable foods and diet-induced obesity similar to exposure to drugs of abuse [92]. Recent review articles have discussed highly processed foods (often high in glycemic index) as impacting neurohormonal and inflammatory signaling pathways in ways that create a vicious cycle of impulsivity, compulsivity, FA, and EDs [93–95]. The Regulatory Model of Addictive Vulnerability (RMAV) proposes that susceptibility to addictive disorders is linked to how well an individual's regulatory system responds to challenges, also referred to as allostasis [96]. According to these authors, both obesity and drug addiction are examples of major disorders characterized by dysregulated control systems. To date, this information has not been integrated into mainstream ED treatment programs, possibly because the translation of these findings contradicts the popular assumption that "it's not about the food." No trials have been conducted using strategies designed to reduce reward-based eating in patients with EDs; however, there are data suggesting that medications commonly used in SUD treatment (naltrexone/bupropion) in conjunction with lifestyle changes can reduce FA severity among those with BED [97]. Prospective research is needed to determine if reduction of highly palatable foods can improve reward dysfunction in people with FA.

3.2. Impulsivity

Impulsivity can be separated into attentional (inability to focus attention or concentrate) and motor (acting without thinking). In a sample of individuals with obesity presenting for bariatric surgery ($n = 193$), FA emerged when both attentional and motor impulsivity levels were elevated [98]. Impulsivity has been identified as a key shared mechanism between BED and addictive disorders [99].

For example, patients with EDs who have problems pursuing tasks to the end and focusing on long-term goals are more likely to develop addiction-like eating patterns [100]. A recent systematic review reported that across 45 studies, impulsivity was consistently associated with FA [101]. Given that FA has been reported as a mediator between impulsivity and obesity [102], it is possible that in certain susceptible individuals, ED behaviors develop along this trajectory to suppress unwanted weight. In a recent study of 145 patients with EDs, those with alcohol and drug abuse symptoms represented a specific phenotype characterized by greater impulsive personality, emotion dysregulation, and problems with executive functioning [103]. Among male military veterans ($n = 106$), impulsivity moderated the relationship between PTSD symptoms and alcohol consumption [104], with relevance discussed in more detail below. In addition to higher levels of impulsivity, individuals with FA are more likely to report a family history of addiction [105] which may be consistent with genetic underpinnings. While addiction research has primarily focused on the mesolimbic dopaminergic projection, impulsivity has also been linked to the serotonin system. Several genetic studies have linked polymorphisms at 5HTTLPR (codes for serotonin transporters) to higher levels of impulsivity among individuals with BN [106,107], with associated aberrations of serotonergic functioning being exacerbated by early life adversity (ELA) [108–110]. However, meta-analysis has linked the 5HTTLPR allele strongest to AN [111] and to date no study has linked this polymorphism to FA. Taken together, assessment of impulsivity in conjunction with assessment of SUD may prove beneficial in separating the FA signal (true positives) from the noise (false positives), but more research is needed before the impulsivity construct can be used in predicting the clinical utility of FA.

4. Trauma and PTSD

The Adverse Childhood Experiences (ACE) study from 1998 highlighted 5- to 10-fold increase in the risk of AUD and SUD following exposure to four or more ACEs in the first 18 years of life [112]. As traumatic stress affects a variety of brain structures and functions, ACEs impact a variety of functions and behaviors therefore have been determined nonspecific [113]. ACEs captured by the various forms of the questionnaire are referred to as a form of ELA; however, it is important to acknowledge there are many other measures used, such as the childhood trauma questionnaire (CTQ) [114,115]. Why is it that some individuals exposed to childhood trauma have a heightened risk for psychiatric disorder while others demonstrate resilience over the lifespan? The Theory of Latent Vulnerability suggests that one's genotype interacts with an adverse environment to create a neurocognitive phenotype, characterized by changes in reward processing (DA), threat processing (amygdala), and memory processing (hippocampus) [116]. One pathway which might in part explain the enduring biological impact of adversity is inflammation. A longitudinal study of adolescent girls ($n = 147$) showed that ELA was associated with greater odds of displaying a proinflammatory phenotype, generating low-level non-resolving inflammation (higher levels of IL-6 and decreased sensitivity to cortisol) [117]. Meta-analysis has linked childhood trauma to cognitive deficits, with the greatest deficits among those with a PTSD diagnosis [118]. If any abuse is identified in children or adolescents, it is likely they have also previously experienced, are currently experiencing, or are at risk for experiencing additional forms of abuse [119], which highlights the importance of social and environmental factors in a biopsychosocial model. While it is outside the scope of this review to clearly distinguish between trauma, adversity, chronic stress, and PTSD, the importance of these events early in life are emphasized as increasing risk for various addictions. Important for the understanding of trauma is that events be differentiated from their effects, which varies based on the experience of the individual [120]. Exposures by themselves do not define PTSD.

4.1. Addictions

Functional magnetic resonance imaging (fMRI) studies have linked ELA to blunted subjective responses to reward-predicting cues and dysfunction in the left basal ganglia regions implicated in reward-related learning and motivation [121]. Other neuroimaging studies have indicated an increase in dopamine transporter (DAT) density in PTSD, which may reflect a higher DA turnover among trauma survivors [122]. Both an increase in the number of traumatic events early in life and an increase in levels of perceived stress were associated with a higher ventral striatal DA response to amphetamine [123]. This evidence supports the biological embedding hypothesis [124] which links ELA to addictive behaviors [125]. ELA can be viewed as nonspecific because it predisposes individuals to a wide range of addictive behaviors. For example, in a sample of healthy young adults (n = 200), greater lifetime stress exposure was related to increased impulsivity and FA [126], suggesting that food is a predictable go-to for self-medication [127]. A nationally representative sample of young adults' (n = 10,813) exposure to multiple forms of maltreatment predicted excessive sugar sweetened beverage consumption [128]. Not surprisingly, childhood physical abuse and childhood sexual abuse both increase risk for FA by approximately 90% [10]. Higher numbers of PTSD symptoms predict increased prevalence of FA and the strength of this association increased when symptom onset occurred at an earlier age [11]. In this study (n = 49,408), the PTSD-FA association did not differ substantially by trauma type, suggesting that all forms of ELA impact reward-related behaviors. Among overweight/obese women (n = 301), the association between FA and childhood trauma was significant after controlling for potential confounders such as socioeconomic status [129]. Compared to women with no addictions, women with FA and with SUD endorsed more depression and PTSD symptoms and had more difficulties with goal-directed behaviors, acceptance of emotions, and impulse control [130]. Taken together, exposure to trauma significantly increases risk for FA and therefore should be considered during comprehensive psychiatric/psychological and nutrition assessments.

4.2. Eating Disorders

All forms of childhood maltreatment are associated with all forms of EDs, although some more than others [131]. The odds of BED following maltreatment is consistently higher than AN [132], yet meta-analysis confirms that, when pooled, the risk for BN is the highest [133]. Given the link between early life trauma and addictive disorders, it is likely that FA is an important pathway on the trajectory toward binge-type EDs. Meanwhile, there are also associations from ELA to EDs which may not include FA as a mediator, capturing a different phenotype with different treatment implications (discussed further below). In one sample of adult patients with EDs from Sweden (n = 853), a quarter had a lifetime diagnosis of PTSD [134]. Other estimates suggest traumatic events occur in over a third of adolescents in ED outpatients (n = 182), and the prevalence is highest among those with BN [135]. A recent review article suggests that the prevalence of comorbid PTSD and EDs ranges from 9% to 24% [136], although estimates are consistently higher when looking specifically at binge-type EDs [137–141]. Several studies have suggested that adverse events experienced early in life predict binge eating symptoms in both men and women [142–144]. Evidence consistently shows that ED symptoms such as anxiety and depression are more severe among those with a PTSD diagnosis [145], and those with the dissociative subtype are even worse off [146]. Some authors believe that it may be helpful to modify current ED treatments to better address the overlapping risk among EDs and obesity among those who have been exposed to trauma [147]. Others posit that any effort to lose weight or restrict food will only make eating problems worse [66,148,149]. In this paper, our aim is to resolve this debate by presenting three clinical vignettes that are fictional yet rooted in extensive clinical experience.

5. Other Psychiatric Diagnoses

5.1. Depression

Multiple lines of evidence suggest that individuals with FA have more depressive symptoms than controls [60,105,130,150–152]. A recent review of studies using YFAS identified depressive symptoms as a clinically relevant correlate [49]. Meta-analysis suggests that FA is significantly correlated to depression (r = 0.459) [4]. The directionality of this relationship remains less clear. While it is likely that depressed individuals may turn to highly palatable foods to alleviate negative affect, several recent studies have suggested that a low-quality diet increases depressive symptoms. A cross-sectional study from the US (n = 16,807) suggests that intakes of total fiber, specifically from fruits and vegetables, was inversely associated with depressive symptoms [153]. In a French cohort of adults (n = 3523) with mean follow-up 12.6 years, diets high in anti-inflammatory properties prevented depressive symptoms, particularly among men, smokers, or physically inactive individuals [154]. In a Spanish cohort of graduate students initially free of depression (n = 14,907), followed for a median 10.3 years, participants with the highest consumption of ultra-processed foods had the highest risk of developing depression, particularly among those with low levels of physical activity [155]. Another large French cohort of adults followed for a mean of 5.4 years demonstrated a positive association between ultra-processed food and the risk of incident depression [156].

While there appears to be preliminary support that low-quality diets can lead to depression, there is also evidence that high-quality diets can mitigate or reverse depressive symptoms. A randomized controlled trial (RCT) showed that dietary support (nutrition counseling by a dietitian) for 12 weeks can improve symptoms [157]. Systematic review and meta-analysis suggest that the most compelling evidence for reducing incident depression exists for the Mediterranean diet, known for its anti-inflammatory properties [158]. Since depressive disorders correlate and cross-associate with EDs, SUDs, and PTSD [138,159,160] the diagnosis may prove important for informing nutrition treatment. While the presence of depressive symptoms might not be informative of whether or not an individual has an actual addiction to food (the signal), it is worth considering the potential role of dietary intake in contributing to symptoms. For example, for a person engaging excess consumption of highly palatable foods, it may be worth experimenting with dietary manipulation before psychiatric medication. Further, if a patient receiving ED treatment with the "all foods fit" philosophy is consistently eating low-fiber foods ("intuitively") and has non-resolving depressive symptoms, it may indicate that a more targeted nutrition strategy is warranted.

5.2. Anxiety

In addition to reducing depressive symptoms, the Mediterranean diet may also be helpful in reducing the odds of anxiety [161]. However, a recent meta-analysis of RCTs concluded that no effect of dietary interventions is observed for anxiety [162]. Meanwhile, anxiety disorders show a dose–response association with worsening diet quality [163]; however, directionality remains unclear. Omega-3 fatty acids have been investigated for their role in anxiety disorders, but results are inconsistent, and data are too sparse to draw conclusions [164,165]. The role of gastrointestinal microbiota has also received attention as a potential mediator linking diet quality to anxiety symptoms [166–169]. Meanwhile, anxiety has been significantly correlated with FA (r = 0.483) [4] which is not surprising given the strong associations between anxiety and SUDs [170]. Anxiety is a well-established risk factor for EDs, SUDs, and PTSD. A recent systematic review suggested that anxiety may mediate the association between PTSD and SUD [171]; therefore, it is biologically plausible that anxiety is on the pathway from ELA to FA, though this has not yet been shown. Among treatment-seeking youth (n = 490), social anxiety predicts binge eating [172]. A rodent model suggests that consumption of a Western diet may lead to long-lasting damage to fear neurocircuitry, particularly during adolescence [173]. In an Australian sample of adults (n = 1344), anxiety sensitivity predicted severe FA [174]. The association between FA and current anxiety disorders has also been reported in bariatric surgery candidates (n = 128) [175]. One study suggested that irrational beliefs may be the source of the anxiety associated with FA [176]. Among adult females with anxiety (n = 51), impulsivity predicted higher intakes of sugar and saturated fat [177], which is consistent with reports of "comfort food" consumption when under stress [178]. Taken together, the presence of an anxiety diagnosis by itself is not likely to be informative of an FA phenotype; however, it may prove beneficial to discern between anxiety that is symptomatic of PTSD/ELA and generalized [145,179] versus other forms of anxiety such as body image disturbance or dysmorphia (likely indicative of dietary restraint). Either way, FA treatment should include positive anxiety management and coping skills [46].

5.3. Attention Deficit Hyperactivity Disorder (ADHD)

ADHD is defined by inattention and/or hyperactivity and is often characterized by impulsivity. Both ADHD and SUDs are characterized by choice impulsivity [180]. There are recent data to support the possibility that choice impulsivity in ADHD results from substance misuse [181]. A popular explanation for the association between ADHD and EDs is that impulsive behavior generates the disordered eating [182,183]. Both conditions rely on a dopaminergic signaling which makes their cooccurrence a logical comorbidity [182]. However, the evidence reviewed above suggests that among those with EDs, impulsivity is also linked to serotonergic genes (i.e., 5HTTLPR). In both sexes, binge eaters have significantly higher prevalence of ADHD [184]. In a nationally representative sample of adults in the US (n = 4719), only the association between ADHD and BN remained significant after confounders were adjusted for [185]. In a sample of patients with obesity (n = 105), adult and childhood ADHD were significantly associated with self-reported FA and binge eating severity [186]. In a recent study of 136 patients with EDs, a positive screen for ADHD related to worse eating symptoms and the presence of high ED levels contributed to treatment dropout [187]. Meanwhile, a large genome-wide association study suggests that higher BMI increases risk of developing ADHD but not the other way around [188]; therefore, directionality remains unclear. It is worth noting that stimulant medications (i.e., amphetamines) often used in the treatment of ADHD can have an impact on appetite, with suppressing effects while using and rebound appetite when not. In one study of undergraduate students (n = 705), nearly 12% reported using prescription stimulants to lose weight [189] however these students were not diagnosed with ADHD. Lisdexamfetamine, which is FDA approved for ADHD as well as BED, works by enhancing dorsofrontal cortex function [190,191]. Meanwhile, it remains unclear whether ADHD symptomatology (e.g., impulsivity) or the effect of ADHD medications (including their discontinuation) drive the potential association with FA. Research is needed to test long-term outcomes of lisdexamfetamine on BED + FA. It may prove important to consider ADHD when conceptualizing FA phenotypes in the context of nutrition strategies.

6. Clinical Vignettes

6.1. Phenotype A

Alma is a 23-year-old, single Columbian female who grew up in a troubled household. Her parents were not married but lived together off and on until she was 10, when her father left. Alma had two older brothers from a different father. Her mother divorced her first husband when the two boys were two and four, right before she met Alma's father, who attempted to parent all three children. However, Alma's father struggled with a severe alcohol use disorder and would be absent for days at a time. Alma's brothers never accepted him as a parent figure. When Alma's father was gone completely, she began to seek attention from boys by playing sports with her brothers. She became athletic and thrived in volleyball. As a freshman in high school, she joined the volleyball team and made many friends among the athletic crowd. Alma loved to play sports and cook food, often referring to herself as a "foodie", known for baking Columbian desserts for her teammates. She grew close to the assistant coach of the girls' volleyball team who had a reputation for drinking with the students after games. Alma never drank alcohol or did drugs because of what she had seen them do to her father. She swore she would never smoke a cigarette. One night the male assistant coach offered to take Alma home and kissed her in the car. Alma felt confused but kept the secret to herself. During the summer after her freshman year, she agreed to visit his home where she was coerced into sex (statutory rape). Alma kept it a secret due to shame, but people close to her knew something had changed.

Alma did not return to the volleyball team for her sophomore year. She became promiscuous with several seniors at her school and some of her brother's friends. She lost interest in sports completely and began binge eating on highly processed foods at night to help her sleep. She often skipped breakfast but never engaged in any compensatory behaviors. Her academic performance began to decline, and she started drinking coffee, soda, and energy drinks throughout the day. Between her sophomore and senior year, Alma gained forty pounds, meanwhile experimenting with a few popular diets that never stuck for more than two days. When she graduated from high school, she moved in with her boyfriend who was 30 years old, owning a small shop that sold electronic cigarettes. Alma began vaping daily. However, she stuck by her commitment to never smoke a cigarette, drink alcohol, or use drugs. They mostly ate fast food and ordered take-out together, but Alma would frequently bake and cook. Alma got a job as an office administrator and slowly stopped responding to texts from her mother and brothers. She never posted any pictures on social media because she did not want people to see how much weight she had gained. Eventually, she learned that her boyfriend was cheating on her and moved back in with her mother after he told her that she had to leave. At this point the mother brought Alma to a psychiatrist for an evaluation, but Alma did not tell the doctor about the rape, in part because she was amnestic for the memories. The doctor identified complex PTSD and a dissociative disorder, prescribing sertraline and trazadone. She was referred to an outpatient psychotherapist who began working with her twice per week, at which point Alma opened up about the sexual abuse. When the trauma therapy started, the bingeing escalated significantly. At this point, Alma was referred to a registered dietitian nutritionist (RDN) specializing in mental and behavioral health. Several assessment tools were administered, including the eating disorder examination questionnaire (EDE-Q) which indicated an absence of dietary restraint and the YFAS 2.0 where she met criteria for severe food addiction (BMI = 36.8).

6.2. Phenotype B

Jeffrey is a 27-year-old, single, half-Taiwanese, half-white male who grew up in a wealthy household as an only child. His father was a cardiologist with mild undiagnosed obsessive compulsive personality disorder (OCPD) and, before getting married, his mother was a swimsuit model with a long history of dieting. Both parents ran marathons together and revered the thin ideal, frequently making negative comments about fat people. Jeffrey's parents were very adamant about their son playing sports and at one point hired a running coach for him. Jeffrey spent a lot of time with nannies and babysitters, including extended periods when his parents vacationed without him. When Jeffrey was nine, he was sent to a psychiatrist for behavioral problems where he was diagnosed with ADHD and prescribed dextroamphetamine/amphetamine. Jeffrey was a straight-A student with the help of the medication and several tutors. Jeffrey also began running with his parents by age 13. His mother told Jeffrey to only eat carbohydrates before, during, and after a run, and to avoid them at all other times. Jeffrey completed his first marathon at age 15 and wore the medal at his private high school the next day, where he was photographed for the cover of the school magazine and website. One of his mother's friends provided an opportunity for Jeffrey to model for a large international fashion company and, at age 17, he was on a billboard in his 6'2" frame with his shirt off. His agent helped him build a following on Instagram, and Jeffrey began to spend more time exercising to prepare for photo shoots. The agreement was that Jeffrey could continue to model as long as he went to college and earned decent grades. He went to a private university as a communications major.

As a freshman in college, Jeffrey was switched from mixed amphetamine salts to a high-dose lisdexamfetamine and was also prescribed clonazepam for anxiety. Jeffrey never told anyone that he spent up to an hour each day looking in the mirror, obsessed with the fat on his abdominal area. During his junior year Jeffrey did a "Freeze the Fat" procedure with the physician who had done several cosmetic surgeries on his mother. He was very disappointed with the results. As Jeffrey continued to get modeling jobs, his performance in school began to decline. Jeffrey continued to run 10 miles per day on a treadmill in the gym at his apartment complex. He also did 30 minutes of abdominal workouts daily and rarely missed a workout. Jeffrey cut out all grains and dairy from his diet and only got small amounts of carbohydrates from fruits, starchy vegetables, and occasionally beans. Jeffrey frequently made negative comments about processed food and did not like to eat at restaurants. Jeffrey had several short-lived relationships with women, but as he became increasingly concerned about his appearance, he lost interest in dating. Jeffrey sought out an RDN to help him lose his stubborn abdominal fat; the dietitian determined that his BMI was 17.2 and contacted the psychiatrist to discuss potential body dysmorphic disorder. The psychiatrist told Jeffrey that being on a stimulant was contraindicated at such a low BMI, discontinuing the lisdexamfetamine and starting him on fluoxetine. At this point Jeffrey starting bingeing on carbohydrates and would "run it off" in his apartment gym, even if it was late at night. One evening, Jeffrey rolled his ankle and due to the sprain was told not to run for several weeks. Jeffrey purged for the first time after ordering Chinese food and eating a whole container of fried rice. He hated the experience of purging but continued to engage that behavior whenever he ate carbohydrates. He began to order food delivery and would often flush the food down the toilet because once he retrieved it from the trash. At the request of the psychiatrist, Jeffrey made another appointment with the RDN and obliged because he was feeling very depressed. Several assessment tools were administered, including the EDE-Q, which indicated high levels of dietary restraint, and the YFAS 2.0, where he met criteria for moderate food addiction (BMI = 17.0).

6.3. Phenotype C

Whitney is a 30-year-old, single, white female, and the oldest of three daughters to happily married parents who had no formal psychiatric diagnoses. Her mother was a professor at a small university and her father a certified public accountant who became obese in his late 40s. Her two sisters looked up to Whitney who was quite popular in middle school. Whitney got a lot of attention from boys but found herself attracted to women. In high school, she had a girlfriend for two years and the relationship made a lot of people in school uncomfortable. Despite becoming somewhat of an outcast, Whitney got good grades and was accepted into a local college as a sociology major. She was passionate about gender studies and started her own blog about sexuality. For a class assignment, Whitney filled out the ACE measure and scored a zero. Some of her friends began frequenting rave parties and taking ecstasy; Whitney fell in love with this culture. Whitney attended the Burning Man festival each year during college and graduated with honors. Whitney's family was proud of her and she maintained successful relationships with her parents and siblings. Everyone in the family loved Whitney's girlfriend. After college, they opened a business selling handmade jewelry, which was a big success in the Burning Man crowd. They eventually moved into a condo together and had two dogs who they took with them on long hikes at nearby trails.

At age 26, Whitney was hit by a drunk driver which killed her partner, witnessing her take her last breath at the scene. Whitney shattered her femur along with several other minor fractures and was in the hospital for two weeks, completely devastated by the loss of her lover. Despite having family by her side constantly and a doctor who gave a positive prognosis of her recovery, Whitney began to express suicidal ideation. She was on heavy doses of opioid medications and everyone assumed her mental health would improve after discharging from the hospital. However, upon returning back to her parents' house, it was obvious that Whitney had PTSD. She was prescribed oxycodone for pain management which she quickly became dependent on. The family found a therapist to do Eye Movement Desensitization and Reprocessing (EMDR), but Whitney would often show up sedated from the medication and the work was not productive. After several months of both physical and emotional therapy, the doctor took her off opioids and prescribed gabapentin. However, Whitney was able to purchase oxycodone on the street and within a matter of months she was buying heroin (which she smoked rather than injected) because it was much more affordable.

Whitney went into her first treatment center for heroin use disorder at age 29. She was prescribed gabapentin, buspirone, methocarbamol, venlafaxine, and quetiapine. During this time, she developed a strong preference for sweets and would eat several bags of candy daily. It was normal for people in her rehab to smoke cigarettes and drink sugary energy drinks, so she did the same. For the first time in her life, Whitney began gaining weight and by six months sober had gained 30 pounds. At this time, she was in a sober living house, which provided restaurant-style catered food. One of her roommates with severe bulimia nervosa taught Whitney how to induce vomiting to lose unwanted pounds. Whitney had never struggled with body image issues until she was sober and on several medications.

She quickly learned that purging was quite soothing and began vomiting daily, yet never tried any specific diets. Sometimes she would purge "healthy foods" simply because it felt relieving to do so. When these behaviors were discovered, her sober living required her to attend an ED outpatient clinic where she was instructed to eat three meals, two snacks, plus dessert every single day. After reaching her highest weight, Whitney relapsed on heroin and, within two weeks, was back in detox, where she began bingeing on ice cream, candy, and grilled cheese sandwiches. Whitney was referred to an RDN specializing in mental and behavioral health. Several assessment tools were administered including the EDE-Q which indicated moderate dietary restraint and the YFAS 2.0 where she met criteria for severe food addiction (BMI = 26.4).

7. Discussion

Phenotype A is a clear example of an FA signal (true positive) not blocked by the noise of dietary restraint (false positive). With an absence of restrictive eating there is little convincing evidence that the addiction is driven by dieting, a relic of internalized weight bias, or other forms of compensation often generated by socially constructed forces such as weight stigma. This case illustrates the link between ELA and FA which is likely mediated by biological mechanisms including altered DA signaling [121,122,192–194]. FA has been independently associated with exposure to early life sexual abuse [195]. Alma's father has AUD, which can be useful in evaluating biological susceptibility to addictive disorders. Furthermore, Alma was a "foodie" prior to the rape incident, suggesting that her tendency to seek highly palatable food may have a genetic basis as well as linked to her early psychosocial environment (and cultural background). The traumatic event did not create the FA but rather exacerbated her symptoms and severity by creating dependence on food for self-medication. Her weight gain may have reinforced incentive salience assigned to food stimuli [196]. Alma did not develop alcohol or drug problems due to important social factors during her upbringing where she witnessed the devastating impact they had on her father. While many people with high susceptibility to addictions struggle with multiple substances, Alma did not cross-addict into intoxicating substances; however, her clinical history indicates evidence of both caffeine and nicotine use disorders. Based on our clinical experience, we have observed that some (not all) of the most severe FA cases develop addictions to food with limited cross-addictions. We recommend considering cross-addiction in discerning the signal from the noise (true versus false positives); however, the absence of cross-addiction does not always indicate a weaker signal. In fact, in some cases it may be more severe because other addictive substances fail to compete with the experience of food. As this phenotype exemplifies FA, it suggests that FA-informed nutritional strategies may be warranted as well as safe (low risk of developing an ED). We suggest that strategies be assessed individually rather than a "one size fits all" approach.

Phenotype B is an example of how "noise" can muddle the FA signal and produce a false positive. In this case, dietary restraint is clearly driving the FA symptoms. Jeffrey is a classic example of how thin ideals can be perpetuated by the family system, become internalized, and eventually become pathological. Jeffrey's modeling career appears influenced by his mother's history of modeling and related social network. There is no AUD/SUD in the immediate family, which can be helpful information when assessing potential FA (reward dysfunction). The fact that Jeffrey never struggled with AUD/SUD is also informative. However, the ADHD diagnosis indicates the potential for higher levels of impulsivity and the stimulant medications may have appetite dysregulating effects [182,189,197]. When Jeffrey was taken off lisdexamfetamine after clinical concerns about under eating and body dysmorphic disorder, the loss-of-control eating began. Binge eating was accompanied by compensatory exercise behaviors, indicating classic ED pathology. The period of time when Jeffrey was depressed and experiencing heightened conflict around food is likely the source of the increased FA scores. He was previously successful in restraining himself with food but eventually lost his ability to do so, which is not uncommon over longer periods of time [34]. This case study exemplifies how an underweight individual can have elevated YFAS scores; however, the diagnosis of moderate FA is not informative for treatment. Rather, FA is a product of restrained eating stemming from body dissatisfaction.

Therefore, intervention strategies should focus on dietary inclusion rather than exclusion, targeting the underlying psychological and family system issues rather than focus on avoiding specific foods (e.g., carbohydrates).

Phenotype C is an example of a case that could be interpreted as an FA signal (true positive), or as a more classic ED presentation (false positive), depending on the training (and bias) of the practitioner. Whitney had no evidence of ELA, although did experience adversity in high school. However, she was resilient to this exposure. She did not develop SUD early on despite regularly using "party drugs" (methylenedioxyamphetamine or MDMA). However, following her serious injury and PTSD warranting opioid medications, she developed an opioid use disorder, implicating trauma as an important risk factor. Once becoming sober and being prescribed several medications, her PTSD symptoms and reward-seeking behavior led to FA and associated distress. Evidence of cross-addiction can be found with caffeine and nicotine. The ED developed after the FA and weight gain, eventually contributing to her relapse with heroin. While body dissatisfaction initially drove the ED behaviors, there was no history of dietary restraint before the SUD. In this case, FA preceded the dietary restraint, meaning that the signal existed before the noise. It is likely that practitioners who do not endorse the clinical utility of FA will observe the PTSD–ED connection and ignore the contribution of addiction-like eating into Whitney's assessment and treatment plan. The best direction for nutrition treatment is not clear and could be effective in multiple ways as long as Whitney had "buy-in" with adequate clinical and social support. Regular inclusion of highly palatable foods appears to be the safest course in order to prevent further progression of restriction and/or purging. However, it is possible that this approach can increase risk for SUD relapse if Whitney continues to gain weight and is unable to accept her body at a higher BMI [75]. Meanwhile, some might argue that FA-informed nutrition strategies that reduce reward-based eating may increase risk for SUD relapse by depriving the brain of DA that it has been conditioned to get from comforting foods. This has been widely endorsed by a "first things first" message from *Alcoholics Anonymous*, suggesting that sweets and chocolate are helpful in early recovery [198], but data to support this are lacking. This is another example of how a nutrition strategy is best assessed on an individual basis. Importantly, the treatment team should be on the same page since consistent messaging from providers appears critical [47].

The three clinical vignettes bring attention to heterogeneity that is possible given an FA diagnosis using the YFAS 2.0. All three cases meet criteria for FA (A and C are severe while B is moderate). However, a comprehensive biopsychosocial assessment identified divergent phenotypes that may warrant different nutrition interventions. While no trials have been reported using targeted nutrition interventions for FA, several studies have shown that non-diet approaches such as intuitive eating can be effective in reducing dietary restraint [199–201]. The present review suggests that it would be effective to identify FA phenotypes based on the presence of other psychiatric disorders such as ED, AUD/SUD, PTSD, depression, anxiety, and ADHD as part of a comprehensive biopsychosocial assessment, and to assign nutrition treatment based on the relative strength of the FA signal amidst the noise (true versus false positive). Recent studies have identified different phenotypic characterizations of the FA construct [60,61,202,203]. However, Table 1 suggests a guide for clinicians to consider in settings where the use of extensive validated instruments is not always practical.

Table 1. Eight Step Process for Clinicians to Discern Food Addiction from Dietary Restraint in Order to Inform Inclusive vs. Exclusive Nutrition Strategies.

Step	Assessment	If Negative	If Positive
1	Food Addiction (FA) • YFAS 2.0 [2] or mYFAS [204]	FA is unlikely to be a relevant construct	⇒ Step 2
2	Dietary Restraint • Examine history of dieting behavior and role of body image as well as internalized weight bias • Can use EDE-Q (long or short) [205] or EAT-26 [206] or similar validated tools	FA is likely to be a relevant construct • Consider ruling out food insecurity since it is also a form of deprivation that may increase FA symptoms [207,208]	Consider if the FA preceded the restraint, or if the restraint created the FA • If FA came first, it is likely to be informative that FA is a relevant construct ⇒ Step 3, and ⇒ Step 7
3	Substance Use Disorder (SUD) • Can use clinical diagnosis or self-report or validated measure • Can assess reward dysfunction by also considering addictions to caffeine and nicotine • Can also assess impulsivity using BIS-11 [209,210] which may help to better understand loss-of-control behavior	Absence of other addictions does not rule out FA. However, concurrent low levels of impulsivity may suggest that the individual is unlikely to have an actual FA. Will want to also consider ADHD when assessing impulsivity ⇒ Step 4, and ⇒ Step 8	FA is likely to be a relevant construct. It is worth considering if the FA or SUD came first • If SUD came first, it may indicate that inclusive nutrition strategies are the most practical ⇒ Step 4
4	PTSD including complex PTSD • Can use clinical diagnosis or validated measure such as PCL-5 [211] • Qualified professionals are required to assess the presence of CPTSD because it can be difficult for some patients to "connect the dots" across multiple life events	If there is an absence of SUD and PTSD, the presence of dietary restraint suggests that FA symptoms are driven by restriction rather than an actual FA. An exception would be if it was clear that FA preceded the restraint; however, in the absence of SUD and PTSD, inclusive nutritional strategies are likely to be the most practical ⇒ Step 6	FA is likely to be a relevant construct regardless of whether there is SUD history. However, history of SUD likely strengthens the confidence in the FA signal ⇒ Step 5
5	Early Life Adversity (ELA) • Can use validated measures such as ACE [112], CTQ [114,115], ETI-SR [212]	Suggests an absence of biological embedding. While later life traumatic experiences can alter physiology, an absence of ELA indicates that inclusive nutritional strategies may be more plausible. There may be some cases of ELA in the absence of PTSD which can indicate high levels of biological resilience, also warranting inclusive nutritional strategies ⇒ Step 6	FA is very likely to be a relevant construct, and in the presence of ELA, PTSD, and SUD and no evidence of dietary restraint as a predisposing risk factor, exclusive/restricted nutritional strategies may be warranted, assuming there are adequate resources including social support and access to nutritious unprocessed foods
6	Depression • Can use clinical diagnosis or self-report or validated measures such as PHQ-9 [213], BDI [214], or CESD [215]	With low levels of depressive symptoms, an inclusive nutritional strategy is likely to be the most practical strategy ⇒ Step 7	If depressive symptoms persist, it may be worth making drastic dietary changes such as the exclusion of highly processed foods in order to improve mood

Table 1. Cont.

Step	Assessment	If Negative	If Positive
7	Anxiety • Can use clinical diagnosis or self-report or validated measures such as the BAI [216], STAI [217], GAD-7 [218] or similar validated tools	Low levels of anxiety indicate that an inclusive nutritional strategy is likely to be most practical ⇒ Step 8	Consider if anxiety is related to body image disturbance. If body image drives anxiety (or vice versa), it may indicate dietary restraint, suggesting an inclusive nutritional strategy. If anxiety is not associated with body image, improving nutritional status by excluding certain foods may be warranted (and safe)
8	ADHD • Can use clinical diagnosis or validated measures such as ASRS [219]	If ADHD is negative but there are high levels of impulsivity, it may indicate higher likelihood of FA	Consider if eating behavior has been altered by the impact of stimulant medications

Legend: YFAS: Yale Food Addiction Scale; FA: Food Addiction; EDE-Q: Eating Disorder Examination Questionnaire; EAT-26: Eating Attitudes Test-26; SUD: Substance Use Disorder; BIS-11: Barratt Impulsiveness Scale-11; ADHD: Attention Deficit Hyperactivity Disorder; PTSD: Post Traumatic Stress Disorder; PCL-5: PTSD Checklist for DSM-5; CPTSD: Complex Post Traumatic Stress Disorder; ELA: Early Life Adversity; ACE: Adverse Childhood Experience; CTQ: Childhood Trauma Questionnaire; ETI-SR: Early Trauma Inventory Self-Report; PHQ-9: Patient Health Questionnaire-9; BDI: Beck Depression Inventory; CESD: Center for Epidemiological Studies Depression; BAI: Beck Anxiety Inventory; STAI: State Trait Anxiety Inventory; GAD-7: General Anxiety Disorder-7; ASRS: Adult ADHD Self-Report Scale.

8. Interventions for Food Addiction

There are few successful interventions for reducing FA in the literature. Likewise, there are no articles describing effective interventions for the treatment of obesity in individuals with a history of ACEs [220] which is likely mediated by FA [9,192]. In a study of 60 women, 12-Step self-help groups for compulsive eating have been shown to reduce anxiety and depression, but not FA [221]. A 14-week group lifestyle modification program including caloric reduction ($n = 178$) significantly reduced addictive eating behaviors [222]. A 6-week integrative group for weight management ($n = 51$) reduced FA from pre to post, with strategies such as mindful eating, keeping a food diary, carrying out an exercise plan, regular weigh-ins, and planning for social eating [223]. In a study of 47 different internet sources, self-perceived sugar addicts shared actional strategies that worked for them, including avoidance, consumption planning, environmental restructuring, professional and social support, addressing underlying issues, and urge management, among others [23]. Qualitative interviews have found that the YFAS does not adequately assess social and situational cues for overeating [224]. Importantly, interventions aimed to reduce weight and FA scores generally do not have strategies in place to mitigate progression into disordered eating. This highlights the difference between dietary restraint that can be helpful for some versus pathological for others. Some authors recommend that if an ED is present in addition to FA, clinicians should first provide evidence-based treatments for those conditions [225]. Notwithstanding, it is worth repeating that among women with BN, patients with higher FA severity at baseline were less likely to obtain abstinence from bingeing/purging episodes after treatment [58]. Thus, it is being suggested to view EDs with co-occurring FA on a continuum rather than as discrete conditions, using the eight-step process as a guide, rather than simply to dichotomize inclusive vs. exclusive nutrition strategies.

It is well established that earlier intervention is beneficial for addressing ED pathology [226]. With respect to reducing FA symptoms and severity, it appears that earlier intervention matters, given that ELA does not lead to obesity immediately but develops over time [227,228]. Recently, there have been recommendations for interventions among adolescents that promote executive functioning in the context of salience and reward processing [196]. Among adolescents with obesity ($n = 18$), an FA-informed mobile health (app) intervention reduced zBMI in a more cost-effective manner than the in-clinic intervention, and there is currently an RCT underway in a larger sample using this approach [229,230]. It has been suggested that the more interactive, engaging and person centered a mobile health treatment is, the more appealing it will be to those suffering from compulsive overeating [231]. Meanwhile, many people with more classic ED training may view these apps as a causal factor to ED pathology, either in the short term or over the life course. It seems that until researchers and clinicians determine who is a good candidate for an FA-based nutrition intervention, FA science will continue to stimulate disagreement. In the meantime, recommended treatments might include abstinence from trigger foods, deliberate inclusion of health-promoting foods, interventions that target impulsivity and habitual patterns of responding, anxiety management, coping mechanisms, positive social connections, spirituality, and deterrence of maladaptive compensatory behaviors [46].

9. Summary

The DEFANG (2017) was the first effort to disentangle FA from more classic ED pathology by incorporating the presence or history of SUD into the nutrition intake process [47]. The current review using three clinical vignettes extends that work by adding trauma and PTSD history, particularly early in life, as well as histories of depression, anxiety, and ADHD to guide treatment. The aim in including psychiatric diagnoses, self-report, scores on validated measures, or even informal assessment (clinical intuition) is to reduce the potential for false FA positives (enhance specificity and sensitivity). We have recognized dietary restraint as a primary contributor of "noise" in the FA signal. Failure to consider restrictive eating patterns is an important criticism of FA that has led many ED professionals to reject the construct altogether [15]. The eight-step process outlined in Table 1 might improve the FA assessment process and help clinicians further integrate FA into ED treatment protocols. Currently, most EDs are treated with an inclusive nutrition strategy aimed to reduce fears around food and desensitize individuals to highly palatable foods through regular consumption. Meanwhile, standard ED treatment is associated with suboptimal results, possibly because existing treatments sometimes fail to recognize impulsivity as part of the eating pathology [232,233]. Our clinical experience suggests that failure to recognize/treat trauma/PTSD is a major contributor to poor outcomes. We have suggested that the proper interpretation of an FA diagnosis may improve treatment for those who would benefit from a different nutritional approach, such as excluding problematic foods like added refined sugars [234]. Evidence supports the validity of FA as a diagnostic construct, particularly as it relates to foods high in added sweeteners and refined ingredients [235]. Similar to how SUD patients exhibit different patterns of abuse, patients with FA may have very different behavioral characteristics such as those that binge versus those that do not. Tailor-made hybrid models between inclusive and exclusive approaches have been useful in our clinical experience but have yet to be formally described or tested. These nutrition interventions usually require some trial-and-error and are best done under the supervision of an RDN and a psychiatrist/psychotherapist who understands EDs, FA, SUDs, trauma, and the associations with other psychiatric diagnoses described herein. A multidisciplinary team approach can be helpful, but it is essential that all team members understand the science of FA.

Emerging data on FA may contribute to reduced stigma around body weight, by clearing up confusion and controversy around why humans consume food beyond physiological need. Better terminology will be important to progressing FA science, with several authors proposing new descriptors such as "food use disorder" [236] among others described earlier. The area of greatest controversy surrounding FA appears to be in those with clinically significant EDs, particularly those with purging behaviors where FA symptoms can become elevated [51]. An understanding of the SUD recovery culture including harm reduction may be useful in helping clinicians integrate FA into ED treatment. However, it will be very challenging to implement divergent nutritional strategies in residential treatment settings where there is comparison on the unit and heightened interest in each other's food plans. Currently, exclusive nutritional strategies might be best conducted in an outpatient setting. These strategies may run the risk of exacerbating restrict–binge patterns, therefore should be supervised by clinicians experienced in EDs as well as in detecting reward dysfunction (through examination of cross-addictions) and impulsivity (with respect to food and other behaviors). Treatment professionals should be aware of the various pathways in which ELA and PTSD can become biologically embedded and alter human physiology. ELA increases vulnerability for FA and obesity later in life [192] and highly palatable foods can become a way to distract from disturbing and intrusive trauma-related thoughts [237]. When food alters DA circuitry, efforts to moderate become more difficult and "intuitive eating" can feel impossible. Trauma-informed care should be applied to recovery systems and providers servicing EDs [238,239].

Future Directions

A large prospective study of individuals meeting criteria for FA separated into a restricted diet group (excluding identified trigger foods) and a non-diet group (including challenging foods) would be informative, timely, and warranted. However, given the heterogeneity associated with FA described herein, it could be more effective to categorize FA phenotypes before implementing nutrition-related treatment. Future research using exclusive nutrition strategies might exclude participants revealing moderate or high levels of dietary restraint in order to assess risk for progression from exclusion into disordered eating, as well as into "orthorexia" [240]. The inclusion of orthorexia into future versions of the DSM might prove useful when conceptualizing treatment strategies and research related to FA. It would be valuable to analyze the benefits vs. risks in reducing reward-based eating in those who meet criteria for FA. Research on medications commonly used on patients with SUD for patients with FA is also needed. There is a growing interest in genetic risk for EDs and it would be valuable to know if genetic counseling would be of benefit [241]. More data on food insecurity and other forms of deprivation as predictors of FA may also elucidate the link between undereating and overeating. The temporal sequence of disorder onset may prove beneficial in terms of case conceptualization with respect to nutrition. Consideration of other psychiatric diagnoses such as obsessive compulsive, bipolar, and borderline personality disorders may prove beneficial for FA treatment as new data becomes available. We have proposed that identifying different phenotypes for FA as well as for EDs might improve nutrition interventions and even modify treatment models. An important question at this time remains unanswered: where does all the dieting stem from in the first place? How have sociocultural influences engrained highly palatable foods into the brain's reward expectancy? Furthermore, can public health interventions aimed at reducing exposure to highly processed foods eventually reduce FA and subsequently reduce chronic dieting?

10. Conclusions

While there is disagreement regarding FA, it appears that much of the controversy pertains to the treatment (lacking data) rather than the existence of the problem (robust data). More specifically, nutrition interventions for individuals with FA and co-occurring ED characterized by high levels of dietary restraint are less clear than for individuals with FA and no history of restrictive ED. Individualized treatment might be helpful based on the existence of FA, but only after it has been determined that the FA signal represents an addiction to food (true positive), rather than a consequence of dietary restraint, food insecurity or insufficiency, or other forms of deprivation or food-related neglect (false positive). Dismissing FA as a clinical entity is ill informed and not helpful. FA may warrant consideration as a distinct category in the DSM, which might lead to additional research at the individual and group level, as well as public health efforts to improve the national food environment. The impact of contemporary Westernized foods may be contributing to poor ED treatment outcomes. Patients may become increasingly distrustful of the message that "there are no bad foods." EDs are far more heterogenous than the transdiagnostic theory originally proposed, and recent data on FA supports this conclusion. Treatment models must be trauma informed. Food philosophies must be dynamic, continually incorporating new findings. In summary, one size will not fit all in FA treatment, and collaboration with the patient is crucial to develop a mutually agreeable/achievable plan. Steps and assessment tools offered herein may improve the clinical utility of FA and, in doing so, improve quality of life in individuals seeking care.

Author Contributions: Conceptualization and first draft preparation (D.W.). Conceptual contribution and draft revisions (T.B.). All authors have read and agreed to the published version of the manuscript.

Funding: This research received no external funding.

Conflicts of Interest: The authors declare no conflict of interest.

References

1. Gearhardt, A.; Corbin, W.; Brownell, K. Preliminary validation of the yale food addiction scale. *Appetite* **2009**, *52*, 430–436. [CrossRef]
2. Gearhardt, A.; Corbin, W.; Brownell, K. Development of the yale food addiction scale version 2.0. *Psychol. Addict. Behav.* **2016**, *30*, 113–121. [CrossRef] [PubMed]
3. Schulte, E.M.; Gearhardt, A.N. Associations of food addiction in a sample recruited to be nationally representative of the united states. *Eur. Eat. Disord. Rev.* **2018**, *26*, 112–119. [CrossRef] [PubMed]
4. Burrows, T.; Kay-Lambkin, F.; Pursey, K.; Skinner, J.; Dayas, C. Food addiction and associations with mental health symptoms: A systematic review with meta-analysis. *J. Hum. Nutr. Diet.* **2018**, *4*, 544–572. [CrossRef] [PubMed]
5. Brunault, P.; Ducluzeau, P.-H.; Bourbao-Tournois, C.; Delbachian, I.; Couet, C.; Réveillère, C.; Ballon, N. Food addiction in bariatric surgery candidates: Prevalence and risk factors. *Obes. Surg.* **2016**, *26*, 1650–1653. [CrossRef]
6. Chao, A.M.; Shaw, J.A.; Pearl, R.L.; Alamuddin, N.; Hopkins, C.M.; Bakizada, Z.M.; Berkowitz, R.; Wadden, T.A. Prevalence and psychosocial correlates of food addiction in persons with obesity seeking weight reduction. *Compr. Psychiatry.* **2017**, *73*, 97–104. [CrossRef]
7. SAMHSA. *Key Substance use and Mental Health Indicators in the United States: Results from the 2018 National Survey on Drug Use and Health [Internet]*; Center for Behavioral Health Statistics and Quality, Substance Abuse and Mental Health Services Administration: Rockville, MD, USA, 2019; (HHS Publication No. PEP19-5068, NSDUH Series H-54). Available online: https://www.samhsa.gov/data (accessed on 1 September 2020).
8. Mies, G.W.; Treur, J.L.; Larsen, J.K.; Halberstadt, J.; Pasman, J.A.; Vink, J.M. The prevalence of food addiction in a large sample of adolescents and its association with addictive substances. *Appetite* **2017**, *118*, 97–105. [CrossRef]
9. Wiss, D.A.; Brewerton, T.D. Adverse childhood experiences and adult obesity: A systematic review of plausible mechanisms and meta-analysis of cross-sectional studies. *Physiol Behav.* **2020**, *223*, 112964. [CrossRef]
10. Mason, S.M.; Flint, A.J.; Field, A.E.; Austin, B.S.; Rich-Edwards, J.W. Abuse victimization in childhood or adolescence and risk of food addiction in adult women. *Obesity* **2013**, *21*, E775–E781. [CrossRef]
11. Mason, S.M.; Flint, A.J.; Roberts, A.L.; Agnew-Blais, J.; Koenen, K.C.; Rich-Edwards, J.W. Posttraumatic stress disorder symptoms and food addiction in women by timing and type of trauma exposure. *JAMA Psychiatry* **2014**, *71*, 1271–1278. [CrossRef]
12. Mason, S.; Santaularia, N.; Berge, J.; Larson, N.; Neumark-Sztainer, D. Is the childhood home food environment a confounder of the association between child maltreatment exposure and adult body mass index? *Prev. Med.* **2018**, *110*, 86–92. [CrossRef] [PubMed]
13. Polk, S.E.; Schulte, E.M.; Furman, C.R.; Gearhardt, A.N. Wanting and liking: Separable components in problematic eating behavior? *Appetite* **2017**, *115*, 45–53. [CrossRef]
14. Linardon, J. The relationship between dietary restraint and binge eating: Examining eating-related self-efficacy as a moderator. *Appetite* **2018**, *127*, 126–129. [CrossRef] [PubMed]
15. Wiss, D.A.; Avena, N.M. *Food Addiction, Binge Eating, and the Role of Dietary Restraint: Converging Evidence From Animal and Human Studies*; Frank, K.W., Berner, L.A., Eds.; Springer Nature: Cham, Switzerland, 2020; pp. 193–209.
16. Meule, A. The psychology of food cravings: The role of food deprivation. *Curr. Nutr. Rep.* **2020**, *9*, 251–257. [CrossRef] [PubMed]
17. Racine, S.E.; Burt, A.S.; Iacono, W.G.; McGue, M.; Klump, K.L. Dietary restraint moderates genetic risk for binge eating. *J. Abnorm. Psychol.* **2011**, *120*, 119. [CrossRef]
18. Freeland-Graves, J.H.; Nitzke, S. Dietetics a of and. position of the academy of nutrition and dietetics: Total diet approach to healthy eating. *J. Acad. Nutr. Diet.* **2013**, *113*, 307–317. [CrossRef]

19. DePierre, J.A.; Puhl, R.M.; Luedicke, J. Public perceptions of food addiction: A comparison with alcohol and tobacco. *J. Subst. Use* **2013**, *19*, 1–6. [CrossRef]
20. Hebebrand, J.; Albayrak, Ö.; Adan, R.; Antel, J.; Diéguez, C.; De Jong, J.; Leng, G.; Menzies, J.; Mercer, J.G.; Murphy, M.; et al. "Eating addiction", rather than "food addiction", better captures addictive-like eating behavior. *Neurosci. Biobehav. Rev.* **2014**, *47*, 295–306. [CrossRef]
21. Schulte, E.M.; Potenza, M.N.; Gearhardt, A.N. A commentary on the "eating addiction" versus "food addiction" perspectives on addictive-like food consumption. *Appetite* **2017**, *115*, 9–15. [CrossRef]
22. Ruddock, H.K.; Hardman, C.A. food addiction beliefs amongst the lay public: What are the onsequences for eating behaviour? *Curr. Addict. Rep.* **2017**, *4*, 110–115. [CrossRef]
23. Rodda, S.N.; Booth, N.; Brittain, M.; McKean, J.; Thornley, S. I was truly addicted to sugar: A consumer-focused classification system of behaviour change strategies for sugar reduction. *Appetite* **2019**, *144*, 104456. [CrossRef]
24. Edwards, S.; Lusher, J.; Murray, E. The lived experience of obese people who feel that they are addicted to food. *Int. J. Psychol. Cogn. Sci.* **2019**, *5*, 79–87.
25. Ruddock, H.K.; Orwin, M.; Boyland, E.J.; Evans, E.H.; Hardman, C.A. Obesity stigma: Is the 'food addiction' label feeding the problem? *Nutrients* **2019**, *11*, 2100. [CrossRef]
26. O'Brien, K.; Puhl, R.M.; Latner, J.D.; Lynott, D.; Reid, J.D.; Vakhitova, Z.I.; Hunter, J.A.; Scarf, D.; Jeanes, R.; Bouguettaya, A.; et al. The Effect of a Food Addiction Explanation Model for Weight Control and Obesity on Weight Stigma. *Nutrients* **2020**, *12*, 294.
27. Latner, J.D.; Puhl, R.M.; Murakami, J.M.; O'Brien, K.S. Food addiction as a causal model of obesity. Effects on stigma, blame, and perceived psychopathology. *Appetite* **2014**, *77*, 79–84. [CrossRef]
28. Cassin, S.E.; Buchman, D.Z.; Leung, S.E.; Kantarovich, K.; Hawa, A.; Carter, A.; Sockalingam, S. Ethical, Stigma, and Policy Implications of Food Addiction: A Scoping Review. *Nutrition* **2019**, *11*, 710. [CrossRef]
29. Moran, A.; Musicus, A.; Soo, J.; Gearhardt, A.N.; Gollust, S.E.; Roberto, C.A. Believing that certain foods are addictive is associated with support for obesity-related public policies. *Prev. Med.* **2016**, *90*, 39–46. [CrossRef] [PubMed]
30. Ifland, J.R.; Preuss, H.; Marcus, M.; Rourke, K.; Taylor, W.; Burau, K.; Jacobs, W.; Kadish, W.; Manso, G. Refined food addiction: A classic substance use disorder. *Med Hypotheses* **2009**, *72*, 518–526. [CrossRef]
31. Ifland, J.; Preuss, H.G.; Marcus, M.T.; Rourke, K.M.; Taylor, W.; Wright, T.H. Clearing the confusion around processed food addiction. *J. Am. Coll. Nutr.* **2015**, *34*, 240–243. [CrossRef]
32. Schulte, E.M.; Avena, N.M.; Gearhardt, A.N. Which foods may be addictive? The roles of processing, fat content, and glycemic load. *PloS ONE* **2015**, *10*, e0117959. [CrossRef]
33. Fildes, A.; Charlton, J.; Rudisill, C.; Littlejohns, P.; Prevost, A.T.; Gulliford, M. Probability of an obese person attaining normal body weight: Cohort study using electronic health records. *Am. J. Public Health* **2015**, *105*, e54–e59. [CrossRef] [PubMed]
34. Fairburn, C.G.; Cooper, Z.; Shafran, R. Cognitive behaviour therapy for eating disorders: A "transdiagnostic" theory and treatment? *Behav. Res. Ther.* **2003**, *41*, 509–528. [CrossRef]
35. Stice, E.; Rohde, P.; Shaw, H.; Desjardins, C. Weight suppression increases odds for future onset of anorexia nervosa, bulimia nervosa, and purging disorder, but not binge eating disorder. *Am. J. Clin. Nutr.* **2020**, nqaa146. [CrossRef]
36. Grilo, C.M.; Masheb, R.M. Onset of dieting vs binge eating in outpatients with binge eating disorder. *Int. J. Obes.* **2000**, *24*, 404–409. [CrossRef]
37. Mussell, M.P.; Mitchell, J.E.; Fenna, C.J.; Crosby, R.D.; Miller, J.P.; Hoberman, H.M. A comparison of onset of binge eating versus dieting in the development of bulimia nervosa. *Int. J. Eat. Disord.* **1997**, *21*, 353–360. [CrossRef]
38. Brewerton, T.D.; Dansky, B.S.; Kilpatrick, D.G.; O'Neil, P.M. Which comes first in the pathogenesis of bulimia nervosa: Dieting or bingeing? *Int. J. Eat. Disord.* **2000**, *28*, 259–264. [CrossRef]
39. Brown-Bowers, A.; Ward, A.; Cormier, N. Treating the binge or the (fat) body? Representations of fatness in a gold standard psychological treatment manual for binge eating disorder. *Health Interdiscip. J. Soc. Study Health Illn. Med.* **2016**, *21*, 21–37. [CrossRef] [PubMed]
40. Dakanalis, A.; Clerici, M. Tackling excess body weight in people with binge eating disorder. *Aust. N. Z. J. Psychiatry* **2019**, *53*, 1027. [CrossRef]

41. Jebeile, H.; Gow, M.L.; Baur, L.A.; Garnett, S.P.; Paxton, S.J.; Lister, N.B. Treatment of obesity, with a dietary component, and eating disorder risk in children and adolescents: A systematic review with meta-analysis. *Obes. Rev.* **2019**, *20*, 1287–1298. [CrossRef]
42. Hunger, J.M.; Smith, J.P.; Tomiyama, A.J. An Evidence-based rationale for adopting weight-inclusive health policy. *Soc. Issues Policy Rev.* **2020**, *14*, 73–107. [CrossRef]
43. Kordy, H.; Krämer, B.; Palmer, R.L.; Papezova, H.; Pellet, J.; Richard, M.; Treasure, J. Remission, recovery, relapse, and recurrence in eating disorders: Conceptualization and illustration of a validation strategy. *J. Clin. Psychol.* **2002**, *58*, 833–846. [CrossRef] [PubMed]
44. Clausen, L. Time to remission for eating disorder patients: A $2\frac{1}{2}$-year follow-up study of outcome and predictors. *Nord. J. Psychiatry* **2009**, *62*, 151–159. [CrossRef] [PubMed]
45. Grilo, C.M.; Pagano, M.; Stout, R.L.; Markowitz, J.C.; Ansell, E.B.; Pinto, A.; Zanarini, M.C.; Yen, S.; Skodol, A.E. Stressful life events predict eating disorder relapse following remission: Six-year prospective outcomes. *Int. J. Eat. Disord.* **2011**, *45*, 185–192. [CrossRef]
46. Treasure, J.; Leslie, M.; Chami, R.; Fernández-Aranda, F. Are trans diagnostic models of eating disorders fit for purpose? A consideration of the evidence for food addiction. *Eur. Eat. Disord. Rev.* **2018**, *26*, 83–91. [CrossRef]
47. Wiss, D.; Brewerton, T.D. Incorporating food addiction into disordered eating: The disordered eating food addiction nutrition guide (DEFANG). *Eat. Weight. Disord. Stud. Anorexia, Bulim. Obes.* **2016**, *22*, 49–59. [CrossRef]
48. Bryant, E.; Rehman, J.; Pepper, L.B.; Walters, E.R. Obesity and Eating Disturbance: The Role of TFEQ Restraint and Disinhibition. *Curr. Obes. Rep.* **2019**, *8*, 363–372. [CrossRef]
49. Meule, A.; Gearhardt, A.N. Ten Years of the Yale Food Addiction Scale: A Review of Version 2.0. *Curr. Addict. Rep.* **2019**, *6*, 218–228. [CrossRef]
50. Meule, A. Food addiction and body-mass-index: A non-linear relationship. *Med. Hypotheses* **2012**, *79*, 508–511. [CrossRef]
51. Granero, R.; Hilker, I.; Agüera, Z.; Jiménez-Murcia, S.; Sauchelli, S.; Islam, M.A.; Fagundo, A.B.; Sanchez, I.; Riesco, N.; Diéguez, C.; et al. Food addiction in a spanish sample of eating disorders: Dsm-5 diagnostic subtype differentiation and validation data. *Eur. Eat. Disord. Rev.* **2014**, *22*, 389–396. [CrossRef]
52. De Vries, S.-K.; Meule, A. Food addiction and bulimia nervosa: New data based on the yale food addiction scale 2.0. *Eur. Eat. Disord. Rev.* **2016**, *24*, 518–522. [CrossRef]
53. Kaye, W.H.; Wierenga, C.E.; Bailer, U.F.; Simmons, A.N.; Wagner, A.; Bischoff-Grethe, A. Does a shared neurobiology for foods and drugs of abuse contribute to extremes of food ingestion in anorexia and bulimia nervosa? *Biol. Psychiatry* **2013**, *73*, 836–842. [CrossRef] [PubMed]
54. Frank, G.K. Altered brain reward circuits in eating disorders: Chicken or egg? *Curr. Psychiatry Rep.* **2013**, *15*, 396. [CrossRef] [PubMed]
55. Hadad, N.A.; Knackstedt, L.A. Addicted to palatable foods: Comparing the neurobiology of bulimia nervosa to that of drug addiction. *Psychopharmacology* **2014**, *231*, 1897–1912. [CrossRef]
56. Donnelly, B.; Touyz, S.W.; Hay, P.; Burton, A.; Russell, J.; Caterson, I. Neuroimaging in bulimia nervosa and binge eating disorder: A systematic review. *J. Eat. Disord.* **2018**, *6*, 3. [CrossRef] [PubMed]
57. Meule, A.; Von Rezori, V.; Blechert, J. Food addiction and bulimia nervosa. *Eur. Eat. Disord. Rev.* **2014**, *22*, 331–337. [CrossRef]
58. Hilker, I.; Sánchez, I.; Steward, T.; Jiménez-Murcia, S.; Granero, R.; Gearhardt, A.N.; Rodríguez-Muñoz, R.C.; Diéguez, C.; Crujeiras, A.B.; Tolosa-Sola, I.; et al. Food Addiction in bulimia nervosa: Clinical correlates and association with response to a brief psychoeducational intervention. *Eur. Eat. Disord. Rev.* **2016**, *24*, 482–488. [CrossRef]
59. Becker, D.F.; Grilo, C.M. Comorbidity of mood and substance use disorders in patients with binge-eating disorder: Associations with personality disorder and eating disorder pathology. *J. Psychosom. Res.* **2015**, *79*, 159–164. [CrossRef]
60. Ivezaj, V.; White, M.A.; Grilo, C.M. Examining binge-eating disorder and food addiction in adults with overweight and obesity. *Obesity* **2016**, *24*, 2064–2069. [CrossRef]
61. Romero, X.; Agüera, Z.; Granero, R.; Sánchez, I.; Riesco, N.; Jiménez-Murcia, S.; Gisbert-Rodriguez, M.; Sánchez-González, J.; Casalé, G.; Baenas, I.; et al. Is food addiction a predictor of treatment outcome among patients with eating disorder? *Eur. Eat. Disord. Rev.* **2019**, *27*, 700–711. [CrossRef]

62. Agüera, Z.; Lozano-Madrid, M.; Mallorquí-Bagué, N.; Jiménez-Murcia, S.; Menchón, J.M.; Fernández-Aranda, F. A review of binge eating disorder and obesity. *Neuropsychiatry* **2020**, 1–11. [CrossRef]
63. Smith, K.E.; Mason, T.B.; Peterson, C.B.; Pearson, C.M. Relationships between eating disorder-specific and transdiagnostic risk factors for binge eating: An integrative moderated mediation model of emotion regulation, anticipatory reward, and expectancy. *Eat. Behav.* **2018**, *31*, 131–136. [CrossRef] [PubMed]
64. Linardon, J.; Messer, M. Assessment of food addiction using the Yale Food Addiction Scale 2.0 in individuals with binge-eating disorder symptomatology: Factor structure, psychometric properties, and clinical significance. *Psychiatry Res. Neuroimaging* **2019**, *279*, 216–221. [CrossRef] [PubMed]
65. Forest, L.N.; Jacobucci, R.C.; Grilo, C.M. Empirically determined severity levels for binge-eating disorder outperform existing severity classification schemes. *Psychol. Med.* **2020**, 1–11. [CrossRef]
66. Andrés, A.; Saldaña, C. Body dissatisfaction and dietary restraint influence binge eating behavior. *Nutr. Res.* **2014**, *34*, 944–950. [CrossRef] [PubMed]
67. Meadows, A.; Higgs, S. Internalized weight stigma and the progression of food addiction over time. *Body Image* **2020**, *34*, 67–71. [CrossRef]
68. Puhl, R.M.; Himmelstein, M.; Pearl, R.L. Weight stigma as a psychosocial contributor to obesity. *Am. Psychol.* **2020**, *75*, 274–289. [CrossRef]
69. Masheb, R.M.; Grilo, C.M. On the relation of attempting to lose weight, restraint, and binge eating in outpatients with binge eating disorder. *Obes. Res.* **2000**, *8*, 638–645. [CrossRef]
70. Canan, F.; Karaca, S.; Sogucak, S.; Gecici, O.; Kuloglu, M. Eating disorders and food addiction in men with heroin use disorder: A controlled study. *Eat. Weight. Disord. Stud. Anorexia Bulim. Obes.* **2017**, *22*, 249–257. [CrossRef]
71. Munn-Chernoff, M.A.; Few, L.R.; Matherne, C.E.; Baker, J.H.; Men, V.Y.; McCutcheon, V.V.; Agrawal, A.; Bucholz, K.K.; Madden, P.A.; Heath, A.C.; et al. Eating disorders in a community-based sample of women with alcohol use disorder and nicotine dependence. *Drug Alcohol Depend.* **2020**, *212*, 107981. [CrossRef]
72. Bahji, A.; Mazhar, M.N.; Hawken, E.; Hudson, C.C.; Nadkarni, P.; MacNeil, B.A. Prevalence of substance use disorder comorbidity among individuals with eating disorders: A systematic review and meta-analysis. *Psychiatry Res.* **2019**, *273*, 58–66. [CrossRef]
73. Tinghino, B.; Lugoboni, F.; Amatulli, A.; Biasin, C.; Araldi, M.B.; Cantiero, D.; Cremaschini, M.; Galimberti, G.L.; Giusti, S.; Grosina, C.; et al. The fodrat study (FOod addiction, DRugs, Alcohol and Tobacco): First data on food addiction prevalence among patients with addiction to drugs, tobacco and alcohol. *Eat Weight Disord.* **2020**, 1–7. [CrossRef] [PubMed]
74. Lu, H.K.; Mannan, H.; Hay, P. Exploring relationships between recurrent binge eating and illicit substance use in a non-clinical sample of women over two years. *Behav. Sci.* **2017**, *7*, 46. [CrossRef] [PubMed]
75. Warren, C.S.; Lindsay, A.R.; White, E.; Claudat, K.; Velasquez, S.C. Weight-related concerns related to drug use for women in substance abuse treatment: Prevalence and relationships with eating pathology. *J. Subst. Abus. Treat.* **2013**, *44*, 494–501. [CrossRef] [PubMed]
76. Bruening, A.B.; Perez, M.; Ohrt, T.K. Exploring weight control as motivation for illicit stimulant use. *Eat. Behav.* **2018**, *30*, 72–75. [CrossRef] [PubMed]
77. Claudat, K.; Brown, T.A.; Anderson, L.; Bongiorno, G.; Berner, L.A.; Reilly, E.E.; Luo, T.; Orloff, N.; Kaye, W.H. Correlates of co-occurring eating disorders and substance use disorders: A case for dialectical behavior therapy. *Eat. Disord.* **2020**, *28*, 1–15. [CrossRef]
78. Cornelis, M.C.; Flint, A.; Field, A.E.; Kraft, P.; Han, J.; Rimm, E.B.; Van Dam, R.M. A genome-wide investigation of food addiction. *Obesity* **2016**, *24*, 1336–1341. [CrossRef] [PubMed]
79. Blum, K.; Sheridan, P.J.; Wood, R.C.; Braverman, E.R.; Chen, T.J.H.; Cull, J.G.; E Comings, D. The D2 dopamine receptor gene as a determinant of reward deficiency syndrome. *J. R. Soc. Med.* **1996**, *89*, 396–400. [CrossRef] [PubMed]
80. Blum, K.; Braverman, E.R.; Holder, J.M.; Lubar, J.F.; Monastra, V.J.; Miller, D.; Lubar, J.O.; Chen, T.J.; Comings, D.E. The reward deficiency syndrome: A biogenetic model for the diagnosis and treatment of impulsive, addictive and compulsive behaviors. *J. Psychoact. Drugs* **2000**, *32*, 1–112. [CrossRef]
81. Blum, K.; Chen, A.L.; Giordano, J.; Borsten, J.; Chen, T.J.; Hauser, M.; Simpatico, T.; Femino, J.; Braverman, E.R.; Barh, D. The addictive brain: All roads lead to dopamine. *J. Psychoact. Drugs* **2012**, *44*, 134–143. [CrossRef]
82. Blum, K. Dopamine genetics and function in food and substance abuse. *J. Genet. Syndr. Gene Ther.* **2013**, *4*, 1–13.

83. Blum, K.; Thanos, P.K.; Wang, G.-J.; Febo, M.; Demetrovics, Z.; Modestino, E.J.; Braverman, E.R.; Baron, D.; Badgaiyan, R.D.; Gold, M.S.; et al. The food and drug addiction epidemic: Targeting dopamine homeostasis. *Curr. Pharm. Des.* **2018**, *23*, 6050–6061. [CrossRef] [PubMed]
84. Hb, C. Common phenotype in patients with both food and substance dependence: Case reports. *J. Genet. Syndr. Gene Ther.* **2013**, *4*, 1–4. [CrossRef] [PubMed]
85. Brunault, P.; Salamé, E.; Jaafari, N.; Courtois, R.; Réveillère, C.; Silvain, C.; Benyamina, A.; Blecha, L.; Belin, D.; Ballon, N. Why do liver transplant patients so often become obese? The addiction transfer hypothesis. *Med. Hypotheses* **2015**, *85*, 68–75. [CrossRef] [PubMed]
86. Kanji, S.; Wong, E.; Aikioyamen, L.; Melamed, O.; Taylor, V. Exploring pre-surgery and post-surgery substance use disorder and alcohol use disorder in bariatric surgery: A qualitative scoping review. *Int. J. Obes.* **2019**, *43*, 1659–1674. [CrossRef] [PubMed]
87. Treur, J.L.; Boomsma, R.I.; Ligthart, L.; Willemsen, G.; Vink, J.M. Heritability of high sugar consumption through drinks and the genetic correlation with substance use. *Am. J. Clin. Nutr.* **2016**, *104*, 1144–1150. [CrossRef]
88. Volkow, N.D.; Wise, R.A.; Baler, R. The dopamine motive system: Implications for drug and food addiction. *Nat. Rev. Neurosci.* **2017**, *18*, 741–752. [CrossRef]
89. Wang, G.-J.; Volkow, N.D.; Logan, J.; Pappas, N.R.; Wong, C.T.; Zhu, W.; Netusll, N.; Fowler, J.S. Brain dopamine and obesity. *Lancet* **2001**, *357*, 354–357. [CrossRef]
90. Wang, G.-J.; Volkow, N.D.; Thanos, P.K.; Fowler, J.S. Similarity between obesity and drug addiction as assessed by neurofunctional imaging. *J. Addict. Dis.* **2004**, *23*, 39–53. [CrossRef]
91. Joutsa, J.; Karlsson, H.K.; Majuri, J.; Nuutila, P.; Helin, S.; Kaasinen, V.; Nummenmaa, L. Binge eating disorder and morbid obesity are associated with lowered mu-opioid receptor availability in the brain. *Psychiatry Res. Neuroimaging* **2018**, *276*, 41–45. [CrossRef]
92. Leigh, S.-J.; Morris, M.J. The role of reward circuitry and food addiction in the obesity epidemic: An update. *Biol. Psychol.* **2016**, *131*, 31–42. [CrossRef]
93. Small, D.M.; DiFeliceantonio, A.G. Processed foods and food reward. *Sciences* **2019**, *363*, 346–347. [CrossRef] [PubMed]
94. Leslie, M.; Lambert, E.R.; Treasure, J. Towards a translational approach to food addiction: Implications for bulimia nervosa. *Curr. Addict. Rep.* **2019**, *6*, 258–265. [CrossRef]
95. Tobore, T.O. Towards a comprehensive theory of obesity and a healthy diet: The causal role of oxidative stress in food addiction and obesity. *Behav. Brain Res.* **2020**, *384*, 112560. [CrossRef] [PubMed]
96. Ramsay, D.S.; Kaiyala, K.J.; Woods, S.C. Individual differences in biological regulation: Predicting vulnerability to drug addiction, obesity, and other dysregulatory disorders. *Exp. Clin. Psychopharmacol.* **2020**, *28*, 388–403. [CrossRef]
97. Carbone, E.A.; Caroleo, M.; Rania, M.; Calabrò, G.; Staltari, F.A.; De Filippis, R.; Aloi, M.; Condoleo, F.; Arturi, F.; Segura-García, C. An open-label trial on the efficacy and tolerability of naltrexone/bupropion SR for treating altered eating behaviours and weight loss in binge eating disorder. *Eat. Weight. Disord. Stud. Anorex. Bulim. Obes.* **2020**, 1–10. [CrossRef]
98. Meule, A.; de Zwaan, M.; Müller, A. Attentional and motor impulsivity interactively predict 'food addiction' in obese individuals. *Compr. Psychiatry* **2017**, *72*, 83–87. [CrossRef]
99. Schulte, E.M.; Grilo, C.M.; Gearhardt, A.N. Shared and unique mechanisms underlying binge eating disorder and addictive disorders. *Clin. Psychol. Rev.* **2016**, *44*, 125–139. [CrossRef]
100. Wolz, I.; Hilker, I.; Granero, R.; Jiménez-Murcia, S.; Gearhardt, A.N.; Diéguez, C.; Casanueva, F.F.; Crujeiras, A.B.; Menchon, J.M.; Fernández-Aranda, F. "Food Addiction" in patients with eating disorders is associated with negative urgency and difficulties to focus on long-term goals. *Front. Psychol.* **2016**, *7*, 61. [CrossRef]
101. Maxwell, A.L.; Gardiner, E.; Loxton, N.J. Investigating the relationship between reward sensitivity, impulsivity, and food addiction: A systematic review. *Eur. Eat. Disord. Rev.* **2020**, *28*, 368–384. [CrossRef]
102. VanderBroek-Stice, L.; Stojek, M.; Beach, S.R.H.; Vandellen, M.R.; MacKillop, J. Multidimensional assessment of impulsivity in relation to obesity and food addiction. *Appetite* **2017**, *112*, 59–68. [CrossRef]
103. Lozano-Madrid, M.; Bryan, D.C.; Granero, R.; Sánchez, I.; Riesco, N.; Mallorquí-Bagué, N.; Jiménez-Murcia, S.; Treasure, J.; Fernández-Aranda, F. Impulsivity, emotional dysregulation and executive function deficits could be associated with alcohol and drug abuse in eating disorders. *J. Clin. Med.* **2020**, *9*, 1936. [CrossRef] [PubMed]

104. Mahoney, C.T.; Cole, H.E.; Gilbar, O.; Taft, C.T. The Role of impulsivity in the association between posttraumatic stress disorder symptom severity and substance use in male military veterans. *J. Trauma. Stress* **2020**, *33*, 296–306. [CrossRef] [PubMed]
105. Wenzel, K.R.; Weinstock, J.; McGrath, A.B. The clinical significance of food addiction. *J. Addict. Med.* **2020**, *1*. [CrossRef]
106. Steiger, H.; Joober, R.; Israël, M.; Young, S.N.; Kin, N.M.K.N.Y.; Gauvin, L.; Bruce, K.R.; Joncas, J.; Torkaman-Zehi, A. The 5HTTLPR polymorphism, psychopathologic symptoms, and platelet [3H-] paroxetine binding in bulimic syndromes. *Int. J. Eat. Disord.* **2004**, *37*, 57–60. [CrossRef] [PubMed]
107. Bruce, K.R.; Steiger, H.; Joober, R.; Kin, N.; Israel, M.; Young, S.N. Association of the promoter polymorphism −1438G/A of the 5-HT2A receptor gene with behavioral impulsiveness and serotonin function in women with bulimia nervosa. *Am. J. Med. Genet. Part B Neuropsychiatr. Genet.* **2005**, *137*, 40–44. [CrossRef] [PubMed]
108. Steiger, H.; Gauvin, L.; Israël, M.; Koerner, N.; Kin, N.M.K.N.Y.; Paris, J.; Young, S.N. Association of serotonin and cortisol indices with childhood abuse in bulimia nervosa. *Arch. Gen. Psychiatry* **2001**, *58*, 837–843. [CrossRef]
109. Steiger, H.; Richardson, J.; Joober, R.; Gauvin, L.; Israel, M.; Bruce, K.R.; Kin, N.M.K.N.Y.; Howard, H.; Young, S.N. The 5HTTLPR polymorphism, prior maltreatment and dramatic–erratic personality manifestations in women with bulimic syndromes. *J. Psychiatry Neurosci.* **2007**, *32*, 354–362.
110. Akkermann, K.; Kaasik, K.; Kiive, E.; Nordquist, N.; Oreland, L.; Harro, J. The impact of adverse life events and the serotonin transporter gene promoter polymorphism on the development of eating disorder symptoms. *J. Psychiatr. Res.* **2012**, *46*, 38–43. [CrossRef]
111. Calati, R.; De Ronchi, D.; Bellini, M.; Serretti, A. The 5-HTTLPR polymorphism and eating disorders: A meta-analysis. *Int. J. Eat. Disord.* **2011**, *44*, 191–199. [CrossRef]
112. Felitti, V.J.; Anda, R.F.; Nordenberg, D.; Williamson, D.F.; Spitz, A.M.; Edwards, V.; Koss, M.P.; Marks, J.S. Relationship of childhood abuse and household dysfunction to many of the leading causes of death in adults. The Adverse Childhood Experiences (ACE) Study. *Am. J. Prev. Med.* **1998**, *14*, 245–258. [CrossRef]
113. Anda, R.F.; Felitti, V.J.; Bremner, J.D.; Walker, J.D.; Whitfield, C.; Perry, B.D.; Dube, S.R.; Giles, W.H. The enduring effects of abuse and related adverse experiences in childhood. *Eur. Arch. Psychiatry Clin. Neurosci.* **2005**, *256*, 174–186. [CrossRef] [PubMed]
114. Bernstein, D.P.; Ahluvalia, T.; Pogge, D.; Handelsman, L. Validity of the Childhood Trauma Questionnaire in an Adolescent Psychiatric Population. *J. Am. Acad. Child Adolesc. Psychiatry* **1997**, *36*, 340–348. [CrossRef] [PubMed]
115. Bernstein, D.P.; Stein, J.A.; Newcomb, M.D.; Walker, E.; Pogge, D.; Ahluvalia, T.; Stokes, J.; Handelsman, L.; Medrano, M.; Desmond, D.; et al. Development and validation of a brief screening version of the Childhood Trauma Questionnaire. *Child Abus. Negl.* **2003**, *27*, 169–190. [CrossRef]
116. McCrory, E.J.; Viding, E. The theory of latent vulnerability: Reconceptualizing the link between childhood maltreatment and psychiatric disorder. *Dev. Psychopathol.* **2015**, *27*, 493–505. [CrossRef]
117. Ehrlich, K.B.; Ross, K.M.; Chen, E.; Miller, G.E. Testing the biological embedding hypothesis: Is early life adversity associated with a later proinflammatory phenotype? *Dev. Psychopathol.* **2016**, *28*, 1273–1283. [CrossRef]
118. Malarbi, S.; Abu-Rayya, H.M.; Muscara, F.; Stargatt, R. Neuropsychological functioning of childhood trauma and post-traumatic stress disorder: A meta-analysis. *Neurosci. Biobehav. Rev.* **2017**, *72*, 68–86. [CrossRef]
119. Ziobrowski, H.N.; Buka, S.L.; Austin, S.B.; Sullivan, A.J.; Horton, N.J.; Simone, M.; Field, A.E. Using latent class analysis to empirically classify maltreatment according to the developmental timing, duration, and co-occurrence of abuse types. *Child Abus. Negl.* **2020**, *107*, 104574. [CrossRef]
120. SAMHSA. *SAMHSA Concept of Trauma and Guidance for a Trauma-Informed Approach*; Substance Abuse and Mental Health Services Administration: Rockville, MD, USA, 2014; (HHS Publication No. (SMA) 14-4884).
121. Dillon, D.G.; Holmes, A.J.; Birk, J.L.; Brooks, N.; Lyons-Ruth, K.; Pizzagalli, D.A. Childhood adversity is associated with left basal ganglia dysfunction during reward anticipation in adulthood. *Biol. Psychiatry* **2009**, *66*, 206–213. [CrossRef]
122. Hoexter, M.Q.; Fadel, G.; Felício, A.C.; Calzavara, M.B.; Batista, I.R.; Reis, M.A.; Shih, M.C.; Pitman, R.K.; Andreoli, S.B.; De Mello, M.F.; et al. Higher striatal dopamine transporter density in PTSD: An in vivo SPECT study with [99mTc]TRODAT-1. *Psychopharmacology* **2012**, *224*, 337–345. [CrossRef]

123. Oswald, L.M.; Wand, G.S.; Kuwabara, H.; Wong, D.F.; Zhu, S.; Brašić, J.R. History of childhood adversity is positively associated with ventral striatal dopamine responses to amphetamine. *Psychopharmacology* **2014**, *231*, 2417–2433. [CrossRef]
124. Hertzman, C. The biological embedding of early experience and its effects on health in adulthood. *Ann. N. Y. Acad. Sci.* **1999**, *896*, 85–95. [CrossRef]
125. Duffy, K.A.; McLaughlin, K.A.; Green, P.A. Early life adversity and health-risk behaviors: Proposed psychological and neural mechanisms. *Ann. N. Y. Acad. Sci.* **2018**, *1428*, 151–169. [CrossRef] [PubMed]
126. McMullin, S.D.; Shields, G.S.; Slavich, G.M.; Buchanan, T.W. Cumulative lifetime stress exposure predicts greater impulsivity and addictive behaviors. *J. Health Psychol.* **2020**. [CrossRef]
127. Brewerton, T.D. Posttraumatic stress disorder and disordered eating: Food addiction as self-medication. *J. Women's Health* **2011**, *20*, 1133–1134. [CrossRef] [PubMed]
128. Cammack, A.L.; Gazmararian, J.A.; Suglia, S.F. History of child maltreatment and excessive dietary and screen time behaviors in young adults: Results from a nationally representative study. *Prev. Med.* **2020**, *139*, 106176. [CrossRef]
129. Imperatori, C.; Innamorati, M.; Lamis, D.A.; Farina, B.; Pompili, M.; Contardi, A.; Fabbricatore, M. Childhood trauma in obese and overweight women with food addiction and clinical-level of binge eating. *Child Abus. Negl.* **2016**, *58*, 180–190. [CrossRef] [PubMed]
130. Hardy, R.; Fani, N.; Jovanovic, T.; Michopoulos, V. Food addiction and substance addiction in women: Common clinical characteristics. *Appetite* **2017**, *120*, 367–373. [CrossRef]
131. Molendijk, M.L.; Hoek, H.W.; Brewerton, T.D.; Elzinga, B.M. Childhood maltreatment and eating disorder pathology: A systematic review and dose-response meta-analysis. *Psychol. Med.* **2017**, *47*, 1402–1416. [CrossRef]
132. Afifi, T.O.; Sareen, J.; Fortier, J.; Taillieu, T.; Turner, S.; Cheung, K.; Henriksen, C.A. Child maltreatment and eating disorders among men and women in adulthood: Results from a nationally representative United States sample. *Int. J. Eat. Disord.* **2017**, *50*, 1281–1296. [CrossRef]
133. Caslini, M.; Bartoli, F.; Crocamo, C.; Dakanalis, A.; Clerici, M.; Carrà, G. Disentangling the association between child abuse and eating disorders. *Psychosom. Med.* **2016**, *78*, 79–90. [CrossRef]
134. Isomaa, R.; Backholm, K.; Birgegård, A. Posttraumatic stress disorder in eating disorder patients: The roles of psychological distress and timing of trauma. *Psychiatry Res.* **2015**, *230*, 506–510. [PubMed]
135. White, A.A.H.; Pratt, K.J.; Cottrill, C.B. The relationship between trauma and weight status among adolescents in eating disorder treatment. *Appetite* **2018**, *129*, 62–69.
136. Rijkers, C.; Schoorl, M.; Van Hoeken, D.; Hoek, H.W. Eating disorders and posttraumatic stress disorder. *Curr. Opin. Psychiatry* **2019**, *32*, 510–517. [PubMed]
137. Dansky, B.S.; Brewerton, T.D.; Kilpatrick, D.G.; O'Neil, P.M. The national women's study: Relationship of victimization and posttraumatic stress disorder to bulimia nervosa. *Int. J. Eat. Disord.* **1997**, *21*, 213–228.
138. Hudson, J.I.; Hiripi, E.; Pope, H.G.; Kessler, R.C. the prevalence and correlates of eating disorders in the national comorbidity survey replication. *Biol. Psychiatry* **2007**, *61*, 348–358.
139. Romans, S.E.; Gendall, K.A.; Martin, J.L.; Mullen, P.E. Child sexual abuse and later disordered eating: A New Zealand epidemiological study. *Int. J. Eat. Disord.* **2001**, *29*, 380–392.
140. Sanci, L.; Coffey, C.; Olsson, C.; Reid, S.; Carlin, J.B.; Patton, G. Childhood sexual abuse and eating disorders in females. *Arch. Pediatr. Adolesc. Med.* **2008**, *162*, 261–267.
141. Johnson, J.G.; Cohen, P.; Kotler, L.; Kasen, S.; Brook, J.S. Psychiatric disorders associated with risk for the development of eating disorders during adolescence and early adulthood. *J. Consult. Clin. Psych.* **2002**, *70*, 1119.
142. Quilliot, D.; Brunaud, L.; Mathieu, J.; Quenot, C.; Sirveaux, M.-A.; Kahn, J.-P.; Ziegler, O.; Witkowski, P. Links between traumatic experiences in childhood or early adulthood and lifetime binge eating disorder. *Psychiatry Res. Neuroimaging* **2019**, *276*, 134–141.
143. Braun, J.; El-Gabalawy, R.; Sommer, J.L.; Pietrzak, R.H.; Mitchell, K.; Mota, N. Trauma Exposure, DSM-5 Posttraumatic Stress, and Binge Eating Symptoms: Results From a Nationally Representative Sample. *J. Clin. Psychiatry* **2019**, *80*, 19m12813.
144. Hazzard, V.M.; Bauer, K.W.; Mukherjee, B.; Miller, A.L.; Sonneville, K.R. Associations between childhood maltreatment latent classes and eating disorder symptoms in a nationally representative sample of young adults in the United States. *Child Abus. Negl.* **2019**, *98*, 104171. [CrossRef] [PubMed]

145. Scharff, A.; Ortiz, S.N.; Ma, L.N.F.; Smith, A.R. Comparing the clinical presentation of eating disorder patients with and without trauma history and/or comorbid PTSD. *Eat. Disord.* **2019**, 1–15. [CrossRef] [PubMed]
146. Gidzgier, P.; Grundmann, J.; Lotzin, A.; Hiller, P.; Schneider, B.; Driessen, M.; Schaefer, M.; Scherbaum, N.; Hillemacher, T.; Schäfer, I. The dissociative subtype of PTSD in women with substance use disorders: Exploring symptom and exposure profiles. *J. Subst. Abus. Treat.* **2019**, *99*, 73–79. [CrossRef] [PubMed]
147. Cuthbert, K.; Hardin, S.; Zelkowitz, R.; Mitchell, K.S. Eating disorders and overweight/obesity in veterans: Prevalence, risk factors, and treatment considerations. *Curr. Obes. Rep.* **2020**, *9*, 98–108.
148. Polivy, J.; Coleman, J.; Herman, C.P. The effect of deprivation on food cravings and eating behavior in restrained and unrestrained eaters. *Int. J. Eat. Disord.* **2005**, *38*, 301–309. [CrossRef]
149. Herman, C.P.; Mack, D. Restrained and unrestrained eating1. *J. Pers.* **1975**, *43*, 647–660. [CrossRef]
150. Racine, S.E.; Hagan, K.E.; Schell, S.E. Is all nonhomeostatic eating the same? Examining the latent structure of nonhomeostatic eating processes in women and men. *Psychol. Assess.* **2019**, *31*, 1220–1233. [CrossRef]
151. Mills, J.G.; Thomas, S.J.; Larkin, T.A.; Deng, C. Overeating and food addiction in Major Depressive Disorder: Links to peripheral dopamine. *Appetite* **2020**, *148*, 104586. [CrossRef]
152. Kiyici, S.; Koca, N.; Sigirli, D.; Aslan, B.B.; Guclu, M.; Kisakol, G. Food addiction correlates with psychosocial functioning more than metabolic parameters in patients with obesity. *Metab. Syndr. Relat. Disord.* **2020**, *18*, 161–167.
153. Xu, H.; Li, S.; Song, X.; Li, Z.; Zhang, D. Exploration of the association between dietary fiber intake and depressive symptoms in adults. *Nutrition* **2018**, *54*, 48–53. [CrossRef]
154. Adjibade, M.; Andreeva, V.A.; Lemogne, C.; Touvier, M.; Shivappa, N.; Hébert, J.R.; Wirth, M.D.; Hercberg, S.; Galan, P.; Julia, C.; et al. The inflammatory potential of the diet is associated with depressive symptoms in different subgroups of the general population. *J. Nutr.* **2017**, *147*, 879–887. [CrossRef] [PubMed]
155. Gómez-Donoso, C.; Sánchez-Villegas, A.; Martínez-González, M.A.; Gea, A.; Mendonça, R.D.D.; Lahortiga-Ramos, F.; Bes-Rastrollo, M. Ultra-processed food consumption and the incidence of depression in a Mediterranean cohort: The SUN Project. *Eur. J. Nutr.* **2019**, *59*, 1093–1103. [CrossRef] [PubMed]
156. Adjibade, M.; Julia, C.; Allès, B.; Touvier, M.; Lemogne, C.; Srour, B.; Hercberg, S.; Galan, P.; Assmann, K.E.; Kesse-Guyot, E. Prospective association between ultra-processed food consumption and incident depressive symptoms in the French NutriNet-Santé cohort. *BMC Med.* **2019**, *17*, 78. [CrossRef]
157. Jacka, F.N.; O'Neil, A.; Opie, R.; Itsiopoulos, C.; Cotton, S.; Mohebbi, M.; Castle, D.; Dash, S.; Mihalopoulos, C.; Chatterton, M.L.; et al. A randomised controlled trial of dietary improvement for adults with major depression (the 'SMILES' trial). *BMC Med.* **2017**, *15*, 23.
158. Lassale, C.; Batty, G.D.; Akbaraly, T. Reply to Veronese and Smith: Healthy dietary indices and risk of depressive outcomes: A systematic review and meta-analysis of observational studies. *Mol. Psychiatry* **2019**, *24*, 1–2. [CrossRef] [PubMed]
159. Davis, L.L.; Uezato, A.; Newell, J.M.; Frazier, E. Major depression and comorbid substance use disorders. *Curr. Opin. Psychiatry* **2008**, *21*, 14–18. [CrossRef] [PubMed]
160. Flory, J.D.; Yehuda, R. Comorbidity between post-traumatic stress disorder and major depressive disorder: Alternative explanations and treatment considerations. *Dialog- Clin. Neurosci.* **2015**, *17*, 141–150.
161. Sadeghi, O.; Keshteli, A.H.; Afshar, H.; Esmaillzadeh, A.; Adibi, P. Adherence to mediterranean dietary pattern is inversely associated with depression, anxiety and psychological distress. *Nutr. Neurosci.* **2019**, 1–12. [CrossRef]
162. Firth, J.; Marx, W.; Dash, S.; Carney, R.; Teasdale, S.B.; Solmi, M.; Stubbs, B.; Schuch, F.B.; Carvalho, A.F.; Jacka, F.; et al. The effects of dietary improvement on symptoms of depression and anxiety. *Psychosom. Med.* **2019**, *81*, 265–280.
163. Gibson-Smith, D.; Bot, M.; Brouwer, I.A.; Visser, M.; Penninx, B.W. Diet quality in persons with and without depressive and anxiety disorders. *J. Psychiatr. Res.* **2018**, *106*, 1–7. [CrossRef]
164. Bozzatello, P.; Rocca, P.; Mantelli, E.; Bellino, S. Polyunsaturated fatty acids: What is their role in treatment of psychiatric disorders? *Int. J. Mol. Sci.* **2019**, *20*, 5257. [CrossRef]
165. Bozzatello, P.; Brignolo, E.; De Grandi, E.; Bellino, S. Supplementation with omega-3 fatty acids in psychiatric disorders: A review of literature data. *J. Clin. Med.* **2016**, *5*, 67. [CrossRef] [PubMed]
166. Cryan, J.F.; O'Riordan, K.J.; Cowan, C.S.M.; Sandhu, K.V.; Bastiaanssen, T.F.S.; Boehme, M.; Codagnone, M.G.; Cussotto, S.; Fulling, C.; Golubeva, A.V.; et al. The microbiota-gut-brain axis. *Physiol. Rev.* **2019**, *99*, 1877–2013. [CrossRef] [PubMed]

167. Cryan, J.F.; Dinan, T.G. Mind-altering microorganisms: The impact of the gut microbiota on brain and behaviour. *Nat. Rev. Neurosci.* **2012**, *13*, 701–712. [CrossRef]
168. Noonan, S.; Zaveri, M.; MacAninch, E.; Martyn, K. Food & mood: A review of supplementary prebiotic and probiotic interventions in the treatment of anxiety and depression in adults. *BMJ Nutr. Prev. Health* **2020**. [CrossRef]
169. Foster, J.A.; Neufeld, K.-A.M. Gut–brain axis: How the microbiome influences anxiety and depression. *Trends Neurosci.* **2013**, *36*, 305–312. [CrossRef]
170. Smith, J.P.; Book, S.W. Anxiety and substance use disorders: A review. *Psychiatric Times.* **2008**, *10*, 19–23.
171. Vujanovic, A.A.; Farris, S.G.; Bartlett, B.A.; Lyons, R.C.; Haller, M.; Colvonen, P.J.; Norman, S.B. Anxiety sensitivity in the association between posttraumatic stress and substance use disorders: A systematic review. *Clin. Psychol. Rev.* **2018**, *62*, 37–55. [CrossRef] [PubMed]
172. Spettigue, W.; Obeid, N.; Santos, A.; Norris, M.; Hamati, R.; Hadjiyannakis, S.; Buchholz, A. Binge eating and social anxiety in treatment-seeking adolescents with eating disorders or severe obesity. *Eat. Weight. Disord. Stud. Anorexia, Bulim. Obes.* **2019**, *25*, 787–793. [CrossRef] [PubMed]
173. Vega-Torres, J.D.; Haddad, E.; Bin Lee, J.; Kalyan-Masih, P.; George, W.I.M.; Pérez, L.L.; Vázquez, D.M.P.; Torres, Y.A.; Santana, J.M.S.; Obenaus, A.; et al. Exposure to an obesogenic diet during adolescence leads to abnormal maturation of neural and behavioral substrates underpinning fear and anxiety. *Brain Behav. Immun.* **2018**, *70*, 96–117. [CrossRef] [PubMed]
174. Burrows, T.L.; Hides, L.; Brown, R.; Dayas, C.V.; Kay-Lambkin, F. Differences in Dietary Preferences, Personality and Mental Health in Australian Adults with and without Food Addiction. *Nutrition* **2017**, *9*, 285. [CrossRef] [PubMed]
175. Benzerouk, F.; Gierski, F.; Ducluzeau, P.-H.; Bourbao-Tournois, C.; Gaubil-Kaladjian, I.; Bertin, E.; Kaladjian, A.; Ballon, N.; Brunault, P. Food addiction, in obese patients seeking bariatric surgery, is associated with higher prevalence of current mood and anxiety disorders and past mood disorders. *Psychiatry Res.* **2018**, *267*, 473–479. [CrossRef] [PubMed]
176. Nolan, L.J.; Jenkins, S.M. Food Addiction Is Associated with Irrational Beliefs via Trait Anxiety and Emotional Eating. *Nutrition* **2019**, *11*, 1711. [CrossRef] [PubMed]
177. Fonseca, N.K.d.O.d.; Molle, R.D.; Costa, M.d.A.; Gonçalves, F.G.; Silva, A.C.; Rodrigues, Y.; Price, M.; Silveira, P.P.; Manfro, G.G. Impulsivity influences food intake in women with generalized anxiety disorder. *Rev. Bras. Psiquiatr.* **2020**, *42*, 382–388. [CrossRef]
178. Tomiyama, A.J.; Dallman, M.F.; Epel, E. Comfort food is comforting to those most stressed: Evidence of the chronic stress response network in high stress women. *Psychoneuroendocrinology* **2011**, *36*, 1513–1519. [CrossRef]
179. Kaplow, J.B.; Widom, C.S. Age of onset of child maltreatment predicts long-term mental health outcomes. *J. Abnorm. Psychol.* **2007**, *116*, 176–187. [CrossRef]
180. Hamilton, K.R.; Mitchell, M.R.; Wing, V.C.; Balodis, I.M.; Bickel, W.K.; Fillmore, M.; Lane, S.D.; Lejuez, C.; Littlefield, A.K.; Luijten, M.; et al. Choice impulsivity: Definitions, measurement issues, and clinical implications. *Pers. Disord. Theory Res. Treat.* **2015**, *6*, 182–198. [CrossRef]
181. Paraskevopoulou, M.; Van Rooij, D.; Schene, A.H.; Scheres, A.P.; Buitelaar, J.K.; Schellekens, A.F.A. Effects of substance misuse and family history of substance use disorder on delay discounting in adolescents and young adults with attention-deficit/hyperactivity disorder. *Eur. Addict. Res.* **2020**, *26*, 295–305. [CrossRef]
182. Ptacek, R.; Stefano, G.B.; Weissenberger, S.; Akotia, D.; Raboch, J.; Papezova, H.; Domkarova, L.; Stepankova, T.; Goetz, M. Attention deficit hyperactivity disorder and disordered eating behaviors: Links, risks, and challenges faced. *Neuropsychiatr. Dis. Treat.* **2016**, *12*, 571–579. [CrossRef]
183. Van Blyderveen, S.; Lafrance, A.; Emond, M.; Kosmerly, S.; O'Connor, M.; Chang, F. Personality differences in the susceptibility to stress-eating: The influence of emotional control and impulsivity. *Eat. Behav.* **2016**, *23*, 76–81. [CrossRef]
184. Brewerton, T.D.; Duncan, A.E. Associations between attention deficit hyperactivity disorder and eating disorders by gender: Results from the national comorbidity survey replication. *Eur. Eat. Disord. Rev.* **2016**, *24*, 536–540. [CrossRef] [PubMed]
185. Ziobrowski, H.; Brewerton, T.D.; Duncan, A.E. Associations between ADHD and eating disorders in relation to comorbid psychiatric disorders in a nationally representative sample. *Psychiatry Res. Neuroimaging* **2018**, *260*, 53–59. [CrossRef]

186. Brunault, P.; Frammery, J.; Montaudon, P.; De Luca, A.; Hankard, R.; Ducluzeau, P.-H.; Cortese, S.; Ballon, N.; Pierre-Henri, P.-H.D.; Nicolas, N.B. Adulthood and childhood ADHD in patients consulting for obesity is associated with food addiction and binge eating, but not sleep apnea syndrome. *Appetite* **2019**, *136*, 25–32. [CrossRef] [PubMed]
187. Testa, G.; Baenas, I.; Vintró-Alcaraz, C.; Granero, R.; Agüera, Z.; Sánchez, I.; Riesco, N.; Jiménez-Murcia, S.; Fernández-Aranda, F. Does ADHD symptomatology influence treatment outcome and dropout risk in eating disorders? A longitudinal study. *J. Clin. Med.* **2020**, *9*, 2305. [CrossRef] [PubMed]
188. Martins-Silva, T.; Vaz, J.S.; Hutz, M.H.; Salatino-Oliveira, A.; Genro, J.P.; Hartwig, F.P.; Moreira-Maia, C.R.; Rohde, L.A.; Borges, M.C.; Tovo-Rodrigues, L. Assessing causality in the association between attention-deficit/hyperactivity disorder and obesity: A Mendelian randomization study. *Int. J. Obes.* **2019**, *43*, 2500–2508. [CrossRef] [PubMed]
189. Jeffers, A.J.; Benotsch, E.G.; Koester, S. Misuse of prescription stimulants for weight loss, psychosocial variables, and eating disordered behaviors. *Appetite* **2013**, *65*, 8–13. [CrossRef]
190. Hudson, J.I.; McElroy, S.L.; Ferreira-Cornwell, M.C.; Radewonuk, J.; Gasior, M. Efficacy of lisdexamfetamine in adults with moderate to severe binge-eating disorder: A randomized clinical trial. *JAMA Psychiatry* **2017**, *74*, 903–910. [CrossRef]
191. McElroy, S.L.; Hudson, J.I.; Mitchell, J.E.; Wilfley, D.; Ferreira-Cornwell, M.C.; Gao, J.; Wang, J.; Whitaker, T.; Jonas, J.; Gasior, M. Efficacy and safety of lisdexamfetamine for treatment of adults with moderate to severe binge-eating disorder. *JAMA Psychiatry* **2015**, *72*, 235–246. [CrossRef]
192. Osadchiy, V.; Mayer, E.A.; Bhatt, R.; Labus, J.S.; Gao, L.; Kilpatrick, L.A.; Liu, C.; Tillisch, K.; Naliboff, B.; Chang, L.; et al. History of early life adversity is associated with increased food addiction and sex-specific alterations in reward network connectivity in obesity. *Obes. Sci. Pr.* **2019**, *5*, 416–436. [CrossRef]
193. McCutcheon, A.R.; Bloomfield, M.A.; Dahoun, T.; Mehta, M.; Howes, O.D. Chronic psychosocial stressors are associated with alterations in salience processing and corticostriatal connectivity. *Schizophr. Res.* **2019**, *213*, 56–64. [CrossRef]
194. Bloomfield, M.A.P.; McCutcheon, R.A.; Kempton, M.; Freeman, T.P.; Howes, O.D. The effects of psychosocial stress on dopaminergic function and the acute stress response. *eLife* **2019**, *8*, e46797. [CrossRef]
195. Nunes-Neto, P.R.; Köhler, C.A.; Schuch, F.B.; Solmi, M.; Quevedo, J.; Maes, M.; Murru, A.; Vieta, E.; McIntyre, R.S.; McElroy, S.L.; et al. Food addiction: Prevalence, psychopathological correlates and associations with quality of life in a large sample. *J. Psychiatr. Res.* **2018**, *96*, 145–152. [CrossRef] [PubMed]
196. Borowitz, M.A.; Yokum, S.; Duval, E.R.; Gearhardt, A.N. Weight-Related differences in salience, default mode, and executive function network connectivity in adolescents. *Obesity* **2020**, *28*, 1438–1446. [CrossRef] [PubMed]
197. Grant, E.J.; Redden, S.A.; Lust, K.; Chamberlain, S.R. Nonmedical use of stimulants is associated with riskier sexual practices and other forms of impulsivity. *J. Addict. Med.* **2018**, *12*, 474–480. [CrossRef] [PubMed]
198. Wilson, B. *Alcoholics Anonymous*; Alcoholics Anonymous World Services, Inc.: New York, NY, USA, 1939.
199. Tylka, T.L.; Wilcox, J.A. Are intuitive eating and eating disorder symptomatology opposite poles of the same construct? *J. Couns. Psychol.* **2006**, *53*, 474–485. [CrossRef]
200. Linardon, J.; Mitchell, S.A. Rigid dietary control, flexible dietary control, and intuitive eating: Evidence for their differential relationship to disordered eating and body image concerns. *Eat. Behav.* **2017**, *26*, 16–22. [CrossRef]
201. Katzer, L.; Bradshaw, A.J.; Horwath, C.C.; Gray, A.; O'Brien, S.; Joyce, J. Evaluation of a "Nondieting" stress reduction program for overweight women: A randomized trial. *Am. J. Health Promot.* **2008**, *22*, 264–274. [CrossRef]
202. Jiménez-Murcia, S.; Agüera, Z.; Paslakis, G.; Munguía, L.; Granero, R.; Sánchez-González, J.; Sánchez, I.; Riesco, N.; Gearhardt, A.N.; Diéguez, C.; et al. Food addiction in eating disorders and obesity: Analysis of clusters and implications for treatment. *Nutrition* **2019**, *11*, 2633. [CrossRef]
203. Fauconnier, M.; Rousselet, M.; Brunault, P.; Thiabaud, E.; Lambert, S.; Rocher, B.; Challet-Bouju, G.; Grall-Bronnec, M. Food addiction among female patients seeking treatment for an eating disorder: Prevalence and associated factors. *Nutrition* **2020**, *12*, 1897.
204. Schulte, E.M.; Gearhardt, A.N. Development of the modified yale food addiction scale version 2.0. *Eur. Eat. Disord. Rev.* **2017**, *25*, 302–308. [CrossRef]

205. Gideon, N.; Hawkes, N.; Mond, J.; Saunders, R.; Tchanturia, K.; Serpell, L. Development and psychometric validation of the ede-qs, a 12 item short form of the eating disorder examination questionnaire (EDE-Q). *PLoS ONE* **2016**, *11*, e0152744. [CrossRef] [PubMed]
206. Garner, D.M.; Olmsted, M.P.; Bohr, Y.; Garfinkel, P.E. The eating attitudes test: Psychometric features and clinical correlates. *Psychol. Med.* **1982**, *12*, 871–878. [CrossRef] [PubMed]
207. Stinson, E.J.; Votruba, S.B.; Venti, C.; Perez, M.; Krakoff, J.; Gluck, M.E. Food Insecurity is associated with maladaptive eating behaviors and objectively measured overeating. *Obesity* **2018**, *26*, 1841–1848. [CrossRef] [PubMed]
208. Rasmusson, G.; Lydecker, J.A.; Coffino, J.A.; White, M.A.; Grilo, C.M. Household food insecurity is associated with binge-eating disorder and obesity. *Int. J. Eat. Disord.* **2018**, *52*, 28–35. [CrossRef] [PubMed]
209. Stanford, M.S.; Mathias, C.W.; Dougherty, D.M.; Lake, S.L.; Anderson, N.E.; Patton, J.H. Fifty years of the Barratt Impulsiveness Scale: An update and review. *Pers. Individ. Differ.* **2009**, *47*, 385–395. [CrossRef]
210. Patton, J.H.; Stanford, M.S.; Barratt, E.S. Factor structure of the barratt impulsiveness scale. *J. Clin. Psychol.* **1995**, *51*, 768–774. [CrossRef]
211. Blevins, C.A.; Weathers, F.W.; Davis, M.T.; Witte, T.; Domino, J.L. The posttraumatic stress disorder checklist for DSM-5 (PCL-5): Development and initial psychometric evaluation. *J. Trauma. Stress* **2015**, *28*, 489–498. [CrossRef]
212. Bremner, J.D.; Bolus, R.; Mayer, E.A. Psychometric properties of the early trauma inventory? Self report. *J. Nerv. Ment. Dis.* **2007**, *195*, 211–218. [CrossRef]
213. Kroenke, K.; Spitzer, R.L.; Williams, J.B.W. The PHQ-9: Validity of a brief depression severity measure. *J. Gen. Intern. Med.* **2001**, *16*, 606–613. [CrossRef]
214. Beck, A.T.; Steer, R.A.; Carbin, M.G. Psychometric properties of the beck depression inventory: Twenty-five years of evaluation. *Clin. Psychol. Rev.* **1988**, *8*, 77–100. [CrossRef]
215. Radloff, L.S. The CES-D Scale. *Appl. Psychol. Meas.* **1977**, *1*, 385–401. [CrossRef]
216. Fydrich, T.; Dowdall, D.; Chambless, D.L. Reliability and validity of the beck anxiety inventory. *J. Anxiety Disord.* **1992**, *6*, 55–61. [CrossRef]
217. Spielberger, C.D. *The Corsini Encyclopedia of Psychology*; John Wiley & Sons: Hoboken, NJ, USA, 2010.
218. Spitzer, R.L.; Kroenke, K.; Williams, J.B.W.; Löwe, B. A brief measure for assessing generalized anxiety disorder. *Arch. Intern. Med.* **2006**, *166*, 1092–1097. [CrossRef] [PubMed]
219. Kessler, R.C.; Adler, L.; Ames, M.; Demler, O.V.; Faraone, S.; Hiripi, E.; Howes, M.J.; Jin, R.; Secnik, K.; Spencer, T.; et al. The world health organization adult ADHD self-report scale (ASRS): A short screening scale for use in the general population. *Psychol. Med.* **2005**, *35*, 245–256. [CrossRef] [PubMed]
220. McDonnell, C.J.; Garbers, S.V. Adverse childhood experiences and obesity: Systematic review of behavioral interventions for women. *Psychol. Trauma: Theory, Res. Pr. Policy* **2018**, *10*, 387–395. [CrossRef]
221. Weinstein, A.M.; Zlatkes, M.; Gingis, A.; Lejoyeux, M. The effects of a 12-step self-help group for compulsive eating on measures of food addiction, anxiety, depression, and self-efficacy. *J. Groups Addict. Recover.* **2015**, *10*, 190–200. [CrossRef]
222. Chao, A.M.; Wadden, T.A.; Tronieri, J.S.; Pearl, R.L.; Alamuddin, N.; Bakizada, Z.M.; Pinkasavage, E.; Leonard, S.M.; Alfaris, N.; Berkowitz, R.I. Effects of addictive-like eating behaviors on weight loss with behavioral obesity treatment. *J. Behav. Med.* **2018**, *42*, 246–255. [CrossRef]
223. Miller-Matero, L.R.; Brescacin, C.; Clark, S.M.; Troncone, C.L.; Tobin, E.T. Why WAIT? Preliminary evaluation of the weight assistance and intervention techniques (WAIT) group. *Psychol. Health Med.* **2019**, *24*, 1029–1037. [CrossRef]
224. Paterson, C.; Lacroix, E.; Von Ranson, K.M. Conceptualizing addictive-like eating: A qualitative analysis. *Appetite* **2019**, *141*, 104326. [CrossRef]
225. Cassin, S.E.; Sijercic, I.; Montemarano, V. Psychosocial interventions for food addiction: A systematic review. *Curr. Addict. Rep.* **2020**, *7*, 9–19. [CrossRef]
226. Romano, K.A.; Heron, K.E.; Amerson, R.; Howard, L.M.; MacIntyre, R.I.; Mason, T.B. Changes in disordered eating behaviors over 10 or more years: A meta-analysis. *Int. J. Eat. Disord.* **2020**, *53*, 1034–1055. [CrossRef]
227. Elsenburg, L.K.; Van Wijk, K.J.E.; Liefbroer, A.C.; Smidt, N. Accumulation of adverse childhood events and overweight in children: A systematic review and meta-analysis. *Obesity* **2017**, *25*, 820–832. [CrossRef] [PubMed]

228. Elsenburg, L.K.; Smidt, N.; Liefbroer, A.C. The longitudinal relation between accumulation of adverse life events and body mass index from early adolescence to young adulthood. *Psychosom. Med.* **2017**, *79*, 365–373. [CrossRef]
229. Vidmar, A.P.; Salvy, S.J.; Pretlow, R.; Mittelman, S.D.; Wee, C.P.; Fink, C.; Fox, D.S.; Raymond, J.K. An addiction-based mobile health weight loss intervention: Protocol of a randomized controlled trial. *Contemp. Clin. Trials* **2019**, *78*, 11–19. [CrossRef]
230. Vidmar, A.P.; Pretlow, R.; Borzutzky, C.; Wee, C.P.; Fox, D.S.; Fink, C.; Mittelman, S.D. An addiction model-based mobile health weight loss intervention in adolescents with obesity. *Pediatr. Obes.* **2018**, *14*, e12464. [CrossRef] [PubMed]
231. Moghimi, E.; Davis, C.; Rotondi, M.A. eHealth treatments for compulsive overeating: A narrative review. *Curr. Addict. Rep.* **2020**, *7*, 395–404. [CrossRef]
232. Bergh, C.; Callmar, M.; Danemar, S.; Hölcke, M.; Isberg, S.; Leon, M.; Lindgren, J.; Lundqvist, A.; Niinimaa, M.; Olofsson, B.; et al. Effective treatment of eating disorders: Results at multiple sites. *Behav. Neurosci.* **2013**, *127*, 878–889. [CrossRef]
233. Manasse, S.M.; Espel, H.M.; Schumacher, L.M.; Kerrigan, S.G.; Zhang, F.; Forman, E.M.; Juarascio, A.S. Does impulsivity predict outcome in treatment for binge eating disorder? A multimodal investigation. *Appetite* **2016**, *105*, 172–179. [CrossRef]
234. Wiss, D.A.; Avena, N.; Rada, P. Sugar addiction: From evolution to revolution. *Front. Psychiatry* **2018**, *9*, 545. [CrossRef] [PubMed]
235. Gordon, E.L.; Ariel-Donges, A.H.; Bauman, V.; Merlo, L.J. What is the evidence for "Food Addiction?" A systematic review. *Nutrition* **2018**, *10*, 477. [CrossRef] [PubMed]
236. Nolan, L.J. Is it time to consider the food use disorder? *Appetite* **2017**, *115*, 16–18. [CrossRef] [PubMed]
237. Brewerton, T.D. Chapter 15 Food addiction and its associations to trauma, severity of illness, and comorbidity. *Compuls. Eat. Behav. Food Addict.* **2019**, 449–468.
238. Brewerton, T.D. An overview of trauma-informed care and practice for eating disorders. *J. Aggress. Maltreatment Trauma* **2018**, *28*, 1–18. [CrossRef]
239. Brewerton, T.D.; Alexander, J.; Schaefer, J. Trauma-informed care and practice for eating disorders: Personal and professional perspectives of lived experiences. *Eat. Weight. Disord. Stud. Anorexia, Bulim. Obes.* **2018**, *24*, 329–338. [CrossRef]
240. Dunn, T.M.; Bratman, S.V. On orthorexia nervosa: A review of the literature and proposed diagnostic criteria. *Eat. Behav.* **2016**, *21*, 11–17. [CrossRef] [PubMed]
241. Michael, J.E.; Bulik, C.M.; Hart, S.J.; Doyle, L.; Austin, J.; Msc, J.E.M. Perceptions of genetic risk, testing, and counseling among individuals with eating disorders. *Int. J. Eat. Disord.* **2020**, *53*, 1496–1505. [CrossRef]

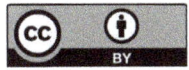

© 2020 by the authors. Licensee MDPI, Basel, Switzerland. This article is an open access article distributed under the terms and conditions of the Creative Commons Attribution (CC BY) license (http://creativecommons.org/licenses/by/4.0/).

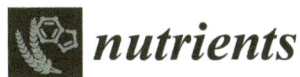

Article

Food Addiction Is Associated with Binge Eating and Psychiatric Distress among Post-Operative Bariatric Surgery Patients and May Improve in Response to Cognitive Behavioural Therapy

Stephanie Cassin [1,2,3,*], Samantha Leung [3,4], Raed Hawa [2,3,4], Susan Wnuk [2,3,4], Timothy Jackson [4,5] and Sanjeev Sockalingam [2,3,4,6,*]

1. Department of Psychology, Ryerson University, Toronto, ON M5B 2K3, Canada
2. Department of Psychiatry, University of Toronto, Toronto, ON M5T 1R8, Canada; raed.hawa@uhn.ca (R.H.); susan.wnuk@uhn.ca (S.W.)
3. Centre for Mental Health, University Health Network, Toronto, ON M5T 2S8, Canada; samantha.leung@uhn.ca
4. Bariatric Surgery Program, Toronto Western Hospital, Toronto, ON M5T 2S8, Canada; timothy.jackson@uhn.ca
5. Division of General Surgery, University Health Network, University of Toronto, Toronto, ON M5T 2S8, Canada
6. Centre for Addiction and Mental Health, Toronto, ON M5S 2S1, Canada
* Correspondence: stephanie.cassin@psych.ryerson.ca (S.C.); sanjeev.sockalingam@camh.ca (S.S.); Tel.: +1-416-979-5000 (ext. 3007) (S.C.); +1-416-535-8501 (ext. 32178) (S.S.)

Received: 2 September 2020; Accepted: 21 September 2020; Published: 23 September 2020

Abstract: The current study examined clinical correlates of food addiction among post-operative bariatric surgery patients, compared the clinical characteristics of patients with versus without food addiction, and examined whether a brief telephone-based cognitive behavioural therapy (Tele-CBT) intervention improves food addiction symptomatology among those with food addiction. Participants ($N = 100$) completed measures of food addiction, binge eating, depression, and anxiety 1 year following bariatric surgery, were randomized to receive either Tele-CBT or standard bariatric post-operative care, and then, repeated the measure of food addiction at 1.25 and 1.5 years following surgery. Thirteen percent of patients exceeded the cut-off for food addiction at 1 year post-surgery, and this subgroup of patients reported greater binge eating characteristics and psychiatric distress compared to patients without food addiction. Among those with food addiction, Tele-CBT was found to improve food addiction symptomatology immediately following the intervention. These preliminary findings suggest that Tele-CBT may be helpful, at least in the short term, in improving food addiction symptomatology among some patients who do not experience remission of food addiction following bariatric surgery; however, these findings require replication in a larger sample.

Keywords: bariatric surgery; food addiction; Yale Food Addiction Scale; cognitive behavioural therapy; telephone therapy

1. Introduction

The increasing prevalence of obesity is a growing global concern [1]. Bariatric surgery remains the most durable intervention for severe obesity, with studies demonstrating significant weight loss and improvements in, or even resolution of, obesity-related comorbidities [2–4]. The period of most significant weight loss occurs within the first 12 months following surgery [5,6]; however, between 20% to 50% of patients experience weight regain during long-term follow-up [7–9]. Bariatric patients' weight change trajectories begin to diverge between 6 and 12 months following surgery [5,6] and different trajectories have an impact on the prevalence of comorbidities and corresponding health care costs [10]. Post-operative binge eating, loss of control eating, and grazing have been shown to predict poorer weight loss outcomes following surgery [11–13].

The concept of food addiction (FA) may help account for the divergent weight change trajectories observed following bariatric surgery. It has been proposed that certain foods (i.e., hyperpalatable foods with refined carbohydrates and/or added fats) share pharmacokinetic properties with drugs of abuse [14], and are capable of activating an addictive-like process in susceptible individuals that can cause weight-promoting eating behaviours such as compulsive overeating and binge eating [15]. Food addiction is not included as a diagnosis in the Diagnostic and Statistical Manual of Mental Disorders, 5th Edition (DSM-5) [16]; however, the term was first coined in the scientific literature in the 1950s [17] and is widely used by health care professionals, researchers, patients, and the general public. The Yale Food Addiction Scale (YFAS) [18] was developed to operationalize food addiction and identify individuals with addictive tendencies towards highly processed foods. Given the similarities between highly processed foods and drugs of abuse, the YFAS adapted the DSM-IV criteria for substance dependence to make them relevant to the consumption of certain foods such as sweets, salty snacks, fatty foods, and sugary drinks (e.g., consuming more of certain foods than intended or over a longer period of time, preoccupation with certain foods, craving or strong urge to consume certain foods, and continued consumption of certain foods despite knowledge of adverse effects).

Rates of food addiction in pre-operative bariatric surgery populations as determined by the YFAS [18] and its subsequent modifications range from 14% to 58% [19]. Food addiction has been found to be associated with increased psychosocial impairment, including higher rates of depression, anxiety, impulsivity, and eating psychopathology, particularly binge eating [20–25]. In fact, food addiction has been conceptualized as a more severe and compulsive subtype of binge eating disorder (BED) [26]. Although food addiction is positively associated with body mass index [25,27], pre-operative YFAS scores do not appear to be significantly associated with percentage total weight loss (% TWL) following surgery [24,28] and food addiction is not considered a contraindication for bariatric surgery [29].

To date, research on food addiction among post-operative bariatric surgery patients remains sparse. Rates of food addiction in post-operative bariatric surgery populations are much lower, ranging from 2% to 14%, with no de novo cases of food addiction identified following bariatric surgery [19]. These improvements in food addiction symptomatology as well as associated problematic eating behaviours have led some researchers to consider whether bariatric surgery could be used as a treatment for food addiction [29]. Despite the improvements in food addiction that generally occur following bariatric surgery, some patients do continue to experience significant food addiction symptomatology. Currently, very little is known about the clinical characteristics of this subgroup of patients; however, they likely represent a subgroup with a particularly severe form of food addiction that may require additional intervention.

A recent systematic review concluded that there are currently no evidence-based psychosocial interventions for food addiction [30]. To our knowledge, no studies conducted to date have examined therapeutic interventions for bariatric patients experiencing food addiction. However, previous studies have shown that a brief telephone-based cognitive behavioural therapy (Tele-CBT) intervention developed specifically for bariatric surgery patients is effective in improving binge eating, emotional eating, depression, and anxiety among both pre- and post-operative patients [31–33]. Given the close association between food addiction, other forms of disordered eating, and psychiatric distress that has been reported in the literature, it is possible that such an intervention may also be effective in improving food addiction symptomatology following surgery.

The current study had three aims: (1) to examine correlates of food addiction among post-operative bariatric surgery patients; (2) to compare the clinical characteristics of patients who meet "diagnosis" for food addiction at 1 year post-surgery to those who do not; and (3) to examine whether Tele-CBT improves food addiction symptomatology among the subset of individuals who meet "diagnosis" for food addiction at 1 year post-surgery. It was hypothesized that: (1) food addiction symptomatology would be strongly correlated with binge eating and moderately correlated with percentage total weight loss and measures of psychiatric distress at 1 year post-surgery; (2) patients meeting "diagnosis" for food addiction would have greater binge eating and psychiatric distress and lower percentage total weight loss compared to those who do not; and (3) patients meeting "diagnosis" for food addiction at 1 year post-surgery who received Tele-CBT would report greater improvements in food addiction symptomatology compared to those receiving standard care.

2. Materials and Methods

2.1. Study Setting

Patients were recruited between 2018 and 2020 from the University Health Network (Toronto Western Hospital) Bariatric Surgery Program (UHN-BSP) and from the Humber River Hospital Bariatric Surgery Program (HRH-BSP) as part of a larger multisite randomized controlled trial examining the efficacy of telephone-based cognitive behavioural therapy 1 year following bariatric surgery. This study was approved by the institutional Research Ethics Boards and all patients provided informed consent before commencing the study; ethical approval code: CTO #0942. Patients were eligible to participate in the study if they were 1 year post-bariatric surgery, fluent in English, and had access to a telephone and a computer with Internet connection to complete the questionnaires. Study exclusion criteria included active suicidal ideation and poorly controlled psychiatric illness that would preclude engaging in Tele-CBT (e.g., psychosis). Participants were between the ages of 18 and 65 years and had a pre-operative body mass index (BMI) of >40 or $\geq$35 kg/m^2 with at least one obesity-related comorbidity. Patients received a Roux-en-Y Gastric Bypass unless a sleeve gastrectomy was surgically indicated (e.g., if there was a history of previous abdominal surgeries resulting in extensive adhesions and/or distorted anatomy).

2.2. Study Procedures

A total of 100 patients completed all study procedures and were included in the analyses. Pre-surgery anthropomorphic data including height and weight were collected by a clinician during pre-surgery appointments. Subsequent post-surgery weights at 1 year post-surgery (henceforth, referred to as "baseline" for the purposes of the present study), post-intervention (1.25 years post-surgery), and follow-up (1.5 years post-surgery) were provided directly from participants via photo or self-report. Percent total weight loss (%TWL) was calculated by dividing the difference in weight at post-intervention by the pre-surgery weight and then multiplying by 100.

All participants completed questionnaires at baseline, post-intervention, and follow-up using Qualtrics (Provo, UT, USA). Upon completion of the baseline questionnaires, participants were randomized to either the Tele-CBT group or the standard care control group using a customized randomization application. Participants randomized to the Tele-CBT group received the intervention described below, whereas those randomized to the control group received standard post-operative care that consisted of routine clinic visits (including post-surgery psychosocial follow-up appointments) and the option of attending a monthly support group. Participants completed questionnaires again at post-intervention and follow-up. The total time interval between the baseline and post-intervention timepoints was 10 weeks.

The Tele-CBT intervention consisted of six 1-hour sessions conducted weekly followed by a 1-hour "booster" session 1 month after the sixth session. Four clinical psychology graduate students who had experience assessing and treating bariatric surgery patients conducted the sessions, and the first author provided clinical supervision. The Tele-CBT intervention introduced participants to a personalized cognitive behavioural model of obesity, and included a variety of clinical strategies such as setting goals, scheduling healthy meals and snacks throughout the day, identifying and planning for difficult eating scenarios, planning pleasurable activities and behavioural alternatives to overeating, engaging in self-care activities, and challenging maladaptive thoughts and solving problems in order to decrease vulnerability to overeating. Participants were asked to complete worksheets for homework between sessions (e.g., food records, thought records) and practice skills that were introduced during the sessions (e.g., engaging in self-care and pleasurable activities) (see full Tele-CBT protocol description) [34]. The final "booster" session served as a check-in for participants to review the skills learned, troubleshoot issues that arose in the month prior, and develop a relapse prevention plan to help maintain the improvements made following surgery.

2.3. Study Measures

The Modified Yale Food Addiction Scale Version 2.0 (mYFAS 2.0) [35] was used to assess food addiction symptoms. The mYFAS 2.0 is a 13-item self-report measure designed to assess indicators of addictive-like eating and is comprised of 11 questions assessing substance use disorders as outlined by the DSM-5 and two questions that evaluate clinically significant impairment and distress. Symptom scores on the mYFAS 2.0 range from 0 to 11, and "diagnosis" scores range from no food addiction (1 or fewer symptoms, or does not meet criteria for clinical significance) to mild (2 or 3 symptoms and clinical significance), moderate (4 or 5 symptoms and clinical significance), or severe food addiction (6 or more symptoms and clinical significance). The YFAS 2.0 has been validated in bariatric surgery patients [36], and the abbreviated version of the YFAS 2.0 (i.e., the mYFAS 2.0) has similar psychometric properties as the full version [35].

The Binge Eating Scale (BES) was used to assess binge eating symptoms [37,38]. The BES is a self-report measure that assesses the presence of binge eating characteristics suggestive of an eating disorder. It was designed for use with individuals with obesity. Total cores on the BES range from 0 to 46. Moderate and severe levels of binge eating correspond to cut-off scores of 18 and 27, respectively.

The Patient Health Questionnaire-9 (PHQ-9) [39] and the Generalized Anxiety Disorder-7 (GAD-7) [40] were used to assess psychological distress. The PHQ-9 is a self-report measure that assesses depressive symptoms on a scale ranging from 0 (not at all) to 3 (nearly every day). Total scores on the PHQ-9 range from 0 to 27. Mild, moderate, moderately severe, and severe levels of depressive symptoms correspond to cut-off scores of 5, 10, 15, and 20, respectively. The GAD-7 is a self-report measure that assesses anxiety symptoms on a scale ranging from 0 (not at all) to 3 (nearly every day). Total scores on the GAD-7 range from 0 to 21. Mild, moderate, and severe levels of anxiety symptoms correspond to cut-off scores of 5, 10, and 15, respectively. Previous studies have used the PHQ-9 and GAD-7 to assess changes in psychological distress among bariatric surgery patients [41–43].

2.4. Statistical Analysis

All statistical analyses were performed using SPSS Statistics for Windows (Version 23.0; SPSS, IBM Corp., Armonk, NY, USA). Descriptive statistics including means, standard deviations, and frequency counts were calculated to describe the participant sample. Bivariate correlational analyses were conducted to examine correlates of food addiction. A Pearson's r effect size of 0.1, 0.3, and 0.5 correspond to a small, medium, and large effect, respectively [44]. Change scores were calculated by comparing post-intervention and follow-up to baseline scores. The Shapiro–Wilk test was used to determine whether the data were normally distributed. Kruskal–Wallis H tests were conducted for clinical variables with non-normally distributed data to assesses differences between groups, and Wilcoxon Signed-Rank tests were conducted for clinical variables with non-normally distributed data to assess differences from baseline (pre-intervention) to post-intervention.

3. Results

3.1. Participant Flow and Characteristics

As mentioned, the current study examining the correlates of food addiction and changes in food addiction in response to cognitive behavioural therapy was part of a larger multisite randomized controlled trial. Of the 136 participants who consented to participate, 122 completed the baseline questionnaires and were randomized to either the Tele-CBT group (n = 61) or control group (n = 61).

Of the remaining participants, eight did not respond to phone calls or emails, two were excluded due to their screening results, and four dropped out due to time constraints. Twelve participants from the Tele-CBT group discontinued treatment due to time constraints and 10 participants from the control group were lost to follow-up due to non-response. Given that this was a pilot study, data analyses for the first and second study aims were conducted with only those who had complete data at baseline ($n = 100$). Participants had a mean age of 48.40 ± 8.51 years, and the majority were female (82%), Caucasian (84%), college or university graduates (68%), were employed full-time (74%), and either married or in a common-law relationship (62%) (see Table 1). Only the subgroup of patients who met "diagnosis" for food addiction at 1 year post-surgery was included in the data analyses for the third study aim (i.e., to examine whether Tele-CBT improves food addiction symptomatology).

Table 1. Participant Characteristics ($n = 100$).

Variable	M (SD) or n (%)
Age (years)	48.40 (8.51)
Gender (female)	82 (82%)
Race/Ethnicity	
Black	4 (4%)
East Asian	1 (1%)
Latin American	3 (3%)
South Asian	1 (1%)
White (Caucasian)	84 (84%)
Other	7 (7%)
Relationship Status	
Married/Common-Law	62 (62%)
Divorced/Separated	13 (13%)
Single	23 (23%)
Widowed	1 (1%)
Occupational status	
Full-Time	74 (74%)
Part-Time	6 (6%)
Retired	7 (7%)
Disability	7 (7%)
Unemployed	6 (6%)
Education	
Some High School	3 (3%)
High School Graduate	7 (7%)
Some College/University	22 (22%)
College or University Graduate	68 (67%)

3.2. Correlates of Food Addiction 1 Year Post-Surgery

The correlates of food addiction are presented in Table 2. As hypothesized, at 1 year post-surgery, mYFAS 2.0 symptom scores were significantly correlated with scores on the BES, PHQ-9, and GAD-7, as well as %TWL. Similarly, mYFAS 2.0 "diagnosis" scores were significantly correlated with scores on the BES, PHQ-9, and GAD-7, as well as %TWL.

Table 2. Correlates of Modified Yale Food Addiction Scale Version 2.0 (mYFAS 2.0) symptom and diagnosis scores at 1 year post-surgery.

Measure	mYFAS 2.0 Symptom Scores		mYFAS 2.0 Diagnosis Scores	
	r	p	r	p
BES	0.633	<0.001	0.365	<0.001
PHQ-9	0.459	<0.001	0.217	0.030
GAD-7	0.372	<0.001	0.239	0.016
%TWL	−0.293	0.003	−0.229	0.022

Note: BES—Binge Eating Scale; PHQ-9—Patient Health Questionnaire 9-Item Scale; GAD-7—Generalized Anxiety Disorder 7-Item Scale; %TWL—Percent Total Weight Loss; mYFAS 2.0 Symptomatology—Modified Yale Food Addiction Scale Version 2.0 Symptomatology Scores.

3.3. Comparison of Participants with versus without Food Addiction 1 Year Post-Surgery

Of the 100 participants in this study, 13 (13%) exceeded the cut-off for food addiction according to the mYFAS "diagnosis" score at 1 year post-surgery. Those who exceeded the cut-off for food addiction reported significantly higher scores on the BES ($p < 0.001$), PHQ-9 ($p = 0.006$), GAD-7 ($p = 0.027$), and mYFAS 2.0 symptoms ($p < 0.001$). Those with food addiction also reported greater %TWL; however, the difference between groups was non-significant ($p = 0.08$). Mean scores (and standard deviations) are presented in Table 3.

Table 3. Clinical characteristics of patients with food addiction (according to the mYFAS2.0), patients without food addiction, and the total sample assessed at 1 year post-surgery. Values represent mean ± standard deviation.

Measure	No Food Addiction ($n = 87$)	Food Addiction ($n = 13$)	Total Sample ($n = 100$)
BES	11.86 ± 7.85	20.46 ± 5.78	12.980 ± 8.12
PHQ-9	5.22 ± 4.60	8.54 ± 3.36	5.65 ± 4.59
GAD-7	4.40 ± 3.96	7.15 ± 4.20	4.76 ± 4.07
%TWL	29.91 ± 9.44	22.09 ± 14.91	28.89 ± 10.55
mYFAS 2.0 Symptomatology	0.72 ± 1.13	3.92 ± 1.44	1.14 ± 1.59

Note: BES—Binge Eating Scale; PHQ-9—Patient Health Questionnaire 9-Item Scale; GAD-7—Generalized Anxiety Disorder 7-Item Scale; %TWL—Percent Total Weight Loss; mYFAS 2.0 Symptomatology—Modified Yale Food Addiction Scale Version 2.0 Symptomatology Scores.

3.4. Changes in Food Addiction Following Tele-CBT

Changes in mYFAS 2.0 scores were examined among the subgroup of patients who met "diagnosis" for food addiction at 1 year post-surgery ($n = 13$). mYFAS 2.0 symptom scores were significantly lower in the Tele-CBT group (1.29 ± 1.38) than the control group (2.33 ± 3.33) at post-intervention ($p = 0.027$). Patients in the Tele-CBT group reported significant improvements in mYFAS 2.0 symptom scores from pre- to post-intervention ($p = 0.027$), whereas those in the control group did not report significant changes over the same period ($p = 0.246$). mYFAS 2.0 symptom scores were not significantly different between the Tele-CBT group (2.00 ± 1.826) and the control group (2.50 ± 2.429) at follow-up ($p = 0.772$). See Figure 1 for changes in mYFAS 2.0 symptom scores across time as a function of group.

Regarding mYFAS 2.0 "diagnosis" scores, only one patient in the Tele-CBT group met "diagnosis" for food addiction at post-intervention and follow-up. Only two patients in the control group met "diagnosis" for food addiction at post-intervention and they no longer met "diagnosis" at follow-up. However, one other patient reported a resurgence of food addiction despite having remitted at post-intervention.

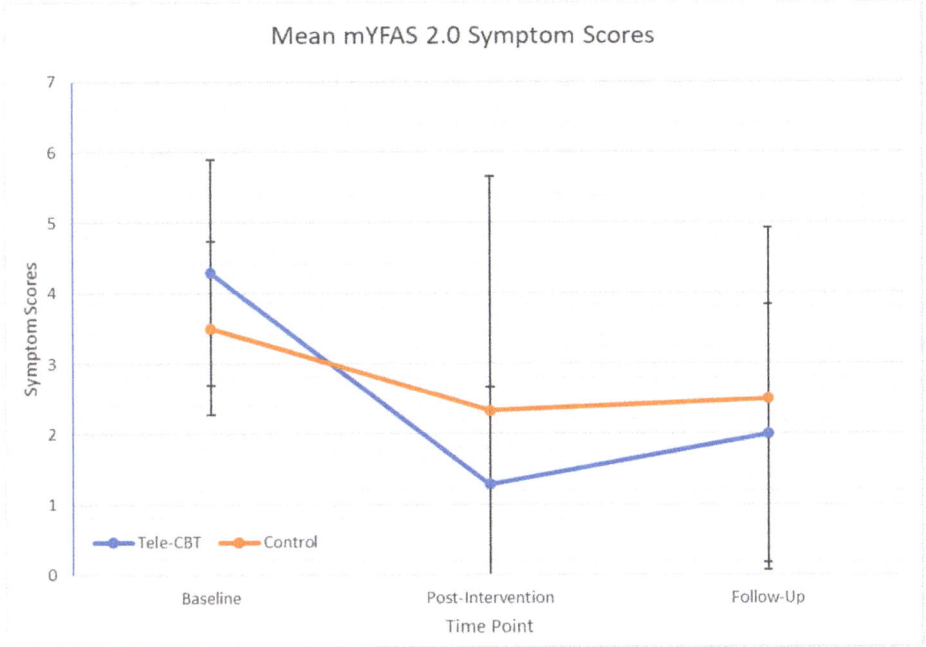

Figure 1. Changes in mYFAS 2.0 symptom scores over time as a function of treatment group among patients meeting "diagnosis" for food addiction at 1 year post-surgery ($n = 13$). Note: Baseline = 1 year post-surgery (prior to CBT); Post-intervention = 15 months post-surgery (immediately following CBT); Follow-up = 18 months post-surgery (3 months following CBT). mYFAS 2.0 Symptomatology—Modified Yale Food Addiction Scale Version 2.0 Symptomatology Scores. Tele-CBT—telephone-based cognitive behavioural therapy.

4. Discussion

The current study sought to examine clinical correlates of food addiction among post-operative bariatric surgery patients, to compare the clinical characteristics of patients with food addiction to those without food addiction, and to examine whether Tele-CBT improves food addiction symptomatology among those with food addiction. Our study hypotheses were largely supported. Consistent with the existing literature [20–25], food addiction symptomatology was strongly correlated with binge eating characteristics and psychiatric distress (i.e., depression and anxiety symptoms). It was also moderately correlated with %TWL. Thirteen percent of patients exceeded the mYFAS 2.0 cut-off for food addiction at 1 year post-surgery, and this subgroup of patients reported greater binge eating characteristics and psychiatric distress compared to patients without food addiction. They also reported almost 8% less total weight loss on average, though the difference was not statistically significantly likely due to the small sample size and variability in weight loss outcomes. Among those with food addiction, Tele-CBT was found to improve YFAS symptomatology immediately following the intervention.

The findings of this study add to the literature demonstrating that food addiction tends to improve following bariatric surgery [29]. The rate of mYFAS 2.0 "diagnosis" of 13% in the current study falls within the range of 2% to 14% that has previously been reported among post-operative patients [45,46], and below the range of 14% to 58% reported among pre-operative patients [19]. The mechanisms underlying this improvement are unclear; however, Koball and colleagues [29] identify a number of changes that occur following surgery, including cravings [47], rewarding properties of food [48], food preference and intolerance [49,50], and regulation of hunger and satiety [51,52], which may help account for improvements in food addiction symptomatology.

The impact of bariatric surgery on food addiction symptomatology is encouraging given the lack of empirical research on treatments for food addiction [30]. The subgroup of patients who meet "diagnosis" for food addiction following bariatric surgery appear to have more persistent and clinically significant binge eating characteristics (falling within the "moderate" range according to BES cut-offs in the current study), which may result in attenuated weight loss outcomes. The very limited research examining the association between post-operative YFAS scores and weight loss outcomes has generated mixed results, with one study reporting that post-operative YFAS score was not associated with the maximum %TWL achieved following surgery but was positively ($r = 0.22$, albeit not significantly, $p = 0.065$) associated with weight regain [53].

To our knowledge, this is the first study to examine the effect of a psychosocial intervention on food addiction symptomatology in a bariatric surgery population. Cognitive behavioural therapy has been suggested as a potential treatment for food addiction among bariatric surgery patients, given its efficacy in the treatment of binge eating disorder and substance use disorders [29,30,54]. Patients receiving Tele-CBT reported significant improvements in food addiction symptomatology immediately following the intervention. They improved to a greater extent than those receiving standard post-operative care alone; however, the group difference was no longer significant 3 months following the intervention. These preliminary findings suggest that Tele-CBT may be helpful, at least in the short term, in improving food addiction symptomatology among some patients who do not experience remission of food addiction following bariatric surgery. It is important to highlight that only one patient in each group met "diagnosis" for food addition at the follow-up assessment, which occurred 1.5 years following surgery. Thus, at least among this small group of study participants, it appears that the prevalence of food addiction may continue to decrease between 1 and 1.5 years post-surgery, even among those receiving standard post-operative bariatric care.

5. Limitations and Future Research Directions

The results of this study must be considered in light of a number of limitations. First and foremost, a relatively low percentage of patients met "diagnosis" for food addiction at 1 year post-surgery. This is a very encouraging finding; however, it meant that the sample size was very small ($n = 13$) to examine the efficacy of the Tele-CBT intervention among the subgroup of patients with food addiction. It will be important to replicate the findings of this pilot study in a much larger sample of patients with food addiction. If Tele-CBT is found to be effective in improving food addiction symptomatology in a larger replication study, it would be informative to examine the mechanisms of change and predictors of response, similar to studies in patients without food addiction [55]. Second, the Tele-CBT intervention did not have an explicit focus on food addiction. It focused predominantly on goal setting, normalized eating, self-care activities, alternative activities to replace overeating, planning for challenging eating situations, and challenging thoughts that may increase vulnerability for maladaptive behaviours, such as binge eating. It is noteworthy that the Tele-CBT intervention resulted in short-term improvements in food addiction symptomatology despite not explicitly addressing food addiction. However, whether incorporating food addiction into the treatment protocol, using models such as those proposed by Wiss and Brewerton [56] and Treasure and colleagues [57], results in larger and sustained improvements in food addiction symptomatology is an important question that could be empirically tested. Third, given that the intervention was delivered by telephone and thus, did not require patients to travel to the bariatric program, the post-operative weight data used to calculate %TWL were collected directly from patients via photo or self-report, which may impact the reliability of those calculations. Finally, the study sample was quite homogeneous with respect to participant ethnicity (Caucasian) and sex (female). Although this is typical of most bariatric surgery programs, the findings may not generalize to male patients and those of diverse racial and ethnic backgrounds. Regarding future research directions, it would also be informative to conduct a longitudinal study examining pre-operative and post-operative predictors of food addiction symptomatology, as well as the mechanisms that might account for improvements in food addiction symptomatology observed from pre- to post-surgery.

6. Conclusions

The findings of this study contribute to the body of literature suggesting that bariatric surgery improves food addiction symptomatology. Patients who continue to experience food addiction after undergoing surgery likely have a more severe form of food addiction that is characterized by greater binge eating characteristics and psychosocial distress. The results of this preliminary study suggest that Tele-CBT may result in short-term improvements in food addiction symptomatology among the subgroup of patients who continue to experience food addiction following surgery.

Author Contributions: Authors S.C., S.S., S.L. and S.W. contributed to the study conception and design, as well as the data analysis. All authors (S.C., S.S., S.L., S.W., R.H., and T.J.) contributed to the data interpretation and manuscript preparation. All authors have read and agreed to the published version of the manuscript.

Funding: This study was funded by the Canadian Institutes of Health Research (Grant No. 317877).

Acknowledgments: The authors would like to thank the patients who participated in the study as well as the Toronto Western Hospital Bariatric Surgery Program team members for their support.

Conflicts of Interest: The authors declare no conflict of interest.

References

1. Arroyo-Johnson, C.; Mincey, K.D. Obesity epidemiology worldwide. *Gastroenterol. Clin. N. Am.* **2016**, *45*, 571–579. [CrossRef]
2. Karlsson, J.; Taft, C.; Ryden, A.; Sjostrom, L.; Sullivan, M. Ten-year trends in health-related quality of life after surgical and conventional treatment for severe obesity: The SOS intervention study. *Int. J. Obes.* **2007**, *31*, 1248–1261. [CrossRef]
3. Puzziferri, N.; Roshek, T.B., III; Mayo, H.G.; Gallagher, R.; Belle, S.H.; Livingston, E.H. Long-term follow-up after bariatric surgery: A systematic review. *JAMA* **2014**, *312*, 934–942. [CrossRef]
4. Sjöström, L.; Lindroos, A.K.; Peltonen, M.; Torgerson, J.; Bouchard, C.; Carlsson, B.; Dahlgren, S.; Larsson, B.; Narbro, K.; Sjöström, C.D.; et al. Lifestyle, diabetes, and cardiovascular risk factors 10 years after bariatric surgery. *N. Engl. J. Med.* **2004**, *351*, 2683–2693. [CrossRef]
5. Courcoulas, A.P.; Christian, N.J.; Belle, S.H.; Berk, P.D.; Flum, D.R.; Garcia, L.; Horlick, M.; Kalarchian, M.A.; King, W.C.; Mitchell, J.E.; et al. Weight change and health outcomes at 3 years after bariatric surgery among individuals with severe obesity. *JAMA* **2013**, *310*, 2416–2425. [CrossRef]
6. Courcoulas, A.P.; King, W.C.; Belle, S.H.; Berk, P.; Flum, D.R.; Garcia, L.; Gourash, W.; Horlick, M.; Mitchell, J.E.; Pomp, A.; et al. Seven-Year Weight Trajectories and Health Outcomes in the Longitudinal Assessment of Bariatric Surgery (LABS) Study. *JAMA Surg.* **2018**, *153*, 427–434. [CrossRef]
7. Dimeglio, C.; Becouarn, G.; Topart, P.; Bodin, R.; Buisson, J.C.; Ritz, P. Weight Loss Trajectories After Bariatric Surgery for Obesity: Mathematical Model and Proof-of-Concept Study. *JMIR Med. Inform.* **2020**, *8*, e13672. [CrossRef]
8. Monaco-Ferreira, D.V.; Leandro-Merhi, V.A. Weight Regain 10 Years After Roux-en-Y Gastric Bypass. *Obes. Surg.* **2017**, *27*, 1137–1144. [CrossRef]
9. Magro, D.O.; Geloneze, B.; Delfini, R.; Pereja, B.C.; Callejas, F.; Pereja, J.C. Longterm weight regain after gastric bypass: A 5-year prospective study. *Obes. Surg.* **2008**, *18*, 648–651. [CrossRef]
10. Davis, J.A.; Saunders, R. Impact of weight trajectory after bariatric surgery on co-morbidity evolution and burden. *BMC Health Serv. Res.* **2020**, *20*, 278. [CrossRef]
11. Devlin, M.J.; King, W.C.; Kalarchian, M.A.; Hinerman, A.; Marcus, M.D.; Yanovski, S.Z.; Mitchell, J.E. Eating pathology and associations with long-term changes in weight and quality of life in the longitudinal assessment of bariatric surgery study. *Int. J. Eat. Disord.* **2018**, *51*, 1322–1330. [CrossRef]
12. Meany, G.; Conceição, E.; Mitchell, J.E. Binge eating, binge eating disorder and loss of control eating: Effects on weight outcomes after bariatric surgery. *Eur. Eat. Disord. Rev.* **2014**, *22*, 87–91. [CrossRef]

13. Pizato, N.; Botelho, P.B.; Gonçalves, V.S.S.; Dutra, E.S.; de Carvalho, K.M.B. Effect of grazing behavior on weight regain post-bariatric surgery: A systematic review. *Nutrients* **2017**, *9*, 1322. [CrossRef]
14. Schulte, E.M.; Avena, N.M.; Gearhardt, A.N. Which foods may be addictive? The roles of processing, fat content, and glycemic load. *PLoS ONE* **2015**, *10*, e0117959. [CrossRef]
15. Gearhardt, A.N.; Davis, C.; Kuschner, R.; Brownell, K.D. The addiction potential of hyperpalatable foods. *Curr. Drug Abuse Rev.* **2011**, *4*, 140–145. [CrossRef]
16. American Psychiatric Association. *Diagnostic and Statistical Manual of Mental Disorders*, 5th ed.; American Psychiatric Association: Arlington, VA, USA, 2013.
17. Randolph, T.G. The descriptive features of food addiction; addictive eating and drinking. *Q. J. Stud. Alcohol.* **1956**, *17*, 198–224. [CrossRef]
18. Gearhardt, A.N.; Corbin, W.R.; Brownell, K.D. Preliminary validation of the Yale Food Addition Scale. *Appetite* **2009**, *52*, 430–436. [CrossRef]
19. Ivezaj, V.; Wiedemann, A.A.; Grilo, C.M. Food addiction and bariatric surgery: A systematic review of the literature. *Obes. Rev.* **2017**, *18*, 1386–1397. [CrossRef]
20. Davis, C.; Curtis, C.; Levitan, R.D.; Carter, J.C.; Kaplan, A.S.; Kennedy, J.L. Evidence that 'food addiction' is a valid phenotype of obesity. *Appetite* **2011**, *57*, 711–717. [CrossRef]
21. Ivezaj, V.; White, M.A.; Grilo, C.M. Examining binge-eating disorder and food addiction in adults with overweight and obesity. *Obesity* **2016**, *24*, 2064–2069. [CrossRef]
22. Benzerouk, F.; Gierski, F.; Ducluzeau, P.-H.; Bourbao-Tournois, C.; Gaubil-Kaladjian, I.; Bertin E' Kaladjian, A.; Ballon, N.; Brunault, P. Food addiction, in obese patients seeking bariatric surgery, is associated with higher prevalence of current mood and anxiety disorders and past mood disorders. *Pyschiatry Res.* **2018**, *267*, 473–479. [CrossRef] [PubMed]
23. Meule, A.; Heckel, D.; Jurowich, C.F.; Vogele, C.; Kubler, A. Correlates of food addiction in obese individuals seeking bariatric surgery. *Clin. Obes.* **2014**, *4*, 228–236. [CrossRef] [PubMed]
24. Koball, A.M.; Clark, M.M.; Collazo-Clavell, M.; Kellogg, T.; Ames, G.; Ebbert, J.; Grothe, K.B. The relationship among food addiction, negative mood, and eating-disordered behaviors in patients seeking to have bariatric surgery. *Surg. Obes. Relat. Dis.* **2016**, *12*, 165–170. [CrossRef] [PubMed]
25. Burrows, T.; Skinner, J.; McKenna, R.; Rollo, M. Food addition, binge eating disorder, and obesity: Is there a relationship? *Behav. Sci.* **2017**, *7*, 54. [CrossRef] [PubMed]
26. Davis, C. From passive overeating to "food addiction": A spectrum of compulsion and severity. *ISRN Obes.* **2013**, *2013*, 435027. [CrossRef]
27. Gearhardt, A.N.; Boswell, R.G.; White, M.A. The association of "food addiction" with disordered eating and body mass index. *Eat. Behav.* **2014**, *15*, 427–433. [CrossRef] [PubMed]
28. Clark, S.M.; Saules, K.K. Validation of the Yale Food Addiction Scale among a weight-loss surgery population. *Eat. Behav.* **2013**, *14*, 216–219. [CrossRef]
29. Koball, A.M.; Ames, G.; Goetze, R.E.; Grothe, K. Bariatric Surgery as a Treatment for Food Addiction? A Review of the Literature. *Curr. Addict. Rep.* **2000**, *7*, 1–8. [CrossRef]
30. Cassin, S.E.; Sijercic, I.; Montemarano, V. Psychosocial Interventions for Food Addiction: A Systematic Review. *Curr. Addict. Rep.* **2020**, *7*, 9–19. [CrossRef]
31. Cassin, S.E.; Sockalingam, S.; Du, C.; Wnuk, S.; Hawa, R.; Parikh, S.V. A pilot randomized controlled trial of telephone-based cognitive behavioural therapy for preoperative bariatric surgery patients. *Behav. Res. Ther.* **2016**, *80*, 17–22. [CrossRef]
32. Sockalingam, S.; Cassin, S.E.; Wnuk, S.; Du, C.; Jackson, T.; Hawa, R.; Parikh, S.V. A Pilot Study on Telephone Cognitive Behavioral Therapy for Patients Six-Months Post-Bariatric Surgery. *Obes. Surg.* **2017**, *27*, 670–675. [CrossRef] [PubMed]
33. Sockalingam, S.; Leung, S.E.; Hawa, R.; Wnuk, S.; Parikh, S.V.; Jackson, T.; Cassin, S.E. Telephone-based cognitive behavioural therapy for female patients 1-year post-bariatric surgery: A pitlo study. *Obes. Res. Clin. Pract.* **2019**, *13*, 499–504. [CrossRef] [PubMed]
34. Cassin, S.E.; Sockalingam, S.; Wnuk, S.; Strimas, R.; Royal, S.; Hawa, R.; Parikh, S.V. Cognitive behavioral therapy for bariatric surgery patients: Preliminary evidence for feasibility, acceptability, and effectiveness. *Cogn. Behav. Pract.* **2013**, *20*, 529–543. [CrossRef]
35. Schulte, E.; Gearhardt, A.N. Development of the Modified Yale Food Addiction Scale Version 2.0. *Eur. Eat. Disord. Rev.* **2017**, *25*, 302–308. [CrossRef] [PubMed]

36. Clark, S.M.; Martens, K.; Smith-Mason, C.E.; Hamann, A.; Miller-Matero, L.R. Validation of the Yale Food Addiction Scale 2.0 among a Bariatric Surgery Population. *Obes. Surg.* **2019**, *29*, 2923–2928. [CrossRef] [PubMed]
37. Gormally, J.; Black, S.; Daston, S.; Rardin, D. The assessment of binge eating severity among obese persons. *Addict. Behav.* **1982**, *7*, 47–55. [CrossRef]
38. Hood, M.M.; Grupski, A.E.; Hall, B.J.; Ivan, I.; Corsica, J. Factor structure and predictive utility of the Binge Eating Scale in bariatric surgery candidates. *Surg. Obes. Relat. Dis.* **2013**, *9*, 942–948. [CrossRef]
39. Kroenke, K.; Spitzer, R.L.; Williams, J.B. The PHQ-9: Validity of a brief depression severity measure. *J. Gen. Intern. Med.* **2001**, *16*, 606–613. [CrossRef]
40. Spitzer, R.L.; Kroenke, K.; Williams, J.B.; Lowe, B. A brief measure for assessing generalized anxiety disorder: The GAD-7. *Arch. Intern. Med.* **2006**, *166*, 1092–1097. [CrossRef]
41. Cassin, S.; Sockalingam, S.; Hawa, R.; Wnuk, S.; Royal, S.; Taube-Schiff, M.; Okrainec, A. Psychometric properties of the Patient Health Questionnaire (PHQ-9) as a depression screening tool for bariatric surgery candidates. *Psychosomatics* **2013**, *54*, 352–358. [CrossRef]
42. Sockalingam, S.; Wnuk, S.; Kantarovich, K.; Meaney, C.; Okrainec, A.; Hawa, R.; Cassin, S. Employment Outcomes One Year after Bariatric Surgery: The Role of Patient and Psychosocial Factors. *Obes. Surg.* **2015**, *25*, 514–522. [CrossRef] [PubMed]
43. Sockalingam, S.; Hawa, R.; Wnuk, S.; Santiago, V.; Kowgier, M.; Jackson, T.; Okrainec, A.; Cassin, S. Psychosocial predictors of quality of life and weight loss two years after bariatric surgery: Results from the Toronto Bari-PSYCH study. *Gen. Hosp. Psychiatry* **2017**, *47*, 7–13. [CrossRef] [PubMed]
44. Rice, M.E.; Harris, G.T. Comparing effect sizes in follow-up studies: ROC area, Cohen's *d*, and *r*. *Law Hum. Behav.* **2005**, *29*, 615–620. [CrossRef] [PubMed]
45. Pepino, M.Y.; Stein, R.I.; Eagon, J.C.; Klein, S. Bariatric surgery-induced weight loss causes remission of food addiction in extreme obesity. *Obesity* **2014**, *22*, 1792–1798. [CrossRef]
46. Sevincer, G.M.; Konuk, N.; Bozkurt, S.; Coskun, H. Food addiction and the outcome of bariatric surgery at 1-year: Prospective observational study. *Psychiatry Res.* **2016**, *244*, 159–164. [CrossRef]
47. Leahey, T.M.; Bond, D.S.; Raynor, H.; Roye, D.; Vithiananthan, S.; Ryder, B.A.; Sax, H.C.; Wing, R.R. Effects of bariatric surgery on food cravings: Do food cravings and the consumption of craved foods "normalize" after surgery? *Surg. Obes. Relat. Dis.* **2012**, *8*, 84–91. [CrossRef]
48. Berthoud, H.R.; Zheng, H.; Shin, A.C. Food reward in the obese and after weight loss induced by calorie restriction and bariatric surgery. *Ann. N. Y. Acad. Sci.* **2012**, *1264*, 36–48. [CrossRef]
49. Le Roux, C.W.; Bueter, M.; Theis, N.; Werling, M.; Ashrafian, H.; Löwenstein, C.; Athanasiou, T.; Bloom, S.R.; Spector, A.C.; Olbers, T.; et al. Gastric bypass reduces fat intake and preference. *Am. J. Physiol. Regul. Integr. Comp. Physiol.* **2011**, *301*, R1057–R1066. [CrossRef]
50. Thomas, J.R.; Marcus, E. High and low fat food selection with reported frequency intolerance following Roux-en-Y gastric bypass. *Obes. Surg.* **2008**, *18*, 282–287. [CrossRef]
51. Schultes, B.; Ernst, B.; Wilms, B.; Thurnheer, M.; Hallschmid, M. Hedonic hunger is increased in severely obese patients and is reduced after gastric bypass surgery. *Am. J. Clin. Nutr.* **2010**, *92*, 277–283. [CrossRef]
52. Thirlby, R.C.; Bahiraei, F.; Randall, J.; Drewnoski, A. Effect of Roux-en-Y gastric bypass on satiety and food likes: The role of genetics. *J. Gastrointest. Surg.* **2006**, *10*, 270–277. [CrossRef] [PubMed]
53. Yanos, B.R.; Saules, K.K.; Schuh, L.M.; Sogg, S. Predictors of lowest weight and long-term weight regain among Roux-en-Y gastric bypass patients. *Obes. Surg.* **2015**, *25*, 1364–1370. [CrossRef] [PubMed]
54. Schulte, E.M.; Joyner, M.A.; Potenza, M.N.; Grilo, C.M.; Gearhardt, A.N. Current conditions regarding food addiction. *Curr. Psychiatry Rep.* **2015**, *17*, 563. [CrossRef] [PubMed]
55. Costa-Dookhan, K.A.; Leung, S.E.; Cassin, S.E.; Sockalingam, S. Psychosocial predictors of response to telephone-based cognitive behavioural therapy in bariatric surgery patients. *Can. J. Diabetes* **2020**, *44*, 236–240. [CrossRef]

56. Wiss, D.A.; Brewerton, T.D. Incorporating food addiction into disordered eating: The disordered eating food addiction nutrition guide (DEFANG). *Eat. Weight Disord.* **2017**, *22*, 49–59. [CrossRef]
57. Treasure, J.; Leslie, M.; Chami, R.; Fernandez-Arand, F. Are trans diagnostic models of eating disorders fit for purpose? A consideration of the evidence for food addiction. *Eur. Eat. Disord. Rev.* **2018**, *26*, 83–91. [CrossRef]

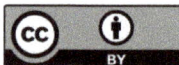

© 2020 by the authors. Licensee MDPI, Basel, Switzerland. This article is an open access article distributed under the terms and conditions of the Creative Commons Attribution (CC BY) license (http://creativecommons.org/licenses/by/4.0/).

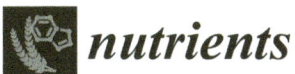

Article

Examining Self-Weighing Behaviors and Associated Features and Treatment Outcomes in Patients with Binge-Eating Disorder and Obesity with and without Food Addiction

Ashley A. Wiedemann [1], Valentina Ivezaj [1], Ralitza Gueorguieva [2], Marc N. Potenza [1,3,4,5,6,*] and Carlos M. Grilo [1]

1. Department of Psychiatry, Yale School of Medicine, New Haven, CT 06511, USA; ashley.wiedemann@yale.edu (A.A.W.); valentina.ivezaj@yale.edu (V.I.); carlos.grilo@yale.edu (C.M.G.)
2. Department of Biostatistics, Yale School of Public Health, New Haven, CT 06511, USA; ralitza.gueorguieva@yale.edu
3. Child Study Center, Yale University School of Medicine, New Haven, CT 06520, USA
4. Connecticut Mental Health Center, New Haven, CT 06519, USA
5. Connecticut Council on Problem Gambling, Wethersfield, CT 06109, USA
6. Department of Neuroscience, Yale University, New Haven, CT 06520, USA
* Correspondence: marc.potenza@yale.edu; Tel.: +1-(203)-737-3553

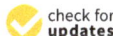

Citation: Wiedemann, A.A.; Ivezaj, V.; Gueorguieva, R.; Potenza, M.N.; Grilo, C.M. Examining Self-Weighing Behaviors and Associated Features and Treatment Outcomes in Patients with Binge-Eating Disorder and Obesity with and without Food Addiction. *Nutrients* 2021, 13, 29. https://doi.org/10.3390/nu13010029

Received: 11 November 2020
Accepted: 15 December 2020
Published: 23 December 2020

Publisher's Note: MDPI stays neutral with regard to jurisdictional claims in published maps and institutional affiliations.

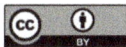

Copyright: © 2020 by the authors. Licensee MDPI, Basel, Switzerland. This article is an open access article distributed under the terms and conditions of the Creative Commons Attribution (CC BY) license (https://creativecommons.org/licenses/by/4.0/).

Abstract: Food addiction (FA) has been linked to clinical features in binge-eating disorder (BED) and obesity. A feature of behavioral weight loss (BWL) treatment involves frequent weighing. However, little is known regarding how frequency of self-weighing and related perceptions are associated with BWL outcomes among individuals with BED and obesity stratified by FA status. Participants (n = 186) were assessed with the Eating Disorder Examination before and after BWL treatment. Mixed effects models examined FA (presence/absence) before and after (post-treatment and 6- and 12-month follow-up) treatment and associations with frequency of weighing and related perceptions (reactions to weighing, sensitivity to weight gain and shape/weight acceptance). Participants with FA reported more negative reactions to weighing and less acceptance of shape/weight throughout treatment and follow-ups, and both variables were associated with greater disordered eating at follow-ups among participants with FA. Sensitivity to weight gain decreased over time independent of FA status. Frequency of weighing was associated with a greater likelihood of achieving 5% weight loss only among those without FA. Reactions to weighing and sensitivity to weight gain are associated with FA and poorer treatment outcomes in individuals with BED and obesity. Targeting these features may improve BWL outcomes among individuals with BED, obesity and FA.

Keywords: food addiction; binge-eating disorder; weighing; obesity; eating disorders; addictive behaviors

1. Introduction

Changes in the food environment have led to greater exposure to obesogenic foods (i.e., highly palatable, processed, relatively low in cost) and a "toxic food environment" (i.e., the modern food environment encouraging consumption of a diet high in fat and calories) [1]. These changes have been posited to contribute to increased rates of obesity; however, there is considerable debate surrounding whether these types of foods have addictive properties [2,3]. Growing interest and scientific study in the area of food addiction has increased substantially during the past two decades [4], concurrent with the development of self-report measures such as the Yale Food Addiction Scale (YFAS) [5].

The YFAS was developed to standardize assessment of symptoms of addictive-like eating based on diagnostic criteria assessing substance use disorders [5]. Importantly, addictive-like eating behaviors are not currently included within any formal diagnostic category or in any nosological system. However, numerous studies find that food addiction (based on the YFAS) is associated with behaviors/conditions linked to poorer health, including disordered eating, binge-eating disorder (BED) and obesity [6–9]. Furthermore, prior work suggests that food addiction is strongly associated with poorer body image, including elevated concerns about weight and shape [10,11]. Despite significant work in the past two decades examining the prevalence and clinical correlates of food addiction, few studies have examined the clinical utility of food addiction, and notably there is a scarcity of research investigating individuals with food addiction while receiving evidence-based treatments [12].

There are, however, preliminary findings that food addiction might attenuate weight-loss outcomes among those in behavioral weight loss (BWL) treatment [13]. BWL is an evidence-based treatment for overweight/obesity with goals of modifying problematic eating by establishing patterns of regular eating, restricting caloric consumption and increasing physical activity. Although BWL produces modest weight loss (i.e., 8–10 kg) among individuals with comorbid obesity/BED [14], prior studies have found that greater symptoms of food addiction at baseline were related to less weight loss following participation in a BWL intervention [13], as well as at 12-month follow-up among adults participating in a dietary intervention [15]. However, in other studies, food addiction did not attenuate weight loss [16,17].

In addition to the equivocal findings regarding the predictive significance of food addiction, even less is known regarding how individuals with food addiction perceive and respond to weight-loss interventions, such as BWL. We are unaware of any studies that have prospectively examined changes in behaviors among individuals with and without food addiction during and after treatment. One key component of BWL includes self-monitoring of weight during treatment, and prior work suggests that more frequent or consistent self-weighing is associated with improved weight-loss outcomes [18–21]. Several prospective studies examining adults during weight-loss treatment found that greater frequency of self-weighing was not associated with adverse psychological outcomes such as binge-eating [22], depression [20,21,23] or other forms of disordered eating, such as compensatory strategies [20,22]. Importantly, however, many of these studies excluded individuals with current or history of eating disorders, and we are unaware of any studies examining self-weighing among those with food addiction.

This present study examined prospectively (during and after BWL treatment) patients with BED with comorbid obesity, with and without food addiction. The first aim was to examine changes in weighing variables, including frequency of self-weighing, reactions to weighing, sensitivity to weight gain and shape/weight acceptance, between groups with and without food addiction during and after BWL treatment. The second aim was to examine associations of weighing variables at post-treatment with binge-eating, disordered eating and weight outcomes following treatment between groups with and without food addiction. We hypothesized that participants with food addiction would endorse greater eating-disorder psychopathology throughout BWL and following treatment compared to those without food addiction. We did not have a priori hypotheses with respect to self-weighing, as no prior studies have assessed the frequency of weighing among those with food addiction.

2. Materials and Methods

2.1. Participants

Participants were 186 adult (ages 18–65 years) patients with BED and obesity recruited from the community in a large university-based medical health-care center in an urban setting (see [24,25] for detailed description of methods and primary outcomes). All participants were diagnosed with DSM-IV-TR [26] criteria for BED and with obesity (criteria included current BMI ≥ 30 and ≤ 50 kg/m^2). Participants currently using antidepressant medications (a contraindication to the study medications involving sibutramine and orlistat), medications known to influence eating/weight or those with severe psychiatric conditions (e.g., schizophrenia, substance use disorder) or medical problems (e.g., cardiac disease, uncontrolled hypertension, thyroid disease or diabetes) were excluded. Participants were on average 48.38 years old (SD = 9.45) and had a mean BMI of 38.88 kg/m^2 (SD = 5.93). The majority of participants were female (71%) and identified as white (84.9%).

2.2. Procedures

This study received approval from the University's Institutional Review Board, and written informed consent was obtained from all participants prior to study procedures. Participants were evaluated by doctoral-level clinicians who were independent assessors with advanced training in eating/weight disorders. Assessors administered the Structured Clinical Interview for DSM-IV Psychiatric Disorders (SCID-I/P; [27]) at baseline to establish a diagnosis of BED and the Eating Disorder Examination Interview (EDE; [28]) to confirm the BED diagnosis at baseline and to comprehensively assess eating-disorder psychopathology at baseline, post-treatment and at 6- and 12-month follow-up assessments. Assessors were blinded to the treatment conditions. Participants completed a battery of self-report questionnaires to characterize associated domains, including food addiction, prior to randomization. Participants were randomly assigned to six-month behavioral weight loss treatment, either an adaptive stepped-care BWL sequential multiple allocation randomized trial (SMART) treatment or "standard" BWL treatment. BWL treatment followed the same protocols in both conditions, which included individual sessions with trained and monitored treatment clinicians following manualized treatment protocols. BWL focuses on making gradual behavioral changes including making moderate increases in physical activity and gradually decreasing caloric consumption. The adaptive SMART stepped-care BWL involved stratifying participants to a different behavioral treatment based on participants' early response in treatment (i.e., reduction in binge eating). The primary outcomes from this trial have previously been reported (including short- and long-term outcomes), and there were no significant overall differences between the conditions [24,25].

2.3. Measures

Weight variables. Following standardized procedures, participant height and weight were measured at participants' first treatment session using a wall-mounted measure and a large-capacity digital scale (MedWeigh MS-4600 High Capacity BMI Platform Scale). Participants were weighed in street clothing without shoes. Current height and weight at baseline were used to calculate participant BMI (kg/m^2). Weight was re-measured at post-treatment and six- and twelve-month follow-ups to calculate percent weight change. Weight loss was also examined categorically based on whether participants achieved greater than or equal to 5% weight loss at post-treatment and follow-ups.

The Eating Disorder Examination Interview (EDE; 16th ed; [29]) is a semi-structured, investigator-based interview designed to assess and diagnose eating disorders and eating-disorder psychopathology. Prior psychometric studies of the EDE support its use with BED [30], including with respect to test-retest reliability [31]. The EDE has been shown to differentiate between case and non-cases of eating disorders [32]. In the present study, the EDE—in addition to serving as the primary measure of binge eating and associated eating-disorder psychopathology (i.e., EDE Global Score)—assessed weighing-related variables of primary focus for the current study. These include frequency of self-weighing (henceforth referenced as Weighing), reaction to weekly weighing (henceforth referenced as Reaction), sensitivity to weight gain (henceforth referenced as Sensitivity) and shape/weight acceptance (henceforth referenced as Acceptance). Table 1 describes the study variables and corresponding item from the EDE, which assesses these constructs. Higher scores are indicative of greater pathology.

Table 1. Weighing and body image variables prospectively examined.

Study Variables	EDE Item	Frequency/Rating
Weighing	"Over the past 4 weeks how often have you weighed yourself?"	Number of times weighed in past 28 days
Sensitivity	"Over the past 4 weeks what amount of weight gain, over a period of 1 week, would have definitely upset you?"	7-point Likert scale based on the number of pounds or kilograms that would generate a marked negative reaction (0 = 7 lbs or 3.5 kg or more to 6 = 1 lb or 0.5 kg).
Reaction	"Over the past 4 weeks how would you have felt if you had been asked to weigh yourself once each week for the subsequent 4 weeks … just once a week; no more often and no less often?"	7-point Likert score ranging from 0 = no reaction to 6 = marked reaction (pronounced reaction which would affect other aspects of the subject's life).
Acceptance	"Over the past 4 weeks, to what extent have you been able to accept your shape and weight—see them as simply being the way you are?"	7-point Likert scale ranging from 0 = complete acceptance to 6 = no acceptance.

Note: EDE = Eating Disorder Examination Interview. Items obtained from the EDE Interview [29].

The EDE also assesses binge-eating episodes, defined as experiencing a subjective sense of loss-of-control while consuming an unusually large amount of food during the past 28 days. Binge-eating episodes were examined as a quantitative variable (number of episodes in past 28 days) and categorically based on binge-eating remission (defined as no binge-eating episodes during the prior 28 days at post-treatment and follow-ups) status. Additionally, the standard EDE global severity (i.e., EDE Global Score) score was calculated, which is comprised the average of four subscales reflecting eating-disorder psychopathology; scores range from 0 to 6, with higher scores reflecting greater severity. It is important to note that none of the weighing variables examined in this study comprise the EDE Global Score. The EDE was administered at pre-treatment, post-treatment and follow-ups.

The Yale Food Addiction Scale (YFAS) [5] is a 25-item self-report measure of food addiction developed in correspondence with substance-dependence criteria from the DSM-IV-TR. The YFAS offers both dimensional (symptom count) and dichotomous (clinical threshold) scoring methods to assess food addiction diagnosis. The YFAS has a one-factor structure and has adequate internal reliability and good convergent validity with measures of problematic eating [5]. For the present study, the dichotomous scoring was used to identify cases with food addiction. The YFAS was administered at pre-treatment, and the pre-treatment assessment was used to determine food addiction status throughout the study period. The Cronbach's alpha in the present study was 0.88.

2.4. Data Analysis

Descriptive statistics were analyzed using SPSS 24.0, and subsequent analyses were conducted in SAS 9.4. To examine changes in weighing variables by food addiction status across the study period, we used mixed effects models with each of the four weighing variables as the response in a separate model, food addiction status (yes/no) and treatment (stepped care vs. BWL) as between-subject factors and time (pre-treatment, post-treatment, 6-month follow-up, 12-month follow-up) as a within-subject factor. Linear mixed models possess several statistical advantages and are considered a robust method for accommodating missing values within longitudinal data. Associations among repeated observations on an individual were modelled using structured variance–covariance matrix with the best structure selected based on the Schwartz Bayesian Criterion (BIC). Transformations were applied prior to analysis in case of non-normality, and residual plots were used to assess the model assumptions. Least square means per food addiction status, treatment and time are shown in all models. Contrasts among least square means were used to explain significant effects. To examine the association of weighing variables at post with dimensional outcomes (i.e., binge-eating frequency, percent weight loss, EDE Global Score) during follow-up, we used mixed effects models with food addiction, time and each weighing variable at post (considered in a separate model) and all their interactions as predictors, controlling for the corresponding outcome at post-treatment as a covariate. Slopes with 95% confidence intervals were estimated when significant effects of weighing variables were observed. For categorical outcomes (i.e., 5% weight loss achieved, binge-eating remission), we fit Generalized Estimating Equations (GEE) models with the same set of predictors as above (without the covariate) and with an exchangeable working correlation structure. Odds ratios with 95% confidence intervals were used to describe significant effects of weighing frequency.

3. Results

Of the $n = 186$ participants, 61.3% ($n = 114$) met criteria for food addiction. The average number of food addiction symptoms endorsed by the total sample was 4.77 ($SD = 1.79$) out of the seven total symptoms assessed. Table 2 summarizes the means and standard deviations among food addiction groups for the weighing variables across the assessment timepoints.

Table 2. Means and standard deviations of weighing variables by Yale Food Addiction Scale Group.

	Pre-Treatment		Post-Treatment		6-Month Follow-Up		12-Month Follow-Up		Sig.
	FA ($n = 114$)	No FA ($n = 72$)	FA ($n = 100$)	No FA ($n = 66$)	FA ($n = 114$)	No FA ($n = 72$)	FA ($n = 91$)	No FA ($n = 63$)	
Weighing	10.63 (15.00)	8.01 (11.10)	9.73 (11.98)	10.18 (17.01)	10.93 (19.32)	8.57 (10.35)	8.66 (10.42)	9.09 (11.63)	ns
Sensitivity	4.31 (1.73)	4.40 (1.63)	4.17 (1.69)	3.92 (1.45)	3.45 (1.80)	3.17 (1.81)	3.68 (1.89)	3.19 (1.62)	0.0001
Reaction	1.46 (1.88)	1.01 (1.64)	1.07 (1.77)	0.61 (1.39)	0.59 (1.41)	0.59 (1.41)	1.14 (1.81)	0.72 (1.59)	0.01
Acceptance	5.28 (1.20)	4.65 (1.20)	4.07 (1.73)	3.27 (1.64)	3.64 (1.87)	3.06 (1.74)	3.89 (1.85)	3.09 (1.67)	0.0001

Note: Means were derived from raw data for ease of interpretation. FA = food addiction. ns = non-significant effects. Weighing = frequency of self-weighing during the past 28 days. Sensitivity = sensitivity to weight gain during the past 28 days. Follow-up scores all significantly different from pre-treatment. Reaction = reaction to prescribed weighing during the past 28 days. Significant main effects for time and FA status. Acceptance = shape/weight acceptance during the past 28 days. Significant main effects for time and FA status.

3.1. Aim 1: Examine Changes in Weighing Variables by Food Addiction Status Over Time

Mixed models analyses of Reaction revealed a significant main effect of food addiction ($F(1,174) = 6.84$, $p = 0.01$). Food addiction was associated with higher Reaction scores across groups and time points (Figure 1).

Mixed models analyses of Acceptance revealed significant main effects of food addiction ($F(1,182) = 16.47$ $p < 0.0001$) and time ($F(3,472) = 37.79$, $p < 0.0001$) (Figure 2). Acceptance scores were more pathological for those with food addiction compared to those without. Acceptance scores improved from pre-treatment to the other time points.

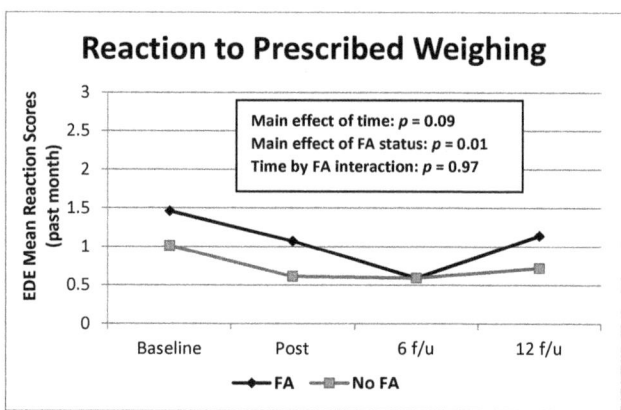

Figure 1. Frequencies of EDE Reaction to prescribed Weighing scores over time by food addiction group. Note: Means were derived from raw data for ease of interpretation. EDE = Eating Disorder Examination; FA = food addiction. Reaction = reaction to prescribed weighing during the past 28 days. Significant main effects were found for food addiction across all time points ($p < 0.01$).

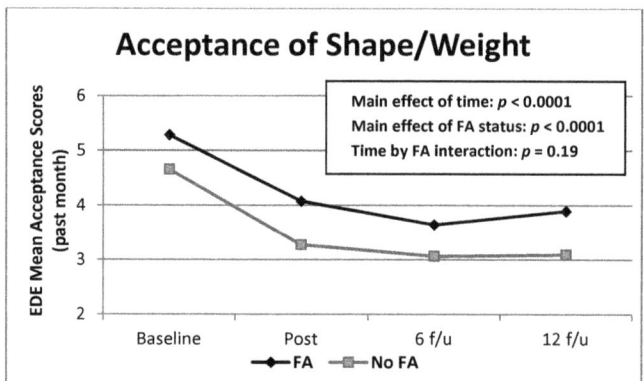

Figure 2. Frequencies of EDE Acceptance of shape/weight scores over time by food addiction group. Note: Means were derived from raw data for ease of interpretation. EDE = Eating Disorder Examination; FA = food addiction. Acceptance = shape/weight acceptance during the past 28 days. Significant main effects were found for food addiction ($p < 0.0001$) and time ($p < 0.0001$). All follow-up scores were significantly different from baseline. Lower scores reflect greater acceptance of shape/weight.

Mixed models analyses of Sensitivity revealed a significant improvement from baseline and post-treatment compared to follow-up across conditions $F(3,465) = 16.94$, $p < 0.0001$, but no significant differences between those with and without food addiction $F(1,178) = 1.59$, $p = 0.21$ and no significant interactions. There were no significant effects when examining Weighing scores (see Figure 3).

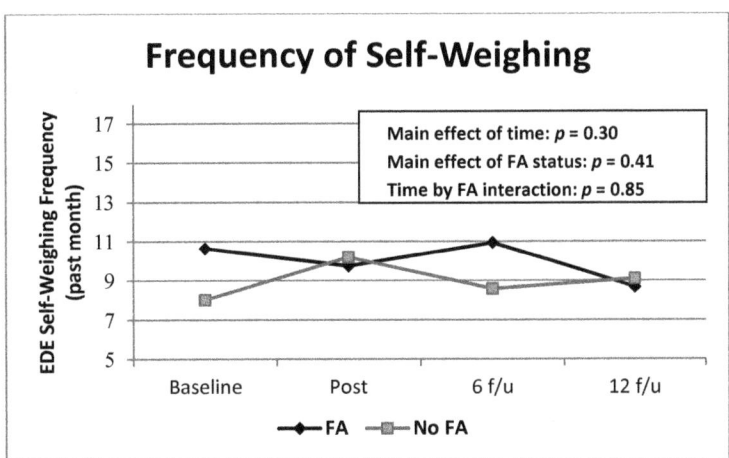

Figure 3. Frequencies of EDE Self-Weighing scores over time by food addiction group. Note. Means were derived from raw data for ease of interpretation. EDE = Eating Disorder Examination; FA = food addiction. All non-significant differences.

3.2. Aim 2: To Examine the Association of Weighing Variables at Post-Treatment with Binge-Eating, Disordered Eating and Weight Outcomes by Food Addiction Groups

Analyses of binge-eating frequency revealed no significant effects of any of the weighing variables, or interaction with food addiction at follow-ups, when examining binge-eating episodes quantitatively (frequency of episodes) or categorically (remission status).

Mixed model analyses of percent weight loss revealed no significant effects of any of the weighing variables or interactions with food addiction at follow-ups. When examining weight loss categorically (achievement of 5% weight loss or more), however, there was a marginally significant interaction between Weighing at post and food addiction ($\chi^2(1) = 3.98$, $p = 0.05$) and significant main effects of Weighing at post ($\chi^2(1) = 10$, $p = 0.002$) and food addiction ($\chi^2(1) = 4.73$, $p = 0.03$). Increasing Weighing frequency by one unit was associated with almost doubling of the odds of 5% weight loss for subjects without food addiction (OR = 1.95, 95% CI: 1.31, 2.90), whereas the effect was not significant in individuals with food addiction (OR = 1.17, 95% CI: 0.84, 1.61). There were no significant effects on 5% weight loss when examining Reaction, Sensitivity and Acceptance.

Mixed models analyses of the EDE Global Score revealed a significant interaction between Acceptance and food addiction ($F(1,147) = 4.24$, $p = 0.04$) and a significant main effect of Acceptance ($F(1,148) = 10.27$, $p = 0.002$). The slope for the relationship between Acceptance and the EDE Global Score was positive in both groups but significantly steeper for individuals with food addiction. Only the slope in the food addiction group was significantly different from 0 (slope = 0.14, $SE = 0.03$, $p < 0.0001$). There was also a significant interaction between Reaction and food addiction ($F(1,149) = 4.89$, $p = 0.03$). The interaction was due to the slope for the relationship between Reaction and EDE Global Score being slightly positive for those with food addiction and slightly negative for those without food addiction, but neither slope was significantly different from zero. There were no significant effects of Weighing or Sensitivity when examining EDE Global Scores.

4. Discussion

This is the first study, to our knowledge, to examine prospectively shape and weight concerns among individuals with and without food addiction participating in weight-loss treatment; more specifically, our study was with patients with BED and comorbid obesity who were subcategorized by food addiction status. Consistent with some of our hypotheses, our findings suggest multiple differences in shape and weight concerns between individuals with and without food addiction, including a stronger negative reaction related to the prospect of weekly weighing, as well as poorer acceptance of shape and weight throughout treatment among those with food addiction. However, no differences in frequency of self-weighing and sensitivity to weight gain were found between groups with and without food addiction.

Furthermore, we found that having a stronger negative reaction to weekly weighing and poorer acceptance of shape/weight following treatment were associated with greater levels of disordered eating following treatment among those with food addiction but were not related to binge-eating or weight-loss treatment outcomes. Sensitivity to weight gain was also unrelated to treatment outcomes and decreased over time across participants. Last, frequency of self-weighing was relatively stable over time and was not related to treatment outcomes (i.e., binge-eating, percent weight loss, disordered eating). However, greater frequency of weighing following treatment was related to a greater likelihood of achieving 5% weight loss following BWL treatment among those without food addiction.

The first aim of this study was to examine changes in weighing variables, including frequency of self-weighing, reactions to weighing, sensitivity to weight and shape/weight acceptance before and after BWL treatment between groups with and without food addiction. There were no significant differences in frequencies of self-weighing and sensitivity to weight gain when comparing those with and without food addiction and no significant changes after BWL treatment. However, participants categorized with food addiction endorsed a stronger negative reaction to weekly weighing and poorer acceptance of shape/weight over time relative to those without food addiction. It is important to note that although the food addiction group endorsed more pathological scores related to the prospect of weekly weighing, both groups endorsed subclinical scores (i.e., scores ≤ 4) throughout the assessment period. Shape/weight acceptance scores, however, were clinically elevated among both groups prior to starting treatment and remained in the clinical range for those with food addiction at the post-treatment assessment. Taken together, these longitudinal findings extend prior cross-sectional work suggesting that the combination of BED and food addiction are associated with elevated eating-disorder psychopathology [10,11,33] and suggest that food addiction, if present in patients with BED, might warrant additional clinical focus during BWL treatment.

The second aim was to examine whether changes in weighing variables (i.e., self-weighing, reaction to weekly weighing, sensitivity to weight gain and shape/weight acceptance) following treatment were associated with treatment outcomes among those with and without food addiction following BWL treatment. Prior work examining self-weighing within adult samples with overweight highlight the significant benefits of consistent self-weighing on weight loss outcomes [18–21], yet individuals with binge-eating or those with a history of eating disorders are often excluded from weight-loss studies. The present findings suggest that frequency of weighing was not significantly related to adverse treatment outcomes, including binge-eating, percent weight loss and eating-disorder psychopathology in a clinical sample of individuals with obesity and BED. Our prospective findings add to the growing literature suggesting that self-weighing in patients with BED with comorbid obesity might not have negative effects [34], and this seems to be the case for those with and without food addiction. Importantly, studies examining individuals with other eating disorders characterized by highly restrictive eating behaviors (i.e., anorexia nervosa, bulimia nervosa) or young adult women and girls, however, have found that more frequent self-weighing is associated with greater eating-disorder psychopathology [34–37]. The present study also found that individuals without food addiction who weighed more often were significantly more likely to achieve 5% weight loss, suggesting some benefit to regularly weighing. However, this result was observed only among those without food addiction. Participants were self-weighing, on average, ten times in a 28-day period, which approximates to weighing 2.5 times per week. An important direction for future research is to determine the threshold at which more frequent self-weighing may become maladaptive in those with BED [38]. Taken together, our findings highlight the benefits of self-weighing to promote weight loss in individuals with BED and obesity without food addiction.

Additionally, we found that endorsing a stronger negative reaction to weekly weighing and poorer acceptance of shape/weight were associated with greater disordered eating following treatment among those with food addiction and BED. Participants with co-occurring food addiction and BED did not self-weigh more often than those with BED without food addiction, yet consistently endorsed a stronger negative reaction to the prospect of weekly weighing. These findings have possible implications for treatments such as BWL and cognitive behavioral therapy (CBT), an evidence-based treatment for BED [39,40]. CBT for BED recommends limiting self-weighing to weekly, as opposed to daily self-weighing, which is common for some BWL treatments. Thus, our findings highlight possible areas for assessment among participants with food addiction, who endorsed a strong reaction to the prospect of weekly weighing. Assessing reactions and perceptions of weekly weighing in patients with food addiction may be helpful to identify potential barriers to weighing interventions in treatments such as BWL and CBT. Additionally, our findings suggest that less acceptance of shape/weight was associated with greater eating-disorder psychopathology in this subgroup. Future studies testing in patients with food addiction the efficacy of CBT, which provides durable and significant improvement in cognitive symptoms for individuals with BED [41], are warranted. Taken together, our findings suggest that certain body image concerns are a negative prognostic indicator among those with food addiction, which highlight important targets for treatment in this subgroup of patients.

There are several limitations to the present study to highlight. Although self-weighing was assessed using a semi-structured diagnostic interview of eating-disorder psychopathology, the frequency of self-weighing is based on participants retrospective report. Future work should assess self-weighing using electronic scales to determine objectively assessed self-weighing. Participants in this study were predominately female and white; thus, generalizability is limited. Future studies should evaluate these outcomes in more diverse samples including larger samples with more male participants. Future studies should also examine these outcomes using the more recent version of the self-report assessment of food addiction (i.e., YFAS 2.0), which corresponds to the DSM-5 definitions of substance use disorders, as the YFAS 2.0 was not yet developed when this study was conducted.

5. Conclusions

In summary, results of the present investigation provide evidence that self-weighing among individuals with BED with comorbid obesity with and without food addiction is not associated with poorer eating-disorder psychopathology or weight outcomes following BWL treatment. Frequency of self-weighing was associated with a marginally greater likelihood of achieving 5% weight loss, but only in those without food addiction. Our findings suggest that individuals categorized with food addiction reported a stronger negative reaction to weekly weighing and poorer acceptance of shape/weight, which were prospectively associated with greater eating-disorder psychopathology but were not related to weight loss outcomes and binge-eating frequency or remission. Clinicians should assess and consider body image concerns in treatment conceptualization and delivery in patients with BED comorbid with obesity who also report food addiction.

Author Contributions: A.A.W., V.I., M.N.P. and C.M.G. conceived the study. A.A.W. and R.G. performed the statistical analysis. All authors contributed to interpretation of the data. A.A.W. drafted the manuscript and all authors contributed to revision of the manuscript. All authors have read and agreed to the published version of the manuscript.

Funding: This research was funded by the National Institutes of Health grants DK049587 and R01 DK121551.

Institutional Review Board Statement: The study was conducted according to the guidelines of the Declaration of Helsinki, and approved by the Institutional Review Board (or Ethics Committee) of Yale School of Medicine (protocol code: 0610001822 and date of approval: 1/25/2012).

Informed Consent Statement: Informed consent was obtained from all subjects involved in the study.

Data Availability Statement: De-identified data will be provided in response to reasonable written request to achieve specified goals in an IRB-approved written proposal. These data are not published available at this time as they continue to be analyzed as part of on-going grant-funded projects.

Conflicts of Interest: The authors report no conflicts of interest with respect to the content of the manuscript. Outside the submitted work, Grilo reports grants from National Institutes of Health, consultant fees from Sunovion and Weight Watchers and royalties from Guilford Press and Taylor and Francis Publishing. Potenza has consulted for and advised the Addiction Policy Forum, Game Day Data, AXA, Idorsia and Opiant/Lakelight Therapeutics; received research support from the Mohegan Sun Casino and the National Center for Responsible Gaming (now the International Center for Responsible Gaming); participated in surveys, mailings, or telephone consultations related to drug addiction, impulse-control disorders or other health topics; consulted for legal and gambling entities on issues related to impulse-control and addictive disorders; performed grant reviews for the National Institutes of Health and other agencies; edited journals and journal sections; has given academic lectures in grand rounds, CME events and other clinical/scientific venues; and generated books or chapters for publishers of mental health texts. Ivezaj reports broader interests including Honoraria for Journal Editorial Role and lectures. The funders had no role in the design of the study; in the collection, analyses, or interpretation of data; in the writing of the manuscript, or in the decision to publish the results.

References

1. Battle, E.K.; Brownell, K.D. Confronting a rising tide of eating disorders and obesity: Treatment vs. prevention and policy. *Addict. Behav.* **1996**, *21*, 755–765. [CrossRef]
2. Fletcher, P.C.; Kenny, P.J. Food addiction: A valid concept? *Neuropsychopharmacology* **2018**, *43*, 2506–2513. [CrossRef] [PubMed]
3. Gordon, E.L.; Ariel-Donges, A.H.; Bauman, V.; Merlo, L.J. What Is the Evidence for "Food Addiction?" A Systematic Review. *Nutrients* **2018**, *10*, 477. [CrossRef] [PubMed]
4. Gearhardt, A.N.; Davis, C.; Kuschner, R.; Brownell, K.D. The addiction potential of hyperpalatable foods. *Curr. Drug Abus. Rev.* **2011**, *4*, 140–145. [CrossRef] [PubMed]
5. Gearhardt, A.N.; Corbin, W.R.; Brownell, K.D. Preliminary validation of the Yale Food Addiction Scale. *Appetite* **2009**, *52*, 430–436. [CrossRef]
6. Gearhardt, A.N.; Boswell, R.G.; White, M.A. The association of "food addiction" with disordered eating and body mass index. *Eat. Behav.* **2014**, *15*, 427–433. [CrossRef]
7. Pedram, P.; Wadden, D.; Amini, P.; Gulliver, W.; Randell, E.; Cahill, F.; Vasdev, S.; Goodridge, A.; Carter, J.C.; Zhai, G.; et al. Food addiction: Its prevalence and significant association with obesity in the general population. *PLoS ONE* **2013**, *8*, e74832. [CrossRef]
8. Schulte, E.M.; Grilo, C.M.; Gearhardt, A.N. Shared and unique mechanisms underlying binge eating disorder and addictive disorders. *Clin. Psychol. Rev.* **2016**, *44*, 125–139. [CrossRef]
9. Taetzsch, A.; Roberts, S.B.; Gilhooly, C.H.; Lichtenstein, A.H.; Krauss, A.J.; Bukhari, A.; Martin, E.; Hatch-McChesney, A.; Das, S.K. Food cravings: Associations with dietary intake and metabolic health. *Appetite* **2020**, *152*, 104711. [CrossRef]
10. Gearhardt, A.N.; White, M.A.; Masheb, R.M.; Morgan, P.T.; Crosby, R.D.; Grilo, C.M. An examination of the food addiction construct in obese patients with binge eating disorder. *Int. J. Eat. Disord.* **2012**, *45*, 657–663. [CrossRef]
11. Frayn, M.; Sears, C.R.; von Ranson, K.M. A sad mood increases attention to unhealthy food images in women with food addiction. *Appetite* **2016**, *100*, 55–63. [CrossRef] [PubMed]
12. Cassin, S.E.; Sijercic, I.; Montemarano, V. Psychosocial interventions for food addiction: A systematic review. *Curr. Addict. Rep.* **2020**, *7*, 9–19. [CrossRef]
13. Burmeister, J.M.; Hinman, N.; Koball, A.; Hoffmann, D.A.; Carels, R.A. Food addiction in adults seeking weight loss treatment. Implications for psychosocial health and weight loss. *Appetite* **2013**, *60*, 103–110. [CrossRef] [PubMed]
14. Grilo, C.M.; Masheb, R.M.; Wilson, G.T.; Gueorguieva, R.; White, M.A. Cognitive-behavioral therapy, behavioral weight loss, and sequential treatment for obese patients with binge-eating disorder: A randomized controlled trial. *J. Consult. Clin. Psychol.* **2011**, *79*, 675–685. [CrossRef] [PubMed]
15. Fielding-Singh, P.; Patel, M.L.; King, A.C.; Gardner, C.D. Baseline Psychosocial and Demographic Factors Associated with Study Attrition and 12-Month Weight Gain in the DIETFITS Trial. *Obesity* **2019**, *27*, 1997–2004. [CrossRef]
16. Lent, M.R.; Eichen, D.M.; Goldbacher, E.; Wadden, T.A.; Foster, G.D. Relationship of food addiction to weight loss and attrition during obesity treatment. *Obesity* **2014**, *22*, 52–55. [CrossRef]
17. Chao, A.M.; Wadden, T.A.; Tronieri, J.S.; Pearl, R.L.; Alamuddin, N.; Bakizada, Z.M.; Pinkasavage, E.; Leonard, S.M.; Alfaris, N.; Berkowitz, R.I. Effects of addictive-like eating behaviors on weight loss with behavioral obesity treatment. *J. Behav. Med.* **2018**. [CrossRef]
18. Brockmann, A.N.; Eastman, A.; Ross, K.M. Frequency and consistency of self-weighing to promote weight-loss maintenance. *Obesity* **2020**, *28*, 1215–1218. [CrossRef]

19. Butryn, M.L.; Phelan, S.; Hill, J.O.; Wing, R.R. Consistent self-monitoring of weight: A key component of successful weight loss maintenance. *Obesity* **2007**, *15*, 3091–3096. [CrossRef]
20. LaRose, J.G.; Fava, J.L.; Steeves, E.A.; Hecht, J.; Wing, R.R.; Raynor, H.A. Daily self-weighing within a lifestyle intervention: Impact on disordered eating symptoms. *Health Psychol.* **2014**, *33*, 297–300. [CrossRef]
21. Wing, R.R.; Tate, D.F.; Gorin, A.A.; Raynor, H.A.; Fava, J.L.; Machan, J. STOP regain: Are there negative effects of daily weighing? *J. Consult. Clin. Psychol.* **2007**, *75*, 652–656. [CrossRef] [PubMed]
22. Jospe, M.R.; Brown, R.C.; Williams, S.M.; Roy, M.; Meredith-Jones, K.A.; Taylor, R.W. Self-monitoring has no adverse effect on disordered eating in adults seeking treatment for obesity. *Obes. Sci. Pr.* **2018**, *4*, 283–288. [CrossRef] [PubMed]
23. Steinberg, D.M.; Tate, D.F.; Bennett, G.G.; Ennett, S.; Samuel-Hodge, C.; Ward, D.S. Daily self-weighing and adverse psychological outcomes: A randomized controlled trial. *Am. J. Prev. Med.* **2014**, *46*, 24–29. [CrossRef] [PubMed]
24. Grilo, C.M.; White, M.A.; Masheb, R.M.; Ivezaj, V.; Morgan, P.T.; Gueorguieva, R. Randomized controlled trial testing the effectiveness of adaptive "SMART" stepped-care treatment for adults with binge-eating disorder comorbid with obesity. *Am. Psychol.* **2020**, *75*, 204–218. [CrossRef]
25. Grilo, C.M.; White, M.A.; Ivezaj, V.; Gueorguieva, R. Randomized controlled trial of behavioral weight loss and stepped care for binge-eating disorder: 12-month follow-up. *Obesity* **2020**, in press. [CrossRef]
26. APA. *Diagnostic and Statistical Manual of Mental Disorders*, 5th ed.; American Psychiatric Association: Arlington, VA, USA, 2013.
27. First, M.B.; Spitzer, R.L.; Gibbon, M.; Williams, J.B.W. *Structured Clinical Interview for DSM-IV Axis I Disorders-Patient Edition (SCID-I/P, Ver 2.0)*; United States Department of Veterans Affairs: New York, NY, USA, 1996.
28. Fairburn, C.G.; Cooper, Z. *The Eating Disorder Examination*, 12th ed.; Fairburn, C.G., Wilson, G.T., Eds.; Guilford Press: New York, NY, USA, 1993.
29. Fairburn, C.G.; Cooper, Z.; O'Connor, M. *Eating Disorder Examination (16.0D) in Cognitive Behavior Therapy and Eating Disorders*; Fairburn, C.G., Ed.; Guilford Press: New York, NY, USA, 2008.
30. Grilo, C.M.; Masheb, R.M.; Wilson, G.T. A comparison of different methods for assessing the features of eating disorders in patients with binge eating disorder. *J. Consult. Clin. Psychol.* **2001**, *69*, 317–322. [CrossRef]
31. Grilo, C.M.; Masheb, R.M.; Lozano-Blanco, C.; Barry, D.T. Reliability of the Eating Disorder Examination in patients with binge eating disorder. *Int. J. Eat. Disord.* **2004**, *35*, 80–85. [CrossRef]
32. Berg, K.C.; Peterson, C.B.; Frazier, P.; Crow, S.J. Psychometric evaluation of the eating disorder examination and eating disorder examination-questionnaire: A systematic review of the literature. *Int. J. Eat. Disord.* **2012**, *45*, 428–438. [CrossRef]
33. Ivezaj, V.; White, M.A.; Grilo, C.M. Examining binge-eating disorder and food addiction in adults with overweight and obesity. *Obesity (Silver Spring)* **2016**, *24*, 2064–2069. [CrossRef]
34. Pacanowski, C.R.; Pisetsky, E.M.; Berg, K.C.; Crosby, R.D.; Crow, S.J.; Linde, J.A.; Mitchell, J.E.; Engel, S.G.; Klein, M.H.; Smith, T.L.; et al. Self-weighing behavior in individuals with eating disorders. *Int. J. Eat. Disord.* **2016**, *49*, 817–821. [CrossRef]
35. Rohde, P.; Arigo, D.; Shaw, H.; Stice, E. Relation of self-weighing to future weight gain and onset of disordered eating symptoms. *J. Consult. Clin. Psychol.* **2018**, *86*, 677–687. [CrossRef]
36. Friend, S.; Bauer, K.W.; Madden, T.C.; Neumark-Sztainer, D. Self-weighing among adolescents: Associations with body mass index, body satisfaction, weight control behaviors, and binge eating. *J. Acad. Nutr. Diet.* **2012**, *112*, 99–103. [CrossRef] [PubMed]
37. Neumark-Sztainer, D.; van den Berg, P.; Hannan, P.J.; Story, M. Self-weighing in adolescents: Helpful or harmful? Longitudinal associations with body weight changes and disordered eating. *J. Adolesc. Health* **2006**, *39*, 811–818. [CrossRef] [PubMed]
38. Pacanowski, C.R.; Crosby, R.D.; Grilo, C.M. Self-weighing in individuals with binge-eating disorder. *Eat. Disord.* **2019**, *1*, 1–8. [CrossRef] [PubMed]
39. Grilo, C.M. Psychological and Behavioral Treatments for Binge-Eating Disorder. *J. Clin. Psychiatry* **2017**, *78* (Suppl. 1), 20–24. [CrossRef] [PubMed]
40. Wilson, G.T.; Grilo, C.M.; Vitousek, K.M. Psychological treatment of eating disorders. *Am. Psychol.* **2007**, *62*, 199–216. [CrossRef] [PubMed]
41. Linardon, J.; Wade, T.D.; de la Piedad Garcia, X.; Brennan, L. The efficacy of cognitive-behavioral therapy for eating disorders: A systematic review and meta-analysis. *J. Consult. Clin. Psychol.* **2017**, *85*, 1080–1094. [CrossRef] [PubMed]

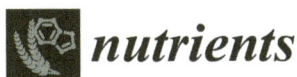

Article

Longitudinal Changes in Food Addiction Symptoms and Body Weight among Adults in a Behavioral Weight-Loss Program

Eliza L. Gordon [1,2,*], Lisa J. Merlo [3], Patricia E. Durning [1] and Michael G. Perri [1]

1 Department of Clinical and Health Psychology, University of Florida, P.O. Box 100165, Gainesville, FL 32610, USA; pdurning@phhp.ufl.edu (P.E.D.); mperri@phhp.ufl.edu (M.G.P.)
2 Division of Physical Medicine & Rehabilitation, University of Utah, 30 N 1900 E (Rm 1B620), Salt Lake City, UT 84132, USA
3 Department of Psychiatry, McKnight Brain Institute, University of Florida College of Medicine, L4-100K, P.O. Box 100256, Gainesville, FL 32611, USA; lmerlo@ufl.edu
* Correspondence: elwarren.22@phhp.ufl.edu

Received: 31 October 2020; Accepted: 27 November 2020; Published: 29 November 2020

Abstract: Interest in food addiction (FA) has increased, but little is known about its clinical implications or potential treatments. Using secondary analyses from a randomized controlled trial, we evaluated the associations between changes in FA, body weight, and "problem food" consumption during a 22-month behavioral weight-loss program consisting of an initial four-month in-person intervention, 12-month extended-care, and six-month follow-up (n = 182). Food addiction was measured using the Yale Food Addiction Scale. "Problem foods" were identified from the literature and self-reporting. Multilevel modeling was used as the primary method of analysis. We hypothesized that reductions in problem food consumption during the initial treatment phase would be associated with long-term (22-month) FA reductions. As expected, we found that reductions in problem foods were associated with greater initial reductions in FA symptoms; however, they were also associated with a sharper rebound in symptoms over time (p = 0.016), resulting in no significant difference at Month 22 (p = 0.856). Next, we hypothesized that long-term changes in FA would be associated with long-term changes in body weight. Although both FA and weight decreased over time (ps < 0.05), month-to-month changes in FA were not associated with month-to-month changes in weight (p = 0.706). Instead, higher overall FA (i.e., mean scores over the course of the study) were associated with less weight loss (p = 0.008) over time. Finally, we hypothesized that initial reductions in problem food consumption would be associated with long-term reductions in weight, but this relationship was not significant (ps > 0.05). Given the complexity of the findings, more research is needed to identify interventions for long-term changes in FA and to elucidate the associations between problem foods, FA, and weight.

Keywords: obesity; food addiction; weight loss; treatment; food

1. Introduction

Prior research has suggested that certain foods (e.g., processed foods high in fat and/or sugar) and eating behaviors (e.g., binge eating) can be associated with addiction-like symptoms. Neurological, genetic, and psychological similarities have been observed between problematic eating behaviors and symptoms of substance use disorders (e.g., excessive consumption, cravings, preoccupation, unsuccessful attempts to limit use of the substance) [1–10]. High-fat and/or high-sugar processed foods, such as ice cream, pizza, potato chips, or chocolate, are most commonly associated with addiction-like changes both behaviorally and neurobiologically [9,11,12]. For example, Gearhardt et al. [12] found that individuals who reported experiencing DSM-IV substance dependence symptoms toward food had greater activation in the anterior cingulate cortex, medial orbitofrontal cortex, and amygdala (brain areas implicated in substance dependence) in response to a chocolate milkshake.

In 2009, Gearhardt et al. [13] published the Yale Food Addiction Scale (YFAS), a validated self-report questionnaire that adapts the DSM-IV substance dependence criteria toward "certain foods" for which respondents may have difficulty controlling their intake. Using this scale, Schulte and Gearhardt [14] estimated that approximately 15% of adults in the United States met the YFAS criteria for food addiction (FA; ≥3 symptoms, plus distress/impairment), with higher prevalence among adults with obesity (19%). In addition to obesity, FA symptoms have been associated with increased risk for disordered eating [8,15–17], depression [15–18], emotional eating [15,17], impulsivity [16], lower self-esteem [16], and poorer quality of life [19].

Despite increased empirical interest in FA, research toward evidence-based treatment is inchoate. A systematic review by Cassin et al. [20] found only eight studies related to FA treatment and concluded that there is not sufficient evidence to support any specific intervention. There is a clear need for research toward evidence-based interventions if FA continues to present as a unique problem [21–23]. Potential treatments could draw on successful approaches used in the substance use disorder and obesity treatment literature. For example, Vella and Pai [24] proposed that techniques commonly used in substance use disorder and obesity treatment—such as problem solving, stimulus control, and cognitive behavioral approaches—could help treat FA by reducing impulsivity, building positive coping skills, and improving distress tolerance.

Behavioral weight-loss treatments represent a logical next step toward identifying evidence-based treatments for FA due to their strong theoretical base, effectiveness in treating obesity, and similarity to substance use disorder treatment. Grounded in cognitive-behavioral theory, these interventions aim to produce healthy weight loss primarily by decreasing caloric consumption, improving diet quality, and increasing physical activity [25]. Often provided in a group setting, these interventions can be a source of health-behavior-specific social support, which is vital to long-term recovery from drug addiction [26], and possibly FA [27].

To our knowledge, only two studies have evaluated changes in FA symptoms among adults participating in behavioral weight-loss programs. In a sample of 90 women, Sawamoto et al. [28] found that "successful" participants (i.e., those who maintained a 10% weight loss at 12- and 24-month follow-ups) in a seven-month behavioral weight-loss program reported fewer symptoms of FA post-treatment compared to "unsuccessful" participants, despite no differences in symptoms at baseline. However, the authors did not report whether changes in FA were statistically significant. Chao et al. [29] analyzed changes in weight and FA symptoms among a sample of 178 adults participating in a 14-week behavioral weight-loss program. They found that, although overall YFAS scores significantly decreased from pre- to post-intervention, neither changes in YFAS scores nor baseline YFAS "diagnosis" significantly predicted weight loss. Taken together, findings from these studies appear to suggest that FA symptoms may decrease in behavioral weight-loss programs.

The current study aimed to describe the associations between early changes in "problem food" consumption, long-term changes in FA symptoms, and long-term weight change. Analyses were conducted using data collected from a multi-site behavioral weight-loss randomized control trial that consisted of a four-month in-person treatment phase (Phase 1; Months 0–4), followed by a 12-month extended-care phase (Phase 2; Months 4–16) and a six-month follow-up phase (Phase 3; Months 16–22). Specifically, we aimed (1) to identify associations between initial (Phase 1) changes in "problem food" consumption (e.g., high-sugar/high-fat processed foods recorded in participant dietary logs) and long-term changes in FA symptoms, and (2) to identify the associations between initial changes in "problem food" consumption, long-term FA symptoms, and long-term weight loss. We hypothesized that (a) Phase 1 reductions in "problem foods" would be associated with a long-term reduction in FA symptoms (Months 0–22), (b) long-term changes in FA symptoms would be associated with long-term changes in body weight, and (c) Phase 1 reductions in problem food consumption would be associated with long-term reductions in body weight.

2. Materials and Methods

The current paper describes a secondary data analysis of data from the Rural Lifestyle Eating and Activity Program (Rural LEAP) [30]. The Rural LEAP project was a randomized controlled trial comparing the effects of three strategies for long-term weight management among 528 women and men (ages 21–75; body mass indexes (BMIs) between 30–45) living in rural north Florida. Approval was obtained from the University of Florida Institutional Review Board (IRB), and all participants gave written informed consent. Participants attended a weekly, in-person behavioral weight-loss program for the first four months of treatment (Phase 1). Those who completed Phase 1 with ≥50% attendance were randomly assigned to 12 months of extended care (Phase 2) delivered via individual or group telephone counseling or an education control program delivered via email. All participants received 18 modules with recommendations for maintaining lost weight. In the phone-based conditions, health coaches provided participants with 18 individual or group sessions focused on problem solving of obstacles to the maintenance of weight loss. Phase 3 (Months 16–22) was a no-contact follow-up period for participants to practice the strategies on their own. Assessments were conducted at baseline (Month 0), post-treatment (Month 4), halfway through the extended-care phase (Month 10), post-extended care (Month 16), and after the final no-contact phase (Month 22).

2.1. Participants

The sample included adult men and women with BMIs between 30–45 kg/m^2 and without medical contraindications for weight loss (see prior publications [30,31] for specific inclusion and exclusion criteria). Although four cohorts ("waves") of volunteers participated in the Rural LEAP program, the YFAS was not added to the study until the third and fourth cohorts; thus, the current study only included participants who completed the program during Waves 3 and 4 (n = 196). In addition, the current study excluded participants if they failed to complete eligible dietary records at the end of Month 4 (i.e., ≥3 days recorded per week; complete information on food types/amounts) or if they did not complete the 22-month assessment. This resulted in a sample size of 182 participants for the current study (see Figure 1 for a flow diagram).

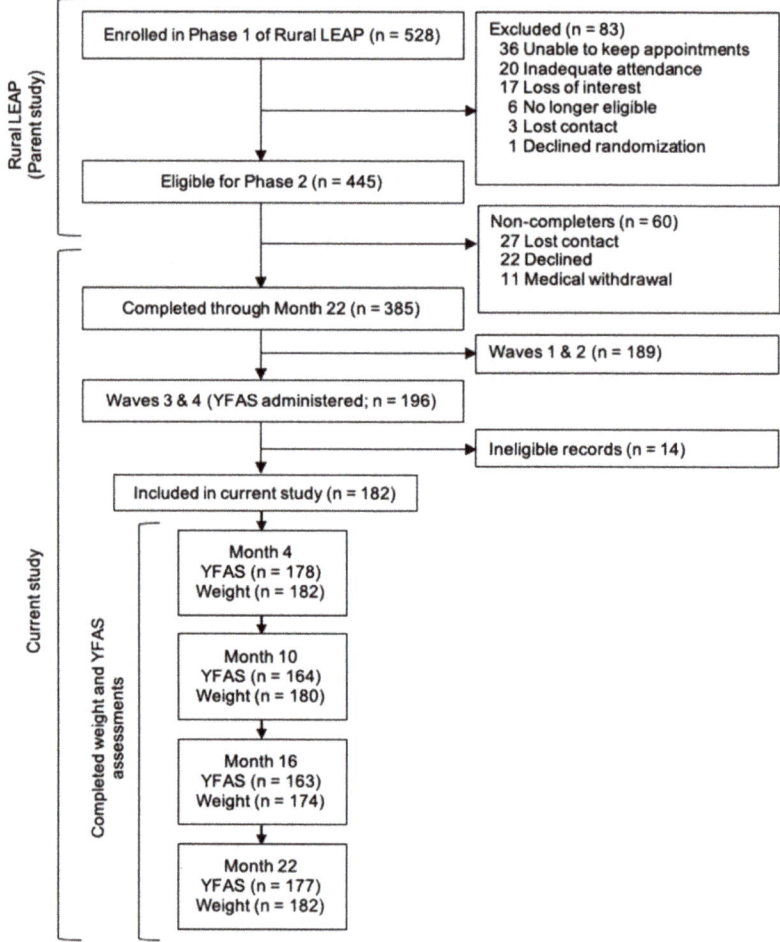

Figure 1. Flow diagram of participants.

2.2. Main Variables

2.2.1. Problem foods

"Problem foods" (i.e., foods more likely to be associated with addiction-like symptoms) were self-identified at baseline using participants' responses to the YFAS. Combined with information from prior literature (e.g., [9,11,32–34]), these responses were used to create a combined "problem foods" variable, which included the following food categories from the USDA's "What We Eat In America" survey [35]: pizza, burgers, savory snacks, sweet bakery products, chocolate, candy, ice cream and frozen desserts, fried potatoes, diet soda, sweetened beverages, sugars, and sugar substitutes. A "problem food consumption" score was calculated for each participant based on the average number of times per day he or she consumed a food item from this list. This was calculated by summing the total number of times participants consumed any item from the "problem food" list in a week (e.g., first week of Month 0; last week of Month 16) and dividing this sum by the number of days recorded that week (e.g., average daily frequency of problem food consumption = total number of times "problem food" consumed that week/number of days recorded that week). Data on food consumption was extracted from participants' dietary records, which they were instructed to keep daily during the course of the intervention. Due to low food record completion rates during Phase 2 (approximately 50%), only food logs from Phase 1 were used for the current study. Data extracted from the logs were entered into the secure Research Electronic Data Capture (REDCap) tool [36], and entries were randomly checked for accuracy and consistency. Food records were excluded if they failed to include accurate or complete information (e.g., no quantities or caloric values), if there were less than three complete days recorded per week, or if the participant had abnormal circumstances that week (i.e., severe illness).

2.2.2. Food Addiction Symptoms

The Yale Food Addiction Scale (YFAS) [13] is a validated self-report instrument, and is currently the most frequently used measure of addiction-like eating behaviors. The original version of this scale was used in the current study. It includes 25 questions, with most presented in either Likert or "yes/no" format. Respondents are instructed to answer questions while keeping in mind "certain foods" for which they have difficulty controlling their intake. Each question contributes to one of seven symptoms (e.g., craving, failure to fulfill major role obligations) or clinical criteria (i.e., distress or impairment). The scale's "diagnostic" threshold is based on the DSM-IV criteria for substance dependence ($\geq$3 symptoms, plus distress or impairment). The questionnaire produces two metrics: a dichotomous "diagnosis" score (meets criteria vs. does not meet criteria) and a continuous "symptom" score (0–7 symptoms). The current study used the symptom score for analyses in order to better quantify the degree of change in symptoms.

The YFAS was administered at all five assessment points (Months 0, 4, 10, 16, and 22). While the original questionnaire asks participants to report on symptoms experienced in the past year, we modified the instructions to read "the past four months" at the Month 4 assessment and "the past six months" at Months 10, 16, and 22 in order to reflect the amount of time between assessments.

2.2.3. Body Weight

Body weight was measured to the nearest 0.1 kg using a calibrated digital scale at all five assessments. Participants wore light indoor clothing and emptied pockets prior to weighing.

2.3. Recruitment and Initial Assessment

Recruitment to the parent study (Rural LEAP) primarily used mailed fliers and brochures presented at community and healthcare organizations. Screening occurred first via telephone and then in person at local county extension offices. At the in-person assessment, participants completed measurements of weight and height, psychosocial questionnaires (e.g., YFAS), and other health-/fitness-related assessments, such as a walking test [30]. Data collection occurred primarily through REDCap [36], which was approved by the University of Florida IRB for HIPAA compliance.

2.4. Intervention

Participants were taught strategies to increase physical activity and reduce caloric intake. Each weekly in-person session consisted of a private weigh-in, reviewing progress, problem-solving challenges, a skills-based lesson, and setting of eating and activity goals. Lessons included topics such as basic nutrition education, physical activity, problem solving, managing cravings, seeking social support, and substituting high-calorie foods for low-calorie foods. All participants were instructed to continue self-monitoring during Phase 2. Details on the study and intervention content have been described in prior publications [30,31].

2.5. Statistical Analyses

Analyses were performed in SPSS version 26 and significance levels were set to $p < 0.05$. Multilevel modeling tests used the full sample ($n = 182$); other tests (e.g., descriptive analyses) did not include participants with missing data (see Figure 1 for sample sizes at each timepoint). One-way analyses of variance (ANOVAs), chi-squared tests, and Kruskal–Wallis tests were used for descriptive and supplementary analyses involving categorical variables. Pearson correlations and related-samples Wilcoxon signed-rank tests were used for analyses involving continuous variables. Bootstrapping to 5000 samples was used to correct for non-normal variables in parametric tests. Bootstrapping is a robust and effective resampling technique for non-parametric and/or smaller samples that does not make parametric assumptions on the distribution [37,38].

Multilevel modeling was used for Aims 1 and 2. The Aim 1 model included FA symptoms at each time point (Level 1) nested within 182 participants (Level 2). The model included the following Level 2 predictors: age, BMI, baseline problem food consumption (PFBaseline), Phase 1 changes in problem food consumption (PFChange), linear time slope (MonthLinear), quadratic time slope (MonthQuad), and the interactions between PFChange and each time slope. Level 1 predictors included: linear time slope (MonthLinear), quadratic time slope (MonthQuad), and BMI. Multilevel modeling also controls for the baseline value of the dependent variable (FA symptoms). In the equation below (Equation (1)), "FA" represents the dependent variable (FA symptoms) for person "i" at timepoint "j". Terms marked with γ represent Level 2 intercepts as labeled after the underscore (e.g., γ_{01}_Age represents the Level 2 intercept for age). The residual is represented by the symbol "ζ_{0i}", and subsequent terms marked with ζ represent individual differences in Level 1 parameters not explained by Level 2 predictors. Age was included as a control variable in Aim 1 due to prior literature suggesting differences in food addiction symptoms by age group [8]. We originally added Phase 2 group randomization as a control variable in our multi-level models because it was significantly related to weight loss in the parent study ($n = 445$) [30]. However, it was ultimately removed from the current study due to worsened fit and no significant effects.

$$FA_{ij} = [\gamma_{00}\_Intercept + \gamma_{01}\_Age + \gamma_{02}\_BMI + \gamma_{03}\_PFBaseline + \gamma_{04}\_PFChange + \gamma_{10}\_MonthLinear + \gamma_{11}\_(MonthLinear*PFChange) + \gamma_{20}\_MonthQuad + \gamma_{21}\_(MonthQuad*PFChange)] + [\zeta_{0i} + \zeta_{1i}\_MonthLinear + \zeta_{2i}\_MonthQuad + \zeta_{3i}\_BMI + \varepsilon_{ij}] \quad (1)$$

The Aim 2 model included body weight at each time point (Level 1) nested within 182 participants (Level 2). The model included the following Level 2 predictors: height, race, baseline problem food consumption (PFBaseline), Phase 1 changes in problem food consumption (PFChange), mean between-person FA symptoms (FAMean), centered within-person FA symptoms (FACent), linear time slope (MonthLinear), quadratic time slope (MonthQuad), and the interactions between PFChange, FAMean, and each time slope. The Level 1 predictors included: linear time slope (MonthLinear), quadratic time slope (MonthQuad), and centered within-person FA symptoms (FACent). Symbol definitions for Equation (2) are the same as for Equation (1). FA was split into Level 1 and Level 2 variables in order to test both within- and between-subject effects. Level 2 effects of FA symptoms were calculated by computing person-means (i.e., averaging each participant's YFAS score across all timepoints). Level 1 effects were calculated by computing person-mean centered values (i.e., subtracting participants' scores at each timepoint from their person-mean). Race was included as a control variable in Aim 2 due to prior literature showing differences in body weight by race [39].

$$Weight_{ij} = [\gamma_{00}\_Intercept + \gamma_{01}\_Height + \gamma_{02}\_Race + \gamma_{03}\_PFBaseline + \gamma_{04}\_PFChange + \gamma_{05}\_FAMean + \gamma_{06}\_FACent + \gamma_{10}\_MonthLinear + \gamma_{11}\_(MonthLinear*PFChange) + \gamma_{12}\_(MonthLinear*FAMean) + \gamma_{20}\_MonthQuad + \gamma_{21}\_(MonthQuad*PFChange) + \gamma_{22}\_(MonthQuad*FAMean)] + [\zeta_{0i} + \zeta_{1i}\_MonthLinear + \zeta_{2i}\_MonthQuad + \zeta_{3i}\_FACent + \varepsilon_{ij}] \quad (2)$$

One-way ANOVA and Bonferroni post-hoc tests were used to evaluate differences between mean values and change scores in FA symptoms and weight (respectively) at each timepoint. Median split graphs were also created to assist in interpreting significant quadratic time interactions.

3. Results

3.1. Demographics

The final study sample included 182 participants (84.6% female) with a mean age of 55.4 ± 9.9 years. Demographic characteristics and YFAS scores are presented in Table 1. At baseline, 24 (13.2%) participants met the YFAS "diagnostic" criteria for FA, and the mean symptom score for the full sample was 2.38 ± 1.58. Non-white participants were more likely to have higher BMIs by about 1.5 kg/m^2 ($p = 0.031$) compared to white participants. No other demographic variables were significantly related to YFAS scores or BMI. YFAS scores were not significantly related to BMI at baseline ($r = 0.061$; $p = 0.410$). There were no significant differences in demographic variables between Waves 1 and 2 (enrolled in the parent study before the YFAS was administered; $n = 215$) and Waves 3 and 4 (from which the current sample was drawn; $n = 230$, $ps > 0.05$). Additionally, there were no significant differences between our sample ($n = 182$) and participants in Waves 3 and 4 who were not eligible for the current study ($n = 48$; $ps > 0.05$).

Table 1. Baseline sample characteristics ($N = 182$).

Characteristic	M (SD)	n (%)
Age (years)	55.4 (9.9)	
Weight (kg)	99.6 (13.9)	
BMI (kg/m^2)	36.6 (3.6)	
YFAS symptom score	2.38 (1.58)	
YFAS clinical cutoff		
≥3 symptoms + distress/impairment		24 (13.2)
<3 symptoms or no distress/impairment		158 (86.8)
Gender		
Female		154 (84.6)
Male		28 (15.4)
Ethnicity		
Non-Hispanic		175 (96.2)
Hispanic		7 (3.8)
Race		
White		146 (80.2)
Black or African American		35 (19.2)
Hispanic or Latino		7 (3.8)
American Indian or Alaskan Native		6 (3.3)
Asian		1 (0.5)
Native Hawaiian or Other Pacific Islander		0 (0.0)
Highest level of education		
<High school		4 (2.2)
High school or GED		89 (48.9)
Associate's degree		21 (11.5)
Bachelor's degree		45 (24.7)
Advanced degree		23 (12.6)
Annual household income		
<$20,000		14 (7.7)
$20,000–$34,999		41 (22.5)
$35,000–$49,999		31 (17.0)
$50,000–$74,999		39 (21.4)
>$75,000		45 (24.7)
Unknown		12 (6.6)

3.2. Phase 1 Problem Food Consumption

Baseline problem food consumption was significantly associated with baseline FA symptoms ($r = 0.230$, $p = 0.002$). During Phase 1, the mean frequency of problem food consumption dropped from 2.5 ± 1.2 times/day to 1.5 ± 0.9 times/day ($p < 0.001$). Decreases in problem food consumption were significantly associated with Phase 1 reductions in FA symptoms ($r = 0.165$, $p = 0.028$), but not weight ($r = 0.119$, $p = 0.115$). However, correlation effect sizes were small. Phase 1 changes in FA symptoms were not significantly associated with weight change ($r = 0.082$, $p = 0.277$).

3.3. Aim 1: Long-Term Changes in Food Addiction Symptoms

Five models (A–E) were tested using YFAS symptoms as the dependent variable and changes in Phase 1 problem food consumption as the independent variable. Body mass index, age, and baseline problem food consumption were included as covariates. Model A tested the unconditional means model, which included only the intercept. Model B tested the unconditional growth model, which added both linear and quadratic time slopes as predictors, both of which were significant (quadratic time, $p = 0.012$; linear time, $p = 0.010$). Model C tested for the fixed effects of baseline problem food consumption (covariate) and Phase 1 changes in problem food consumption (independent variable) on FA symptoms over time. Fixed effects test the association of a predictor with the intercept (in this study, baseline value) of the dependent variable. Neither predictor had a significant fixed effect.

Model D added the interaction of changes in problem food consumption with both linear and quadratic time, respectively. A variable's interaction effect with time looks at its association with subsequent changes in the dependent variable across time (as opposed to at the intercept only). We found that the quadratic time interaction with problem food change was significant ($p = 0.012$), suggesting that Phase 1 decreases in problem food consumption were initially associated with a slightly sharper decline in FA symptoms, followed by a slightly sharper rebound. The interaction between problem food changes and linear time was not significant, indicating that Phase 1 problem food changes were not associated with long-term changes in FA scores. Model E included our remaining control variables (BMI and age), both of which had significant fixed effects ($p < 0.001$ and $p = 0.043$, respectively). The random effect of BMI was not significant ($p = 0.321$; see Figures 2 and 3 and Table 2).

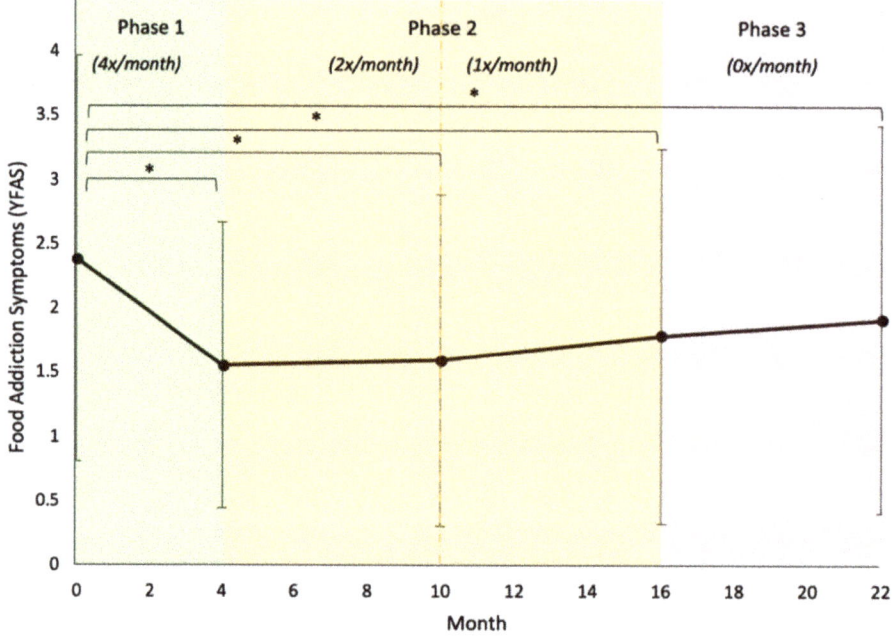

Figure 2. Model-implied trend of food addiction symptoms over time. Shaded areas mark Phases 1, 2, and 3 of the study, with the frequency of intervention sessions noted in italics. * = $p < 0.05$.

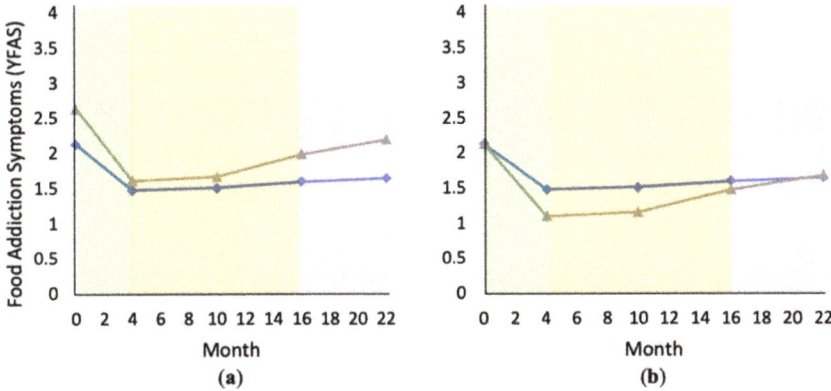

Figure 3. Changes in food addiction (FA) symptoms over time, comparing subjects with greater versus smaller Phase 1 reductions in problem food consumption (based on median split: greater reduction = gray triangles, smaller reduction = blue diamonds): (**a**) graph using original data; (**b**) graph correcting for baseline differences in Yale Food Addiction Scale (YFAS) scores for comparison.

Table 2. Aim 1 results of the model tests (food addiction symptoms as outcome).

	Par	Model A	Model B	Model C	Model D	Model E
Fixed effects						
Initial status						
Intercept	γ_{00}	0.007 (0.058)	−0.216 ** (0.062)	−0.217 *** (0.061)	−0.135 * (0.062)	−0.134 * (0.062)
PF Change	γ_{04}			−0.117 (0.080)	−0.026 (0.084)	−0.026 (0.085)
PF Baseline	γ_{03}			0.088 (0.080)	0.098 (0.080)	0.088 (0.080)
BMI	γ_{02}					0.262 *** (0.049)
Baseline Age	γ_{01}					−0.113 * (0.056)
Rate of change						
Time (linear)	γ_{10}		−0.082 ** (0.026)	−0.083 ** (0.026)	−0.040 (0.026)	−0.039 (0.026)
X PF Change	γ_{11}				−0.003 (0.025)	−0.005 (0.025)
Time (quad)	γ_{20}		0.214 *** (0.031)	0.215 *** (0.031)	0.135 *** (0.034)	0.135 *** (0.033)
X PF Change	γ_{21}				−0.078 * (0.031)	−0.074 * (0.031)
Random effects						
Level 1						
Residual	ε_{ij}	0.496 *** (0.027)	0.385 *** (0.028)	0.389 *** (0.028)	0.360 *** (0.026)	0.352 *** (0.028)
BMI	ζ_{3i}					0.041 (0.042)
Level 2						
Intercept	ζ_{0i}	0.503 *** (0.064)	0.468 *** (0.063)	0.437 *** (0.059)	0.443 *** (0.060)	0.420 *** (0.059)
Time (linear)	ζ_{1i}		0.034 * (0.013)	0.034 * (0.013)	0.034 ** (0.013)	0.033 ** (0.013)
Time (quad)	ζ_{2i}		0.042 * (0.017)	0.036 * (0.016)	0.041 * (0.016)	0.036 * (0.016)
Fit Statistics						
Deviance		2165.464	2099.093	2087.688	2046.568	2041.203
AIC		2171.464	2113.093	2105.688	2070.568	2069.203
BIC		2185.749	2146.424	2148.542	2127.693	2135.849

Estimates are presented with standard errors between parentheses. * $p < 0.05$, ** $p < 0.01$, *** $p < 0.001$. PF = problem foods; BMI = body mass index; AIC = Akaike information criterion; BIC = Bayesian information criterion.

3.4. Aim 2: Long-Term Changes in Body Weight

Five models (A–E) were tested using body weight as the dependent variable and both FA symptoms and changes in Phase 1 problem food consumption as independent variables. Height, race (white vs. not white), and baseline problem food consumption were covariates. Model A was the unconditional means model and Model B was the unconditional growth model. In Model B, both linear and quadratic time slopes were significant ($ps < 0.001$).

Model C included the fixed effects of both FA symptoms and problem food consumption (baseline values and change scores); of these, only the fixed effects of within-person (Level 1, person-mean centered) FA symptoms were significant in Model C ($p < 0.001$). Model D added four interaction terms: Phase 1 changes in problem food consumption by time and person-mean (between-subject) FA symptoms by time. Of these, only the interaction between FA symptoms and linear time was significant ($p = 0.008$), such that higher mean FA scores were associated with less long-term weight loss. Model E added the remaining covariates (height and race), both of which had significant fixed effects ($ps \leq 0.001$). The fixed effect of between-person (Level 2, person-mean) FA symptoms also became significant ($p = 0.009$) in this model, such that individuals with higher mean YFAS scores were more likely to have a higher baseline body weight. The quadratic time by person-mean FA interaction also became significant ($p = 0.045$), such that higher mean FA scores were associated with a slightly shallower weight-loss curve and a slightly steeper rate of weight regain (see Figures 4 and 5 and Table 3).

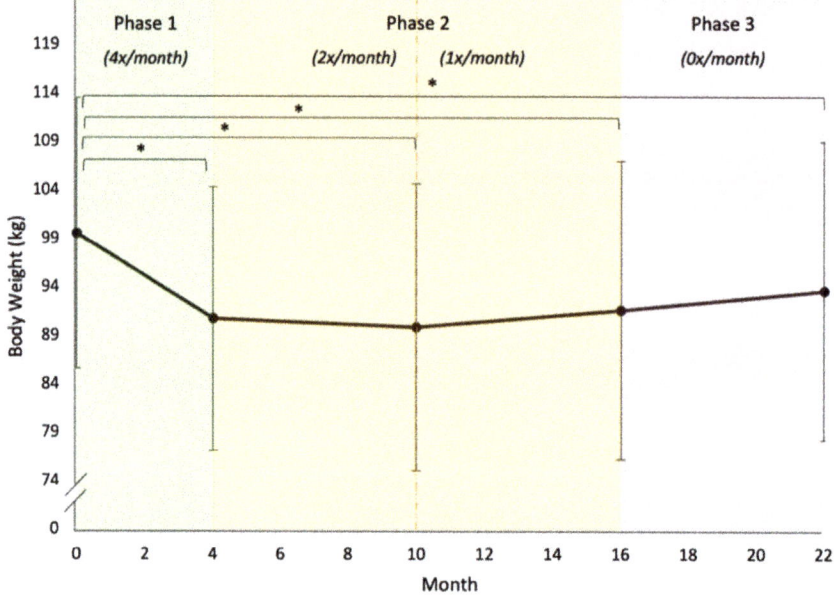

Figure 4. Model-implied trend of body weight over time. Shaded areas mark Phases 1, 2, and 3 of the study, with the frequency of intervention sessions noted in italics. * = $p < 0.05$.

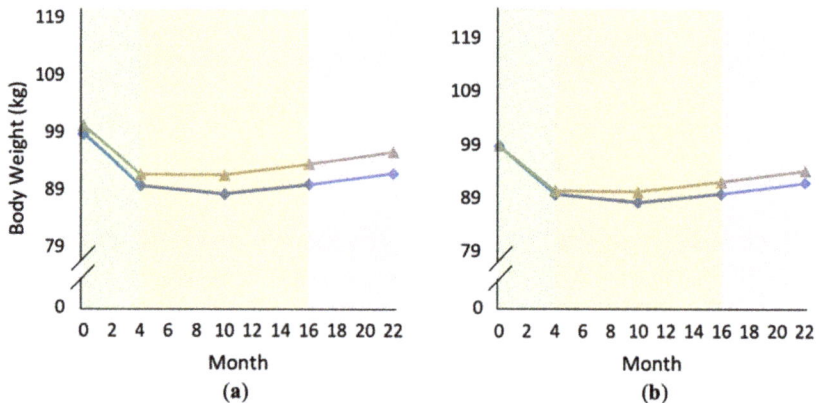

Figure 5. Changes in body weight over time, comparing subjects with higher versus lower person-mean YFAS scores (based on median split: higher YFAS scores = gray triangles; lower YFAS scores = blue diamonds): (**a**) graph using original data; (**b**) graph correcting for baseline differences in body weight for comparison.

Table 3. Aim 2 results of the model tests (body weight as outcome).

	Par	Model A	Model B	Model C	Model D	Model E
Fixed effects						
Initial status						
Intercept	γ_{00}	0.003 (0.069)	−0.235 ** (0.070)	−0.228 ** (0.070)	−0.228 ** (0.070)	−0.230 *** (0.052)
FA (M)	γ_{05}			0.083 (0.091)	0.105 (0.092)	0.181 ** (0.069)
FA (C)	γ_{06}			0.101 *** (0.016)	0.101 *** (0.015)	0.101 *** (0.016)
PF Change	γ_{04}			−0.107 (0.101)	−0.104 (0.101)	−0.063 (0.075)
PF Baseline	γ_{03}			0.005 (0.100)	0.005 (0.100)	−0.015 (0.075)
Height	γ_{01}					0.610 *** (0.052)
White race	γ_{02}					−0.170 ** (0.052)
Rate of change						
Time (linear)	γ_{10}		−0.123 *** (0.015)	−0.121 *** (0.015)	−0.120 *** (0.014)	−0.120 *** (0.014)
X FA (M)	γ_{12}				0.051 ** (0.019)	0.050 ** (0.019)
X PF Change	γ_{11}				0.002 (0.015)	0.002 (0.015)
Time (quad)	γ_{20}		0.238 *** (0.013)	0.224 *** (0.013)	0.224 *** (0.013)	0.224 *** (0.013)
X FA (M)	γ_{22}				−0.033 (0.017)	−0.033 * (0.016)
X PF Change	γ_{21}				−0.005 (0.014)	−0.005 (0.013)
Random effects						
Level 1						
Residual	ε_{ij}	0.147 *** (0.008)	0.049 *** (0.004)	0.044 *** (0.004)	0.044 *** (0.004)	0.046 *** (0.004)
FA (C)	ζ_{3i}			0.002 (0.004)	0.001 (0.003)	0.001 (0.004)
Level 2						
Intercept	ζ_{0i}	0.846 *** (0.092)	0.874 *** (0.093)	0.843 *** (0.090)	0.844 *** (0.090)	0.457 *** (0.050)
Time (linear)	ζ_{1i}		0.030 *** (0.004)	0.028 *** (0.004)	0.027 *** (0.004)	0.026 *** (0.004)
Time (quad)	ζ_{2i}		0.013 *** (0.003)	0.013 *** (0.003)	0.013 *** (0.003)	0.010 ** (0.003)
Fit Statistics						
Deviance		1443.129	1013.281	944.070	933.623	825.881
AIC		1449.129	1027.281	968.070	965.623	861.881
BIC		1463.536	1060.898	1025.195	1041.790	947.569

Estimates are presented with standard errors between parentheses. * $p < 0.05$, ** $p < 0.01$, *** $p < 0.001$. FA = food addiction symptoms; M = mean; C = centered; PF = Problem foods; AIC = Akaike information criterion; BIC = Bayesian information criterion.

3.5. ANOVAs and Bonferroni Post-Hocs: Food Addiction Symptoms and Body Weight

3.5.1. Food Addiction

Finally, one-way ANOVA and Bonferroni tests detected statistically significant differences between baseline (Month 0) FA symptoms and each subsequent timepoint, respectively (all $ps < 0.05$). Months 4–22 were not significantly different from each other. Changes in FA symptoms between Months 0–4 (Phase 1) were significantly different from Months 4–10, 10–16, and 16–22 (first half of Phase 2, second half of Phase 2, and Phase 3, respectively; $ps < 0.001$). None of the subsequent phases were significantly different from each other ($ps > 0.05$).

3.5.2. Body Weight

There were statistically significant differences between baseline (Month 0) body weight and each subsequent timepoint (all $ps < 0.05$). Months 4–22 were not significantly different from each other. Phase 1 changes in body weight were significantly different from all other timepoints ($ps < 0.001$), as were the changes during the first half of Phase 2 (Months 4–10; $ps < 0.001$; see Table 4).

Table 4. Means and change slopes for main variables by timepoint.

Timepoint M ± SD	YFAS Score	Body Weight (kg)	Timepoint M ± SD	Change in YFAS Score	Change in Weight (kg)
Month 0	2.39 ± 1.58 [b,c,d,e] N = 182	99.57 ± 13.95 [b,c,d,e] N = 182	Months 0–4 (Phase 1)	−0.882 ± 1.47 [g,h,i] N = 178	−8.83 ± 4.75 [g,h,i] N = 182
Month 4	1.56 ± 1.1 [a] N = 178	90.74 ± 13.56 [a] N = 182	Months 4–10 (Phase 2, 1st half)	0.044 ± 1.23 [f] N = 161	−0.789 ± 4.51 [f,h,i] N = 180
Month 10	1.60 ± 1.29 [a] N = 164	89.90 ± 14.8 [a] N = 180	Months 10–16 (Phase 2, 2nd half)	0.252 ± 1.10 [f] N = 153	1.93 ± 3.08 [f,g] N = 174
Month 16	1.79 ± 1.46 [a] N = 163	91.65 ± 15.38 [a] N = 174	Months 16–22 (Phase 3)	0.073 ± 1.11 [f] N = 161	1.80 ± 3.79 [f,b] N = 174
Month 22	1.92 ± 1.51 [a] N = 177	93.67 ± 15.38 [a] N = 182	-	-	-

Significance evaluated at $p < 0.05$ using One-way analysis of variance (ANOVA) and bootstrapped T-tests. Key: [a] = significantly different from Month 0, [b] = significantly different from Month 4, [c] = significantly different from Month 10, [d] = significantly different from Month 16, [e] = significantly different from Month 22; [f] = significantly different from Months 0–4, [g] = significantly different from Months 4–10, [h] = significantly different from Months 10–16, [i] = significantly different from Months 16–22.

4. Discussion

The primary goal of this study was to evaluate long-term changes in food addiction (FA) symptoms and weight loss among a sample of adults participating in a behavioral weight-loss program. We hypothesized that reductions in problem food consumption during the initial phase of treatment would be associated with long-term reductions in FA symptoms, that long-term changes in FA would be associated with long-term changes in body weight, and that initial reductions in problem food consumption would be associated with long-term reductions in body weight.

4.1. Food Addiction and Problem Foods

We found that changes in problem food consumption during the initial in-person treatment phase were not associated with changes in FA symptoms from the baseline to Month 22. Rather, reductions in problem food consumption were associated with a different pattern of change, suggesting sharper initial reductions in FA symptoms followed by a sharper rebound after the in-person phase. While future research is needed to clarify the relationship between problem food consumption and FA symptoms, our findings suggest that decreasing problem food consumption (in the context of a behavioral weight loss program) may be associated with improvements in FA symptoms in the short term, but that these changes may not last in the long term.

Many have proposed that, similarly to drug addiction treatment models, the goal of FA treatment should be either abstinence [40], moderation [23], or harm reduction [41] in regard to problem food consumption. Others have implied that non-dieting approaches may be beneficial [42–45]. However, few studies have tested the efficacy of any FA treatment. The FA studies identified by Cassin et al. [20] examined a variety of different approaches, including abstinence, cognitive-behavioral therapy, exposure and response prevention, intuitive eating, and mindfulness. However, only two of the included studies specifically targeted FA as a primary outcome. The authors concluded that more research is needed to compare the effects of potential interventions, particularly those drawn from evidence-based treatments for substance use or eating disorders [20].

4.2. Food Addiction and Weight

We found that both FA symptoms and body weight decreased over time, and that higher average YFAS scores over the course of the study were associated with less weight loss. These findings are consistent with several studies that have shown an association between FA symptoms and body weight both cross-sectionally and across time [8,15,28]. However, others have failed to find an association [29,46,47]. Despite some inconsistency, most prior research has shown significant reductions in FA symptoms following weight-loss treatment [28,29,46,48,49]. These findings require further exploration, but it is possible that the connection between FA symptoms and weight may become more apparent over periods of time that extend beyond the length of typical intervention studies (i.e., 4–6 months), and/or that both FA and body weight are influenced or caused by an external factor.

4.3. Problem Foods and Weight

We did not find a significant association between early changes in problem food consumption and long-term changes in weight. This finding was contrary to our hypotheses, and also contrary to some prior cross-sectional and behavioral weight-loss studies [50–54]. One possible explanation could be that participants in our intervention were instructed to reduce calories rather than reduce problem foods specifically; the results may have been different had problem food consumption been directly targeted. Another possible explanation could be that our measure of problem food consumption (number of times consumed per day) did not provide enough power given its seemingly restricted range. However, at least one other study has reported a similarly unexpected finding: Nikiforova and associates [55] found that, among their sample of 300 laparoscopic sleeve gastrectomy patients, there was a 12.9% increase in the number of patients who reported a diet rich in "sweets" and an 8.9% increase in the number of patients who reported a diet rich in "snacks" three years after surgery, despite a significant reduction in BMI. They concluded that while consumption of these foods increased post-surgery, they did not appear to have a negative effect on BMI. Further research is required to clarify the association between high-fat and/or high-sugar foods and body weight, especially while controlling for caloric consumption.

4.4. Implications and Future Directions

Some have proposed that FA causes weight gain through the overconsumption of high-calorie foods (e.g., [56]), while others have suggested that obesity may cause FA symptoms via brain chemistry changes that lead to overeating (e.g., [57]). An additional question to consider is whether FA and obesity may both be symptoms of an external factor. For example, it has been well established that both obesity and FA symptoms are associated with increased depression and anxiety, lower self-esteem, and poorer quality of life [16,19,58–62]. In addition to psychosocial factors, biological contributors, such as gut microbiota and genetics, have also been associated with weight and addiction-like eating [63–66]. Future studies should prospectively analyze the relationships between neurobiological and psychosocial factors, body weight, and FA in order to predict which factors may put individuals at risk of developing either or both of these conditions.

If FA leads to weight gain through the overconsumption of high-calorie, highly palatable foods, reducing consumption of these foods should lead to weight loss. However, the current study's findings did not support an association between changes in problem food consumption and either concurrent (Phase 1) or subsequent (long-term) changes in body weight. Future studies should evaluate long-term changes in problem food consumption simultaneously with both FA symptoms and weight in order to elucidate these relationships. Future studies should also evaluate the long-term effects of problem food consumption on both body weight and FA symptoms by specifically targeting problem food consumption without caloric restriction.

4.5. Strengths and Limitations

The results should be interpreted in light of this study's limitations. First, the analyses conducted cannot demonstrate causal relationships between the variables, nor determine the direction of the association between FA and body weight. Second, the study sample was primarily female and had sociodemographic characteristics similar to adults in the rural southeastern United States, which may limit generalizability to other populations. Additionally, the proportion of participants in the current study who met YFAS criteria for FA (13.2%) was less than the estimated prevalence for adults with overweight/obesity (approximately 25%) [8]. This may be due to the fact that ours was a treatment-seeking sample, as other behavioral weight-loss studies have also reported relatively low

FA prevalence rates (e.g., 19% [15]; 6.7% [29]; 15.2% [47]). Third, dietary records were based on self-reporting and were not independently verified, and problem food consumption was coded post hoc for secondary data analyses. Additionally, we were unable to evaluate long-term changes in problem food consumption due to the low rates of self-monitoring after Phase 1. Fourth, the current sample size may have been insufficient to detect certain differences, such as the effects of Phase 2 group randomization and problem food consumption on weight change. Finally, the present results were consistent with previous research regarding the direction of change in problem food consumption [52,53,67,68]; however, differences in methodology (i.e., using measures of quantity vs. frequency) precluded our ability to compare the clinical significance of the change with that observed in prior studies e.g., [52,53,67,68]. Nevertheless, this is the first study to our knowledge that has evaluated long-term changes in FA symptoms in the context of a behavioral weight-loss program. The above findings regarding the associations between problem food consumption, FA symptoms, and body weight over time have important implications for future research.

5. Conclusions

Despite increased interest in the concept of food addiction, there is a dearth of research regarding its clinical implications and potential treatments. The current study examined long-term (two-year) changes in food addiction symptoms and their association with changes in body weight and "problem food" (i.e., highly palatable food) consumption among adults in a behavioral weight-loss program. The findings suggest that food addiction symptoms improve during behavioral weight-loss treatment and that reducing problem food consumption is associated with short-term improvements in FA symptoms. Despite some evidence for a negative association between food addiction symptoms and weight loss, more research is needed to elucidate the complex interplay of food addiction symptoms, body weight, and problem food consumption. A greater understanding of these relationships may inform the development of effective interventions for long-term changes in FA.

Author Contributions: Conceptualization, data curation, data analysis, and writing—original draft preparation and review/editing, E.L.G.; writing—review/editing, L.J.M.; data curation and writing—review/editing, P.E.D.; supervision, project administration, funding acquisition, and writing—review/editing, M.G.P. All authors have read and agreed to the published version of the manuscript.

Funding: This research was funded by the National Heart, Lung, and Blood Institute, grant number HL112720.

Conflicts of Interest: The authors declare no conflict of interest.

References

1. Avena, N.M.; Rada, P.; Hoebel, B.G. Evidence for sugar addiction: Behavioral and neurochemical effects of intermittent, excessive sugar intake. *Neurosci. Biobehav. Rev.* **2008**, *32*, 20–39. [CrossRef] [PubMed]
2. Carter, A.; Hendrikse, J.; Lee, N.; Yücel, M.; Verdejo-Garcia, A.; Andrews, Z.B.; Hall, W. The neurobiology of "food addiction" and its implications for obesity treatment and policy. *Annu. Rev. Nutr.* **2016**, *36*, 105–128. [CrossRef] [PubMed]
3. Gordon, E.L.; Ariel-Donges, A.H.; Bauman, V.; Merlo, L.J. What Is the Evidence for "Food Addiction?" A Systematic Review. *Nutrients* **2018**, *10*, 477. [CrossRef] [PubMed]
4. Gordon, E.L.; Lent, M.R.; Merlo, L.J. The Effect of Food Composition and Behavior on Neurobiological Response to Food: A Review of Recent Research. *Curr. Nutr. Rep.* **2020**, *9*, 75–82. [CrossRef] [PubMed]
5. Ifland, J.R.; Preuss, H.G.; Marcus, M.T.; Rourke, K.M.; Taylor, W.C.; Burau, K.; Jacobs, W.S.; Kadish, W.; Manso, G. Refined food addiction: A classic substance use disorder. *Med. Hypotheses* **2009**, *72*, 518–526. [CrossRef]
6. Meule, A.; Gearhardt, A.N. Food addiction in the light of DSM-5. *Nutrients* **2014**, *6*, 3653–3671. [CrossRef] [PubMed]
7. Olsen, C.M. Natural rewards, neuroplasticity, and non-drug addictions. *Neuropharmacology* **2011**, *61*, 1109–1122. [CrossRef]

8. Pursey, K.M.; Stanwell, P.; Gearhardt, A.N.; Collins, C.E.; Burrows, T.L. The prevalence of food addiction as assessed by the Yale Food Addiction Scale: A systematic review. *Nutrients* **2014**, *6*, 4552–4590. [CrossRef]
9. Pursey, K.M.; Davis, C.; Burrows, T.L. Nutritional Aspects of Food Addiction. *Curr. Addict. Rep.* **2017**, *4*, 142–150. [CrossRef]
10. Ruffle, J.K. Molecular neurobiology of addiction: What's all the (Δ) FosB about? *Am. J. Drug Alcohol Abus.* **2014**, *40*, 428–437. [CrossRef]
11. Schulte, E.M.; Avena, N.M.; Gearhardt, A.N. Which foods may be addictive? The roles of processing, fat content, and glycemic load. *PLoS ONE* **2015**, *10*, e0117959. [CrossRef] [PubMed]
12. Gearhardt, A.N.; Yokum, S.; Orr, P.T.; Stice, E.; Corbin, W.R.; Brownell, K.D. Neural correlates of food addiction. *Arch. Gen. Psychiatry* **2011**, *68*, 808–816. [CrossRef] [PubMed]
13. Gearhardt, A.N.; Corbin, W.R.; Brownell, K.D. Preliminary validation of the Yale food addiction scale. *Appetite* **2009**, *52*, 430–436. [CrossRef] [PubMed]
14. Schulte, E.M.; Gearhardt, A.N. Associations of Food Addiction in a Sample Recruited to Be Nationally Representative of the United States. *Eur. Eat. Disord. Rev.* **2017**, *26*, 112–119. [CrossRef] [PubMed]
15. Burmeister, J.M.; Hinman, N.; Koball, A.; Hoffmann, D.A.; Carels, R.A. Food addiction in adults seeking weight loss treatment. Implications for psychosocial health and weight loss. *Appetite* **2013**, *60*, 103–110. [CrossRef]
16. Gearhardt, A.N.; White, M.A.; Masheb, R.M.; Morgan, P.T.; Crosby, R.D.; Grilo, C.M. An examination of the food addiction construct in obese patients with binge eating disorder. *Int. J. Eat. Disord.* **2012**, *45*, 657–663. [CrossRef]
17. Masheb, R.M.; Ruser, C.B.; Min, K.M.; Bullock, A.J.; Dorflinger, L.M. Does food addiction contribute to excess weight among clinic patients seeking weight reduction? Examination of the Modified Yale Food Addiction Survey. *Compr. Psychiatry* **2018**, *84*, 1–6. [CrossRef]
18. Long, C.G.; Blundell, J.E.; Finlayson, G. A systematic review of the application and correlates of YFAS-diagnosed 'food addiction' in humans: Are eating-related 'addictions' a cause for concern or empty concepts? *Obes. Facts* **2015**, *8*, 386–401. [CrossRef]
19. Brunault, P.; Ducluzeau, P.H.; Bourbao-Tournois, C.; Delbachian, I.; Couet, C.; Réveillère, C.; Ballon, N. Food addiction in bariatric surgery candidates: Prevalence and risk factors. *Obes. Surg.* **2016**, *26*, 1650–1653. [CrossRef]
20. Cassin, S.E.; Sijercic, I.; Montemarano, V. Psychosocial Interventions for Food Addiction: A Systematic Review. *Curr. Addict. Rep.* **2020**, *7*, 9–19. [CrossRef]
21. Davis, C. A commentary on the associations among 'food addiction', binge eating disorder, and obesity: Overlapping conditions with idiosyncratic clinical features. *Appetite* **2017**, *115*, 3–8. [CrossRef] [PubMed]
22. McKenna, R.A.; Rollo, M.E.; Skinner, J.A.; Burrows, T.L. Food Addiction Support: Website Content Analysis. *JMIR Cardio* **2018**, *2*, e10. [CrossRef] [PubMed]
23. Schulte, E.M.; Joyner, M.A.; Potenza, M.N.; Grilo, C.M.; Gearhardt, A.N. Current considerations regarding food addiction. *Curr. Psychiatry Rep.* **2015**, *17*, 19. [CrossRef] [PubMed]
24. Vella, S.L.C.; Pai, N.B. A narrative review of potential treatment strategies for food addiction. *Eat. Weight Disord.-Stud. Anorex. Bulim. Obes.* **2017**, *22*, 387–393. [CrossRef] [PubMed]
25. Foster, G.D.; Makris, A.P.; Bailer, B.A. Behavioral treatment of obesity. *Am. J. Clin. Nutr.* **2005**, *82*, 230S–235S. [CrossRef] [PubMed]
26. Laudet, A.B.; Savage, R.; Mahmood, D. Pathways to long-term recovery: A preliminary investigation. *J. Psychoact. Drugs* **2002**, *34*, 305–311. [CrossRef]
27. Farrow, C.; Tarrant, M.; Khan, S. Using social identity to promote health. In *Addiction, Behavioral Change and Social Identity: The Path to Resilience and Recovery*; Buckingham, S.A., Best, D., Eds.; Routledge: New York, NY, USA; Abington, UK, 2016.
28. Sawamoto, R.; Nozaki, T.; Nishihara, T.; Furukawa, T.; Hata, T.; Komaki, G.; Sudo, N. Predictors of successful long-term weight loss maintenance: A two-year follow-up. *Biopsychosoc. Med.* **2017**, *11*, 14. [CrossRef]
29. Chao, A.M.; Wadden, T.A.; Tronieri, J.S.; Pearl, R.L.; Alamuddin, N.; Bakizada, Z.M.; Pinkasavage, E.; Leonard, S.M.; Alfaris, N.; Berkowitz, R.I. Effects of addictive-like eating behaviors on weight loss with behavioral obesity treatment. *J. Behav. Med.* **2019**, *42*, 246–255. [CrossRef]

30. Perri, M.G.; Shankar, M.N.; Daniels, M.J.; Durning, P.E.; Ross, K.M.; Limacher, M.C.; Janicke, D.M.; Martin, A.D.; Dhara, K.; Bobroff, L.B.; et al. Effect of Telehealth Extended Care for Maintenance of Weight Loss in Rural US Communities: A Randomized Clinical Trial. *JAMA Netw. Open* **2020**, *3*, e206764. [CrossRef]
31. Perri, M.G.; Ariel-Donges, A.H.; Shankar, M.N.; Limacher, M.C.; Daniels, M.J.; Janicke, D.M.; Ross, K.M.; Bobroff, L.B.; Martin, D.; Radcliff, T.A.; et al. Design of the Rural LEAP randomized trial: An evaluation of extended-care programs for weight management delivered via group or individual telephone counseling. *Contemp. Clin. Trials* **2019**, *76*, 55–63. [CrossRef]
32. Burrows, T.; Hides, L.; Brown, R.; Dayas, C.V.; Kay-Lambkin, F. Differences in dietary preferences, personality and mental health in Australian adults with and without food addiction. *Nutrients* **2017**, *9*, 285. [CrossRef] [PubMed]
33. Lemeshow, A.R.; Rimm, E.B.; Hasin, D.S.; Gearhardt, A.N.; Flint, A.J.; Field, A.E.; Genkinger, J.M. Food and beverage consumption and food addiction among women in the Nurses' Health Studies. *Appetite* **2018**, *121*, 186–197. [CrossRef] [PubMed]
34. Pursey, K.M.; Collins, C.E.; Stanwell, P.; Burrows, T.L. Foods and dietary profiles associated with 'food addiction' in young adults. *Addict. Behav. Rep.* **2015**, *2*, 41–48. [CrossRef] [PubMed]
35. USDA Agricultural Research Service. Available online: https://www.ars.usda.gov/northeast-area/beltsville-md-bhnrc/beltsville-human-nutrition-research-center/food-surveys-research-group/docs/dmr-food-categories/ (accessed on 27 July 2020).
36. Harris, P.A.; Taylor, R.; Thielke, R.; Payne, J.; Gonzalez, N.; Conde, J.G. Research electronic data capture (REDCap)—A metadata-driven methodology and workflow process for providing translational research informatics support. *J. Biomed. Inform.* **2009**, *42*, 377–381. [CrossRef] [PubMed]
37. Preacher, K.J.; Hayes, A.F. SPSS and SAS procedures for estimating indirect effects in simple mediation models. *Behav. Res. MethodsInstrum. Comput.* **2004**, *36*, 717–731. [CrossRef] [PubMed]
38. Preacher, K.J.; Hayes, A.F. Asymptotic and resampling strategies for assessing and comparing indirect effects in multiple mediator models. *Behav. Res. Methods* **2008**, *40*, 879–891. [CrossRef]
39. Petersen, R.; Pan, L.; Blanck, H.M. Racial and ethnic disparities in adult obesity in the United States: CDC's tracking to inform state and local action. *Prev. Chronic Dis.* **2019**, *16*, 1–6. [CrossRef]
40. Meule, A. A critical examination of the practical implications derived from the food addiction concept. *Curr. Obes. Rep.* **2019**, *8*, 11–17. [CrossRef]
41. Schulte, E.M.; Joyner, M.A.; Schiestl, E.T.; Gearhardt, A.N. Future directions in "food addiction": Next steps and treatment implications. *Curr. Addict. Rep.* **2017**, *4*, 165–171. [CrossRef]
42. Corwin, R.L. The Face of Uncertainty Eats. *Curr. Drug Abus. Rev.* **2011**, *4*, 174–181. [CrossRef]
43. Corwin, R.L.; Babbs, R.K. Rodent models of binge eating: Are they models of addiction? *ILAR J.* **2012**, *53*, 23–34. [CrossRef] [PubMed]
44. Fletcher, P.C.; Kenny, P.J. Food addiction: A valid concept? *Neuropsychopharmacology* **2018**, *43*, 2506–2513. [CrossRef] [PubMed]
45. Webber, K.H.; Mellin, L.; Mayes, L.; Mitrovic, I.; Saulnier, M. Pilot Investigation of 2 Nondiet Approaches to Improve Weight and Health. *Altern. Ther. Health Med.* **2018**, *24*, 16–20. [PubMed]
46. Sevinçer, G.M.; Konuk, N.; Bozkurt, S.; Coşkun, H. Food addiction and the outcome of bariatric surgery at 1-year: Prospective observational study. *Psychiatry Res.* **2016**, *244*, 159–164. [CrossRef] [PubMed]
47. Lent, M.R.; Eichen, D.M.; Goldbacher, E.; Wadden, T.A.; Foster, G.D. Relationship of food addiction to weight loss and attrition during obesity treatment. *Obesity* **2014**, *22*, 52–55. [CrossRef] [PubMed]
48. Murray, S.M.; Tweardy, S.; Geliebter, A.; Avena, N.M. A Longitudinal Preliminary Study of Addiction-Like Responses to Food and Alcohol Consumption Among Individuals Undergoing Weight Loss Surgery. *Obes. Surg.* **2019**, *29*, 2700–2703. [CrossRef]
49. Pepino, M.Y.; Stein, R.I.; Eagon, J.C.; Klein, S. Bariatric surgery-induced weight loss causes remission of food addiction in extreme obesity. *Obesity* **2014**, *22*, 1792–1798. [CrossRef]
50. Wing, R.R.; Hill, J.O. Successful weight loss maintenance. *Annu. Rev. Nutr.* **2001**, *21*, 323–341. [CrossRef]
51. San-Cristobal, R.; Navas-Carretero, S.; Celis-Morales, C.; Brennan, L.; Walsh, M.; Lovegrove, J.A.; Daniel, H.; Saris, W.H.; Traczyk, I.; Manios, Y.; et al. Analysis of dietary pattern impact on weight status for personalised nutrition through on-line advice: The Food4Me Spanish cohort. *Nutrients* **2015**, *7*, 9523–9537. [CrossRef]

52. Hutchesson, M.J.; Collins, C.E.; Morgan, P.J.; Watson, J.F.; Guest, M.; Callister, R. Changes to dietary intake during a 12-week commercial web-based weight loss program: A randomized controlled trial. *Eur. J. Clin. Nutr.* **2014**, *68*, 64–70. [CrossRef]
53. Kong, A.; Beresford, S.A.; Alfano, C.M.; Foster-Schubert, K.E.; Neuhouser, M.L.; Johnson, D.B.; Duggan, C.; Wang, C.Y.; Xiao, L.; Jeffery, R.W.; et al. Self-monitoring and eating-related behaviors are associated with 12-month weight loss in postmenopausal overweight-to-obese women. *J. Acad. Nutr. Diet.* **2012**, *112*, 1428–1435. [CrossRef] [PubMed]
54. Vidmar, A.P.; Pretlow, R.; Borzutzky, C.; Wee, C.P.; Fox, D.S.; Fink, C.; Mittelman, S.D. An addiction model-based mobile health weight loss intervention in adolescents with obesity. *Pediatric Obes.* **2019**, *14*, e12464. [CrossRef] [PubMed]
55. Nikiforova, I.; Barnea, R.; Azulai, S.; Susmallian, S. Analysis of the Association between Eating Behaviors and Weight Loss after Laparoscopic Sleeve Gastrectomy. *Obes. Facts* **2019**, *12*, 618–631. [CrossRef] [PubMed]
56. Lennerz, B.; Lennerz, J.K. Food addiction, high-glycemic-index carbohydrates, and obesity. *Clin. Chem.* **2018**, *64*, 64–71. [CrossRef] [PubMed]
57. Cope, E.C.; Gould, E. New evidence linking obesity and food addiction. *Biol. Psychiatry* **2017**, *81*, 734–736. [CrossRef]
58. Burrows, T.; Kay-Lambkin, F.; Pursey, K.; Skinner, J.; Dayas, C. Food addiction and associations with mental health symptoms: A systematic review with meta-analysis. *J. Hum. Nutr. Diet.* **2018**, *31*, 544–572. [CrossRef]
59. Chu, D.T.; Nguyet, N.T.M.; Nga, V.T.; Lien, N.V.T.; Vo, D.D.; Lien, N.; Ngoc, V.T.N.; Le, D.H.; Nga, V.B.; Van Tu, P.; et al. An update on obesity: Mental consequences and psychological interventions. *Diabetes Metab. Syndr. Clin. Res. Rev.* **2019**, *13*, 155–160. [CrossRef]
60. Jorm, A.F.; Korten, A.E.; Christensen, H.; Jacomb, P.A.; Rodgers, B.; Parslow, R.A. Association of obesity with anxiety, depression and emotional well-being: A community survey. *Aust. N. Z. J. Public Health* **2003**, *27*, 434–440. [CrossRef]
61. Kamody, R.C.; Thurston, I.B.; Decker, K.M.; Kaufman, C.C.; Sonneville, K.R.; Richmond, T.K. Relating shape/weight based self-esteem, depression, and anxiety with weight and perceived physical health among young adults. *Body Image* **2018**, *25*, 168–176. [CrossRef]
62. Strine, T.W.; Mokdad, A.H.; Dube, S.R.; Balluz, L.S.; Gonzalez, O.; Berry, J.T.; Manderscheid, R.; Kroenke, K. The association of depression and anxiety with obesity and unhealthy behaviors among community-dwelling US adults. *Gen. Hosp. Psychiatry* **2008**, *30*, 127–137. [CrossRef]
63. Bell, C.G.; Walley, A.J.; Froguel, P. The genetics of human obesity. *Nat. Rev. Genet.* **2005**, *6*, 221–234. [CrossRef] [PubMed]
64. Davis, C.; Loxton, N.J.; Levitan, R.D.; Kaplan, A.S.; Carter, J.C.; Kennedy, J.L. Food addiction' and its association with a dopaminergic multilocus genetic profile. *Physiol. Behav.* **2013**, *118*, 63–69. [CrossRef] [PubMed]
65. Osadchiy, V.; Labus, J.S.; Gupta, A.; Jacobs, J.; Ashe-McNalley, C.; Hsiao, E.Y.; Mayer, E.A. Correlation of tryptophan metabolites with connectivity of extended central reward network in healthy subjects. *PLoS ONE* **2018**, *13*, e0201772. [CrossRef] [PubMed]
66. Santacruz, A.; Marcos, A.; Wärnberg, J.; Martí, A.; Martin-Matillas, M.; Campoy, C.; Moreno, L.A.; Veiga, O.; Redondo-Figuero, C.; Garagorri, J.M.; et al. Interplay between weight loss and gut microbiota composition in overweight adolescents. *Obesity* **2009**, *17*, 1906–1915. [CrossRef]
67. Huseinovic, E.; Winkvist, A.; Bertz, F.; Brekke, H.K. Changes in food choice during a successful weight loss trial in overweight and obese postpartum women. *Obesity* **2014**, *22*, 2517–2523. [CrossRef]
68. Assunção, M.C.F.; Gigante, D.P.; Cardoso, M.A.; Sartorelli, D.S.; Santos, I.S. Randomized, controlled trial promotes physical activity and reduces consumption of sweets and sodium among overweight and obese adults. *Nutr. Res.* **2010**, *30*, 541–549. [CrossRef]

Publisher's Note: MDPI stays neutral with regard to jurisdictional claims in published maps and institutional affiliations.

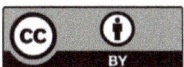

© 2020 by the authors. Licensee MDPI, Basel, Switzerland. This article is an open access article distributed under the terms and conditions of the Creative Commons Attribution (CC BY) license (http://creativecommons.org/licenses/by/4.0/).

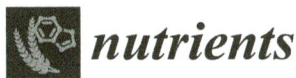

Article

Ultraprocessed Food: Addictive, Toxic, and Ready for Regulation

Robert H. Lustig [1,2,3]

1. Department of Pediatrics, University of California, San Francisco, CA 94143, USA; Robert.Lustig@ucsf.edu
2. Institute for Health Policy Studies, University of California, San Francisco, CA 94143, USA
3. Department of Research, Touro University-California, Vallejo, CA 94592, USA

Received: 27 September 2020; Accepted: 23 October 2020; Published: 5 November 2020

Abstract: Past public health crises (e.g., tobacco, alcohol, opioids, cholera, human immunodeficiency virus (HIV), lead, pollution, venereal disease, even coronavirus (COVID-19) have been met with interventions targeted both at the individual and all of society. While the healthcare community is very aware that the global pandemic of non-communicable diseases (NCDs) has its origins in our Western ultraprocessed food diet, society has been slow to initiate any interventions other than public education, which has been ineffective, in part due to food industry interference. This article provides the rationale for such public health interventions, by compiling the evidence that added sugar, and by proxy the ultraprocessed food category, meets the four criteria set by the public health community as necessary and sufficient for regulation—abuse, toxicity, ubiquity, and externalities (How does your consumption affect me?). To their credit, some countries have recently heeded this science and have instituted sugar taxation policies to help ameliorate NCDs within their borders. This article also supplies scientific counters to food industry talking points, and sample intervention strategies, in order to guide both scientists and policy makers in instituting further appropriate public health measures to quell this pandemic.

Keywords: processed food; nutrition; non-communicable disease; metabolic syndrome; diabetes; addiction; policy

---

1. Introduction: Pandemics and Public Health

We are in the midst of two pandemics. The COVID-19 pandemic had an identifiable start in January 2020. Yet despite media attention and warnings from scientists, many countries are experiencing a "second wave"; here in the United States, we never even cleared the first wave. There is no cure, at least not yet; all we have to mitigate this pandemic are public health efforts—social distancing, handwashing, and face masks—which do not seem to work very well voluntarily, unless made mandatory by authorities. The second pandemic, of non-communicable diseases (NCDs; type 2 diabetes, cardiovascular disease, fatty liver disease, hypertension, heart disease, stroke, cancer, and dementia), has been more insidious, slowly building over a 50-year time frame [1]. There is also no cure for this pandemic; all we have are educational efforts such as voluntary "diet and exercise", which do not seem to work very well either.

NCDs now account for 72% of deaths [2] and 75% of health care dollars in the United States [3] and globally [2]; and the morbidity, mortality, and economic costs continue to climb. In the U.S., Medicare is expected to be insolvent by 2026, and Social Security will be broke by 2034 [4], due to both the loss of economic productivity combined with increased healthcare expenditures. Without young and healthy people paying into the system, old and infirm people cannot take out. The cost of these diseases is not limited to the U.S. [5], and NCDs have been declared a global health crisis by the United Nations (U.N.) [6]. Thus, NCDs pose an existential threat to the survival of each country, and indeed the entire planet. Identifying the cause(s) of NCDs, and upstream policy initiatives to mitigate them is of paramount importance.

Nonetheless, the world has recently faced down two other chronic disease pandemics, tobacco and ethanol; both caused by hedonic substances readily available for purchase, and both responsive to public health regulatory interventions. It was not until the U.S.'s Master Settlement Agreement and the World Health Organization (WHO) Framework Convention on Tobacco Control that we saw a reduction in cigarette consumption and reduction in lung cancer [7]. For alcohol, individual countries have passed their own public health ethanol regulatory efforts, with clear improvements [8].

2. Criteria for Public Health Regulation

The question for public health officials is whether there is something specific and identifiable that could be regulated on a global scale that could help to mitigate the pandemic of NCDs. While some behaviors can be mandated (e.g., mask-wearing), most are left up to each individual (e.g., exercise). Rather, targeting a substance or class of causative substances would be more effective, as predicted by the *Iron Law of Public Health*, which states that reducing availability of a substance reduces consumption, which reduces health harms [9]. Public health officials have identified the four criteria which must be met in order to be considered for public health regulation [10]:

- Abuse (why can't you stop?)
- Toxicity (why do you get sick?)
- Ubiquity (why can't you escape it?)
- Externalities (why does your consumption harm me?)

To generate enthusiasm for any public health regulatory effort, the science and the logic of each of these criteria must be obvious and inescapable. The goal of this treatise is to provide the science that ultraprocessed food in general, and sugar in particular, meet all four criteria, and should be considered as targets for regulation of the NCD pandemic by the public health community and by policymakers.

However, first we must deal with the "elephant in the room"; the mythology that calories are the cause of obesity, and obesity is the cause of NCDs. If this were the case, then the processed food industry can use the mantra that "any calorie can be part of a balanced diet", and thus deflect criticisms of their products. In order to provide evidence for the specific roles of sugar and ultraprocessed food in the pandemic of NCDs, we must first confront and dispel this mythology, by demonstrating that obesity is not a cause of NCDs because normal-weight individuals get NCDs as well. We must also demonstrate that the effects of sugar and ultraprocessed food on NCD prevalence and severity are exclusive of inherent calories, and independent of effects on obesity [11].

3. Obesity Is a 'Marker', Not a Cause of Non-Communicable Diseases (NCDs)

Most clinicians mistakenly attribute the growing rise of NCDs to growing prevalence of obesity because of the *quantity of the food* ingested. This is untrue, for five separate reasons. (a) While obesity prevalence and diabetes prevalence correlate, they are not concordant [12]. There are countries that are obese without being diabetic (such as Iceland, Mongolia, and Micronesia), and there are countries that are diabetic without being obese, such as India, Pakistan, and China (they manifest a 12% diabetes rate). This is further elaborated looking at years of life lost from diabetes vs. obesity [13]. (b) Twenty percent of individuals with obesity are metabolically healthy and have normal life spans [14–16], while up to 40% of normal weight adults harbor metabolic perturbations similar to those in obesity, including type 2 diabetes mellitus (T2DM), dyslipidemia, non-alcoholic fatty liver disease (NAFLD), and cardiovascular disease (CVD) [17,18]. Indeed, in the U.S. 88% of adults exhibit metabolic dysfunction [19], while only 65% are overweight or obese—some normal weight people are metabolically ill as well. (c) The "Little Women of Loja" are a founder-effect cohort in Ecuador who are growth hormone-receptor deficient, and who become markedly obese yet are protected from chronic metabolic disease such as diabetes and heart disease [20]. (d) The secular trend of diabetes in the U.S.

from 1988 to 2012 has demonstrated a 25% increase in prevalence in both the obese *and* the normal weight population [21]. (e) The aging process does not explain T2DM, as children as young as the first decade now manifest these same biochemical processes [22,23]. Now children get two diseases that were never seen before in this age group—T2DM and fatty liver disease. These two diseases used to be prevalent only in the elderly, or in those who abused ethanol.

These five lines of reasoning argue that obesity is a "marker" for the pathophysiology of NCDs (e.g., insulin resistance), but not a primary cause—because a percentage of normal weight people get NCDs as well, while a percentage of people with obesity are metabolically healthy. If obesity was a cause of NCDs, then one could by extension make the case that "eating is addictive"—but clearly neither are true. That young and normal weight people can contract these diseases suggests an exposure, rather than a behavior, at the root of the NCD pandemic, and that the *quantity of the food is not the cause*.

4. Ultraprocessed Food Is the Cause of NCDs

Rather, *the quality of the food is the cause*. Ultraprocessed food, defined as industrial formulations typically with 5 or more ingredients [24], is the category of food that drives NCDs [25], such as obesity [26,27], diabetes [28], heart disease [29], and cancer [30]. In particular, added sugar (i.e., any fructose-containing sweetener; sucrose, high-fructose corn syrup, maple syrup, honey, agave) is the prevalent, insidious, and egregious component of ultraprocessed food that drives that risk.

In this article, using scientific and legal evidence, I will elaborate three related arguments. First, I will demonstrate that ultraprocessed food is addictive because of the sugar that is added to it, and that the food industry specifically adds sugar because of its addictive properties. Second, I will highlight the specific mechanisms by which sugar is toxic to the liver, which leads to NCDs. Lastly, I will argue that added sugar is more appropriately defined as a *food additive* rather than as a *food*. In so doing, I will argue that added sugar, and by extension the entire ultraprocessed food category, meets these criteria established by the public health community for regulation of a substance (abuse, toxicity, ubiquity, externalities) [9].

5. Added Sugar Is Abused

The seminal role of the Western Diet in the pandemic of NCDs is unchallenged [31]. For instance, ultraprocessed food consumption correlates with body mass index (BMI) in the U.S. [26] and in 19 European countries [27]. As market deregulation policies of the 1990s took hold, fast food sales increased incrementally in all countries and cultures to which it has been introduced, along with commensurate increases in BMI [32]. Indeed, every country that has adopted the Western diet is burdened with the development of NCDs and their resultant costs [33]. However, the food industry continues to promulgate the argument that it is the quantity, not the quality of the foods that are to blame. This is not a semantic argument. Quantity is determined by the end user, a personal responsibility issue; while quality is determined by manufacturers, a public health issue. But what if the quality altered the quantity? Those that favored either view over the other would thus appear to be justified within their own stance. Indeed, this debate seems to have drawn to an academic stalemate [34–36]. This must be answered before any form of societal intervention can be contemplated.

5.1. 'Food Addiction' versus 'Eating Addiction'

Recent revelations in the popular literature have alluded to the addictiveness of the Western diet [37,38], driving excessive consumption. Physiologic [39,40] and neuroanatomic [41] overlap between obesity and addiction pathways have been elucidated. Some investigators have argued that specific components of processed food, and in particular those in "fast food", are addictive in a manner similar to cocaine and heroin [42,43]. The Yale Food Addiction Scale (YFAS) logs specific foods as having addictive properties [44], and a children's YFAS also reveals that food addiction is common, especially in obese youth [45].

However, not everyone subscribes to this expanded view of specific foods having addicting properties. For instance, a group of academics in Europe called NeuroFAST does not accept the concept of food addiction, rather calling it "eating addiction" [46]. This group has proffered its own "eating addiction scale" in which all foods are treated similarly [47], and it is the behavior that distinguishes the phenomenon. These investigators state that even though specific foods can generate a reward signal, they cannot be addicting because they are essential to survival. In their own words:

"In humans, there is no evidence that a specific food, food ingredient or food additive causes a substance-based type of addiction (the only currently known exception is caffeine which via specific mechanisms can potentially be addictive). Within this context we specifically point out that we do not consider alcoholic beverages as food, despite the fact that one gram of ethanol has an energy density of 7 kcal [48]".

NeuroFAST recognizes caffeine as addictive, but gives it a pass. Xanthine alkaloids are present naturally in many foods, yet caffeine is classified by the U.S. Food and Drug Administration (FDA) as a food additive. It is also a drug; we give it to premature newborns with underdeveloped nervous systems to stimulate the central nervous system (CNS) to prevent apnea. NeuroFAST also recognizes ethanol as addictive, and also gives it a pass. Natural yeasts constantly ferment fruit while still on the vine or tree, causing it to ripen [49], yet NeuroFAST acknowledges that purified ethanol is not a food. Rather, ethanol is a drug; we used to give it to pregnant women to stop premature labor.

Recently, another European group with food industry ties assessed the effects of specific foodstuffs on "eating dependence" in a cohort of university students, using weight gain as the metric of food addiction. In their study, they found no difference between fats and sugars as cause for weight gain [50]. However, as stated earlier, using weight gain as the metric of food addiction is inherently flawed.

In order to assess mechanism of effects of food on the addiction pathway in the brain, our group at UCSF studied a cohort of postmenopausal women with obesity who received orally the mu-opioid receptor antagonist naltrexone as a probe of the brain's reward system. We found that the amplitude of cortisol responses and nausea generation in response to naltrexone correlated with symptoms of craving for sweet palatable foods in these women. These data suggest that naltrexone interfered with endogenous opioid peptide (EOP) tone that mediated these cravings. In so doing, we have discerned a phenomenon of "Reward Eating Drive" (RED), which belies those individuals with obesity who appear to respond excessively to hedonic food cues [51–53], and which is tied to the opioidergic component of the reward system in the brain, which is driven by sweet foods. Furthermore, using functional magnetic resonance imaging (fMRI) studies, other investigators have defined the prefrontal cortex as responsible for the response of sweet tastes as being "attractive" or "unattractive" [54].

5.2. Addictive Potential of Food Components

If there was a class of consumables that was uniquely addictive, it would have to be "fast food". But is it just the calories, or is there something specific about fast food that generates an addictive response? Fast food contains four components whose hedonic properties have been examined: salt, fat, caffeine, and sugar [37,42].

5.2.1. Salt

In humans, salt intake has traditionally been conceived as a learned preference [55] rather than as an addiction. The preference for salty foods is likely learned early in life. Four- to six-month-old infants establish a salt preference based on the sodium content of breast milk, water used to mix formula, and diet [56]. Because energy-dense fast foods are relatively high in salt [57], in part as a preservative to reduce depreciation, the preference for salty foods is associated with higher calorie intake. For example, a study in Korean teens showed a correlation between frequent fast food intake and preference for saltier versions of traditional foods [58]. Another study examined 27 subjects undergoing opiate (mostly oxycodone) withdrawal and showed significant increases in fast food intake and weight gain over 60 days [59], suggesting "addiction transfer". On the other hand, studies show that people can 'reset' their preference for less salty items. This has been demonstrated in adolescents deprived of salty pizza on their school lunch menu, and hypertensive adults who were retrained to consume a lower sodium diet over 8 to 12 weeks [55]. Furthermore, at low levels, salt intake is well known to be tightly regulated. For example, patients with salt-losing congenital adrenal hyperplasia who lack the mineralocorticoid aldosterone modulate have an obligatory salt loss, which modulates their salt intake [60], until appropriate doses of fludrocortisone are supplemented. The notion that human sodium intake is "physiologically fixed" had been used to criticize recent public health efforts to reduce sodium intake so drastically [61]. Nonetheless, the U.K. government engaged in a secret mass campaign to reduce public salt consumption by 30%, and saw a 40% reduction in hypertension and stroke without signs of withdrawal [62].

5.2.2. Fat

The high fat content of fast food is vital to its rewarding properties. Indeed, there may be a "high-fat phenotype" among human subjects, characterized by a preference for high-fat foods and weak satiety in response to them, which acts as a risk factor for obesity [63]. However, so-called "high-fat foods" preferred by people are almost always also high in carbohydrate (e.g., potato chips, pizza, or cookies). Indeed, adding sugar significantly enhances preference for high-fat foods among normal weight human subjects; yet there was no limit for preference with increasing fat content [64]. Thus, the synergy of high fat along with high sugar is likely to be more effective at stimulating addictive overeating than fat alone. However, these rewarding properties of fat appear to be strictly dependent on simultaneous ingestion of carbohydrate, as low-carbohydrate high-fat (LCHF) [65] and ketogenic diets [66] consistently result in reduced caloric intake, significant weight loss, and resolution of metabolic syndrome. In other words, fat increases the salience of fast food, but does not appear to be addictive in and of itself.

5.2.3. Caffeine

Caffeine is a "model drug" of dependence in humans [67], meeting the DSM-IV and DSM-5 criteria for tolerance, physiologic withdrawal, and psychological dependence in children [68], adolescents [69], and adults [70]. Headache [70], fatigue, and impaired task performance [68] have been demonstrated during withdrawal. While adolescents and children get their caffeine from soft drinks and hot chocolate, adults get most of their caffeine from coffee and tea [71]. These drinks average 239 calories and provide high amounts of sugar [72]. Soft drink manufacturers identify caffeine as a flavoring agent in their beverages, but only 8% of frequent soda drinkers can detect the difference in a blinded comparison of a caffeine-containing and caffeine-free cola [73]. Thus, the most likely function of the caffeine in soda is to increase the salience of an already highly rewarding (high sugar) beverage. These drinks may be acting as a gateway for caffeine-dependent customers to visit a fast food restaurant and purchase fast food [74].

5.2.4. Sugar

Other than caffeine, the component with the highest score on the YFAS is sugar [44]. Adding a soft drink to a fast food meal increases the sugar content 10-fold. Multivariate analysis of fast food transactions demonstrate that only soft drink intake is correlated with changes in BMI; not animal fat products [32]. While soda intake has been shown to be independently related to obesity and the diseases of metabolic syndrome [75,76], fast food eaters clearly consume more soft drinks. Sugar has been used for its analgesic effect in neonatal circumcision [77], suggesting a link between sugar and EOP tone. Indeed, anecdotal reports from self-identified food addicts describe sugar withdrawal as feeling "irritable", "shaky", "anxious" and "depressed" [78]; symptoms also seen in opiate withdrawal. Other studies demonstrate the use of sugar to treat psychological dependence [79]. Sugar craving can vary widely by age, menstrual cycle and time of day [80].

Sugar is added to food either as sucrose, high-fructose corn syrup (HFCS), honey, maple syrup, or agave. In general, each are assumed to consist of half fructose, half glucose; although this percentage has recently come into question when an analysis of store-bought sodas in Los Angeles revealed a fructose content as high as 65% [81]. This difference may be relevant, as fructose appears to generate a greater reward response and more toxicity than does glucose (see below).

5.3. Correlates of Addiction in Animals Exposed to Sucrose

In rodents, oral sucrose administration uniquely induces the acute reactant *c-fos* in the ventral tegmental area, implying activation of the reward pathway [82]. Furthermore, sucrose infusion directly into the nucleus accumbens reduces dopamine and μ-opioid receptors similar to morphine [83], and fMRI studies demonstrate the establishment of hard-wired pathways for craving [84]. Furthermore, sucrose administration to rodents induces behavioral alterations consistent with dependence; i.e., bingeing, withdrawal, craving, and cross-sensitization to other drugs of abuse [85]. Indeed, in one oft-quoted rat study, sweetness surpassed cocaine as reward [86].

5.4. Differential Effects of Fructose vs. Glucose vs. Fat on the Human Brain

Despite being calorically equivalent (4.1 kcal/gm), fructose and glucose are metabolized differently. Glucose is the energy of life. Glucose is so important that if you do not consume it, your liver makes it from amino acids and fatty acids (gluconeogenesis). Conversely fructose, while an energy source, is otherwise vestigial; there is no biochemical reaction in any eukaryote that requires it. Our research has shown that when provided in excess of the liver's capacity to metabolize fructose via the tricarboxylic acid cycle, the rest is turned into liver fat, promoting insulin resistance, and resultant NCDs [87–89].

Physiologically, chronic fructose administration promotes fasting hyperinsulinemia and hypertriglyceridemia [90], which blocks leptin's ability to cross the blood brain barrier [91], and attenuates leptin's ability to extinguish mesolimbic dopamine signaling in rodents [92] and humans [93], thus promoting tolerance and withdrawal [94]. Furthermore, fructose does not suppress the stomach-derived hunger hormone ghrelin [95]. Through these pathways, fructose fosters overconsumption independent of energy need [96]. A comparison of the two monosaccharides demonstrates increased risk for bingeing with fructose (similar to sucrose) as opposed to glucose [97], suggesting the fructose molecule is the moiety that generates both reward and addiction responses.

Neuroanatomically, human fMRI studies show that acute glucose vs. fructose administration exert effects on different sites in the brain. One study infused each monosaccharide intravenously, and measured blood oxygenation level-dependent (BOLD) fMRI signal in cortical areas of the brain; glucose increased the BOLD signal in cortical executive control areas, whereas fructose suppressed the signal coming from those same areas [98]. Another study examined regional cerebral blood flow (rCBF) after oral glucose vs. fructose. With glucose, rCBF within the hypothalamus, thalamus, insula, anterior cingulate, and striatum (appetite and reward regions) was reduced, while fructose reduced rCBF in the thalamus, hippocampus, posterior cingulate cortex, fusiform, and visual cortex [99]. Consistent with other studies, fructose demonstrated lack of satiety or fullness in comparison to glucose. Furthermore, glucose increased "functional connectivity" of the caudate, putamen, precuneus, and lingual gyrus (basal ganglia) more than fructose; whereas fructose increased functional connectivity of the amygdala, hippocampus, parahippocampus, orbitofrontal cortex and precentral gyrus (limbic system) more than glucose [100]. In obese youth, the effects of oral fructose on dopamine activation of the nucleus accumbens is severely attenuated, suggesting down-regulation of dopamine receptors [101]. Lastly, the effects of fat and sugar both separately and together (adjusting for calories) on fMRI signaling have been assessed [102]. High-fat milkshakes increased brain activity in the caudate and oral somatosensory areas (postcentral gyrus, hippocampus, inferior frontal gyrus); while sugar increased activity in the insula extending into the putamen, the Rolandic operculum, and thalamus (gustatory regions). Furthermore, increasing sugar caused greater activity in those regions, but increasing fat content did not alter this activation. In other words, the fat increases the salience of the sugar, but it is the sugar that effectively recruits reward and gustatory circuits.

To summarize, added sugar (and specifically the fructose moiety) is unique in activating reward circuitry; fructose works both directly and indirectly to increase consumption; and that both obesity and chronic fructose exposure down-regulate dopamine receptors, requiring greater and greater stimuli to enact a reward-signaling effect (tolerance), a primary component of addiction.

5.5. 'Food' Addiction Is Really 'Food Additive' Addiction, and 'Added Sugar' Is a Food Additive

In the past, the concept of food addiction was not embraced by psychiatrists. For instance, the DSM-IV published in 1993 listed "substance use disorder" as requiring both tolerance and withdrawal as necessary criteria for the definition of addiction, and (apart from caffeine and ethanol) no foodstuff elicited withdrawal. However, as the public health difficulties stemming from addiction expanded, the definition, of necessity, expanded. The DSM-5 published in 2013 reclassified the field so as to include "behavioral addictions", such as gambling (internet gaming was included in the Appendix as "requiring further study"). Thus, a revised set of criteria related to psychological dependence was proffered [103], including:

1. Craving or a strong desire to use;
2. Recurrent use resulting in a failure to fulfill major role obligations (work, school, home);
3. Recurrent use in physically hazardous situations (e.g., driving);
4. Use despite social or interpersonal problems caused or exacerbated by use;
5. Taking the substance or engaging in the behavior in larger amounts or over a longer period than intended;
6. Attempts to quit or cut down;
7. Time spent seeking or recovering from use;
8. Interference with life activities;
9. Use despite negative consequences.

However, food addiction was not codified in the DSM-5. Nonetheless, systematic reviews of the literature demonstrate that ultraprocessed foods have the highest addictive potential due to their added sugar content [104]. While sugar itself does not exhibit the DSM-IV criteria of classic tolerance and withdrawal, sugar clearly meets the DSM-5 requirements of tolerance and dependence (use despite conscious knowledge and recognition of their detriment).

Coca leaves are medicinal in Bolivia, yet cocaine is a drug, and regulated. Opium poppies are also medicinal, but morphine is a drug, and regulated. Caffeine is found in coffee (medicinal for many), yet concentrated caffeine is a drug, and regulated. In ancient times, sugar was a spice. Through the Industrial Revolution it was a condiment. Now it is purified, and it is a drug. Refined sucrose is the same compound found in fruit, but the fiber has been removed, and it has been crystallized for purity. This process of purification has turned sugar from "food" into "drug" [105]. Like these other addictive consumables, it can be present in low dose in nature and not exert toxic effects; but when purified and added to food, it becomes addictive.

Drugs are a luxury, food is a necessity. NeuroFAST asks how can foods that are necessary to survival also be addicting? Because certain "foods" are *not* necessary for survival. Of the hedonic substances found in food, only alcohol, caffeine, and sugar are addictive. But these are food additives, not foods. Some form of sugar has been added to 74% of the food supply [106], because the food industry knows that when they add it, we buy more [107]. For instance, the tobacco industry manipulated nicotine levels in cigarettes specifically to keep users consuming, and to convert as many as possible into "heavy users" [108]. The food industry has engaged in similar practices, which has increased the percent of calories as added sugar (58%) in ultraprocessed foods [27]. In fact, sugar's allure is a big reason why the processed food industry's current profit margin is 5% (it used to be 1%) [109]. The addictive nature of sugar is also revealed in its economics. For instance, coffee is price-inelastic, i.e., increasing price does not reduce consumption much. When prices jumped in 2014 due to decreased supply, Starbuck's sales remained constant, owing to its hedonic effects [110]. As consumables go, soft drinks are the second most price-inelastic, just below fast food [107]. When the price is raised by 10% (e.g., with taxes), consumption dropped only 7.6%, mostly among the poor, as was seen in Mexico [111]. Thus, sugar consumption is only minimally responsive to either its economic or caloric value, consistent with its addictive properties.

6. Added Sugar Is Toxic

Toxicity is defined as "the degree to which a substance can damage an organism". Such detrimental effects must be exclusive of caloric equivalence, or else *all* calories are toxic, which is clearly not true. Just because a substance is an energy source does not mean that it is not toxic. For instance, alcohol possesses a caloric equivalence (7 kcal/gm), yet we humans have an upper limit of hepatic and brain metabolism, beyond which toxicity becomes manifest, either acute (mental status changes) or chronic (fatty liver disease progressing to cirrhosis, insulin resistance). Alcohol is not dangerous because of its calories or its effects on weight. Alcohol is dangerous because it is alcohol [112]; the biochemistry of the molecule in the liver confers its toxicity. Alcohol exerts its negative effects on liver metabolism through two mechanisms: (1) liver mitochondrial overload with diversion of substrate to the process of *de novo* lipogenesis (DNL; new fat-making), with subsequent hepatic fat accumulation and insulin resistance [113]; and (2) the non-enzymatic binding of the intermediate metabolite acetaldehyde to liver proteins, known as the Maillard or "aging" reaction, with subsequent "carbonyl" stress (see Section 6.1.2), protein denaturation, subsequent inflammation, and cell death.

6.1. Detrimental Effects of Fructose on Liver Metabolism

The metabolic perturbations associated with fructose consumption exclusive of its caloric equivalence are well documented by numerous investigators [114,115]. There are no biochemical reactions that require dietary fructose. The same two primary molecular mechanisms of alcohol delineate the toxicity of fructose apart from its caloric equivalence [105].

6.1.1. *De Novo* Lipogenesis

Only the liver metabolizes fructose for energy, and a fructose bolus (e.g., a soft drink) absorbed across the intestinal lining delivers the majority of the fructose via the portal vein to the liver. Fructose is particularly lipogenic, as the glycolytic intermediate acetyl-CoA is delivered to the liver mitochondria in an unregulated fashion, driving hepatic DNL, which will either be exported as triglyceride (which contributes to heart disease); or possibly overwhelming the liver's lipid export capacity, leading to intrahepatic lipid deposition and hepatic steatosis, resulting in liver insulin resistance, which is a driving force behind all the NCDs [89]. The intermediate metabolic pathways have been elucidated elsewhere [116].

6.1.2. Carbonyl Stress—The Maillard Reaction

Carbonyl stress occurs when the reactive aldehyde or keto-group of a carbohydrate molecule binds non-enzymatically to the amino-group of a protein, leading to the Maillard or the "browning reaction" [117]. This is why bananas brown as they age. This is also why humans get wrinkles as they age. This is also why patients with diabetes check their hemoglobin A1c measurement (which is a carbohydrate molecule bound to position 1 of the globin chain), to determine if their diabetes is out of control. Every time this reaction occurs, the protein becomes less flexible (leading to cell dysfunction), and an oxygen radical is produced, which if not quenched by an antioxidant, can lead to protein or lipid peroxidation, cell damage, and death.

Due to its unique stereochemistry, the ring form of fructose (a five-membered furan with axial hydroxymethyl groups) is under a great deal of ionic strain, which favors the linear form of the molecule, exposing the reactive 2-keto position, which engages in the fructosylation of exposed amino-moieties of proteins via the Maillard reaction, and 7 times faster than the 1-aldehyde position of glucose reacts with those same proteins. Each Maillard reaction generates one oxygen radical, which must be quenched by an antioxidant, or else cellular damage can ensue. Thus, due to its chemical makeup, fructose leads to increased cellular damage [118] and disease progression compared to glucose, and unrelated to its caloric equivalence.

6.1.3. Tying Two Pathophysiologic Mechanisms Together—Methylglyoxal

Recently, our UCSF/Touro research group has determined that methylglyoxal, a specific intermediate in the glycolytic pathway, is likely the nidus of both of these toxic phenomena within the liver [119]. Methylglyoxal is a transient metabolic intermediate of the process of anaerobic glycolysis, whose production is dependent on the availability of excess substrate (either glucose or fructose) in the liver; but, because virtually 100% fructose load is handled by the liver, compared to only 20% of glucose, then fructose is the primary driver of its formation. Methylglyoxal is an alpha-dicarbonyl; it is both a reactive aldehyde (like glucose) and a reactive ketone (like fructose) at the same time. Therefore, it engages in the Maillard reaction 35 times faster than fructose, and 250 times faster than glucose, generating 250 times the oxygen radicals. Methylglyoxal is detoxified to the byproduct D-lactate, which can be measured in the blood, and serves as a proxy of the rate of methylglyoxal formation. D-lactate levels are higher in obese adolescents [120], and reductions in D-lactate levels by fructose restriction in obese children correlate with improvements in DNL, liver fat content, and insulin sensitivity [121], all unrelated to caloric equivalence or obesity. These findings argue that fructose is a chronic, dose-dependent hepatotoxin, which drives progression of NCDs.

6.2. Dissociating Added Sugar from Its Calories and Effects on Weight

The food industry often tries to divert the public health conversation toward obesity [50,122]. Sugar ranks below potato chips and French fries as a cause of weight gain [123]; the data correlating sugar consumption to obesity are weak, accounting for only about 10% of the observed effect [124]. If sugar is only one of many causes of weight gain, it can iterate its mantra, 'a calorie is a calorie'. However, a new study demonstrates that the correlation between added sugar consumption and population obesity obeys a slightly more complex function, taking into account both current and previous consumption of added sugar [125]. This model predicts the effects of added sugar on obesity quite accurately.

But, as stated before, obesity is the wrong metric. Obesity and diabetes are discordant; there are countries where diabetes rates are high yet obesity rates are low, such as India, Pakistan, and China; while their sugar consumption has increased by 15% in the past 6 years alone [126]. When weight and calories are factored out, the correlation between sugar consumption and type 2 diabetes is even stronger [12,127]. To date, the food industry refuses to engage in a discussion on the role of added sugar in chronic metabolic diseases, exclusive of obesity.

There are many case-control studies (reviewed in [128,129]) which point to dietary fructose consumption as a primary cause of T2DM, but such studies are not controlled for calories or weight. In order to prove that fructose (and, therefore, added sugar) is specifically toxic, the molecule must be dissociated from its inherent calories and its effects on weight. Furthermore, standard cross-sectional or correlational studies without a time-factor analysis component are not acceptable, as they cannot distinguish reverse or intermediate causality; it is like the snapshot rather than the movie. Lastly, the food industry is quick to point out that most fructose studies are done in rodents, with large doses over a short period of time. In defense, a recent study in rats shows that sugar at normal levels of consumption can cause morbidity and mortality [130], and a primate study demonstrates similar detrimental effects [131]. Nonetheless, in order to prove toxicity, this section will be limited to human studies using doses of added sugar routinely consumed.

6.2.1. Prospective Association Studies

Three recent studies, all controlled for calories and adiposity and with a time analysis, support sugar as a specific and direct causative agent in T2DM. First, a prospective cohort analysis of the European EPIC-Interact study found that sugar-sweetened beverage (SSB) consumption increased risk for development of diabetes over a 10-year period. The multivariate modeling, which adjusted for both energy intake (EI) and for adiposity (BMI), demonstrated that each SSB consumed increased the hazard risk (HR) ratio by 1.29 (95% CI 1.02, 1.63) exclusive of energy intake (calories) or BMI (obesity) [132]. In the U.S., we are currently consuming the equivalent of 2.5 servings of SSB's per day; so our HR ratio is 1.68.

Second, a meta-analysis of studies isolated consumption of soda ($n = 17$) and fruit juice ($n = 13$) separately, while controlling for calories and adjusting for adiposity [76]. This meta-analysis showed that both soda and fruit juice significantly increased the relative risk (RR) ratio for diabetes (1.27, 1.10, respectively) over time. Furthermore, this study specifically took into account the fact that food industry-sponsored studies frequently demonstrate publication and information bias, and calibrated for these biases.

Third, our UCSF group evaluated the National Health and Nutrition Examination Survey (NHANES) adolescent database across three cycles 2005–2012, to determine nutritional consumption and any changes within the American diet within that interval. We then binned subjects into quintiles based on added sugar consumption, and after controlling for caloric intake and BMI, determined what aspects of the diet predicted the prevalence of metabolic syndrome [133]. We set the HR ratio for metabolic syndrome in the 1st quintile (median added sugar consumption = 30 gm/day) at 1.0; by the 4th quintile (median added sugar consumption = 125 gm/day), the HR ratio for metabolic syndrome had increased to 9.7.

6.2.2. Econometric Analyses

One econometric analysis [134] of 156 countries over the period 1995–2014 demonstrated that global availability of sugar and sweeteners was correlated with diabetes prevalence, health care costs per diabetic, and health care costs per capita; demonstrating both personal and societal harm related to added sugar consumption. This analysis also showed that this correlation occurred in both developed and developing countries. However, this study did not account for calories or obesity, and could not account for other aspects of the diet.

Our UCSF/Stanford group performed an econometric analysis to assess what foods were specifically implicated in altered diabetes rates over time [12]. We melded three freely available databases together; (1) the Food and Agriculture Organization statistics database (FAOSTAT; a branch of the World Health Organization), which lists by food availability per person by country, by year 2000–2010, and by line item (total calories, fruits excluding wine, meats, oils, cereals, fiber-containing foods, and sugar/sweeteners); (2) the International Diabetes Federation (IDF) database which lists diabetes prevalence by country by year 2000–2010; and (3) the World Bank World Development Indicators Database for the years 2000–2010, in which Gross Domestic Product is expressed in purchasing power parity in 2005 US dollars for comparability among countries to control for poverty. It also controls for urbanization, aging, physical activity, and obesity. We asked what food(s) availability predict change in diabetes prevalence country by country over the decade? We performed this analysis using generalized estimating equations with a conservative fixed-effects approach (Hausman test), a hazard model to control for selection bias (Heckman selection test), and period effects controlled for secular trends that may have occurred as a result of changes diabetes detection capacity or importation policies. Most importantly, we examined longitudinal data between 2000 and 2010, which allowed us to determine what dietary changes preceded the changes in diabetes prevalence (Granger causality test).

We demonstrated that retrospective changes in sugar availability predicted the prevalence of diabetes during the decade 2000–2010, exclusive of total calories, other foodstuffs, aging, obesity, physical activity, or income. For every 150 calories per day in excess, diabetes prevalence increased

0.1%, but if those 150 calories happened to be a can of soda, diabetes prevalence increased 11-fold, by 1.1% [12]. These data meet the Bradford Hill criteria for "causal medical inference", because we demonstrate dose (more sugar, more diabetes), duration (longer sugar exposure, more diabetes), directionality (the few countries where sugar availability went down experienced a reduction in diabetes), and precedence (we noted a three-year lag between increase in sugar availability and increase in diabetes prevalence; in a prospective modeling study we noticed a three-year lag between sugar reduction and decrease in diabetes prevalence [3]).

This econometric analysis has been criticized for two reasons. First, it is an "ecological study", which by convention is hierarchically considered of low quality. Rather, this econometric analysis is more rigorous and of higher quality than all studies except randomized controlled trials [135], as it assesses multiple points in time, discerns complex relationships between internal and external motivating factors (adjusted over time), and allows for determination of causation (Granger causality test). Second, the FAOSTAT database assesses country-specific food availability rather than consumption, and waste is not taken into account. Rather, assessing availability is a positive feature rather than a negative, as availability is more accurate, easily quantifiable, not subject to the vicissitudes of individual recall, and independent of food wastage.

6.2.3. Interventional Starch-for-Sugar Exchange

Our UCSF/Touro research group documented the effects of isocaloric substitution of sugar with starch in 43 Latino and African-American children with metabolic syndrome over a 10-day period [87–89]. We performed food questionnaires and interviews using sophisticated software to assess their total caloric consumption, as well as specific macronutrient and fiber intake. On Day 0, we assessed their metabolic health on their home diet using: (1) baseline analyte levels; (2) oral glucose tolerance testing; and (3) dual-emission X-ray absorptiometry (DEXA) scanning. Then, for the next 9 days, we catered their meals, to provide the same caloric content, the same fat, protein, and fiber content, and the same amount of total carbohydrate; but we reduced the percent calories from dietary sugar from a mean of 28% to 10%, and the percent calories from fructose from 12% to 4%. They were allowed fruit, but not fruit juice. We gave them a scale to take home and called them every day. If their weight was declining, we made them eat more, and they were given extra snacks to prevent weight loss. Then we studied them again 10 days later.

Every aspect of their metabolic health improved, with essentially no change in weight. Blood pressure reduced by 5 mmHg, triglycerides by 33 mg/dL, low-density lipoproteins (LDL) by 10 mg/dL, glucose levels reduced by 5 mg/dL, glucose area under the curve dropped by 8%, fasting insulin dropped by 10 mU/L, insulin area under the curve dropped 25%, on the same number of calories and without weight loss, just by removing the added sugar and substituting with starch. Furthermore, subcutaneous fat did not change (as there was no weight loss), but visceral fat reduced by 7%, and most importantly liver fat was reduced by 22%. We also showed that insulin dynamics improved markedly, thus reversing their predisposition to T2DM.

Taken together with the aforementioned studies [12,136,137], Koch's Postulates for causation of NCDs by added sugar are fulfilled. Sugar is a chronic, dose-dependent liver toxin unrelated to calories or obesity, similar to ethanol, because fructose and ethanol exert similar effects on the liver and the brain [112].

7. Added Sugar Is Ubiquitous

Sugar has become ubiquitous in the Western diet, increasing from 15 gm/day at the beginning of the 20th century to 94 gm/day at the beginning of the 21st century [138,139]. In the U.S. 56% of the diet is now ultra-processed food, 62% of sugar in the American diet is in this category [28], and some form of sugar has been added to 74% of the items in the American grocery store [106], because the food industry knows that when they add it, we buy more. Similarly, world sugar consumption tripled 1960–2010 while the world population doubled over the same time [140], arguing that most of the world's population has experienced a significant increase in added sugar consumption in the 50 years that NCDs have become prominent [140]. For instance, changes in consumption of Coca-Cola over the interval 1993–2006 correlated with changes in diabetes prevalence in both China and Mexico. During this interval, the consumer price index for sugared beverages increased 50% vs. food, and 25% vs. fruits and vegetables [141]. The introduction of high-fructose corn syrup in 1975 reduced cost the cost of sugar by 50%, which allowed serving size to rise, and sugar to be added to foods that previously did not contain it. For instance, 50% of milk sales in elementary and middle schools are for flavored milk (chocolate, strawberry). Furthermore, in most developing nations, soda is cheaper than water, which has increased consumption of added sugar around the world. Processed foods and sugared beverages are marketed heavily as they are extremely profitable; in 2006, food marketers spent USD $1.05 billion on marketing to children and adolescents; half of which were for sugared beverages [142].

Marketing practices by tobacco and food companies are highly congruent [143]. Big Tobacco in the past, and Big Food currently, have used "commercial speech" provided by the First Amendment to cull favor with the public through advertising and sponsorships. For instance, both have in the past engaged in vigorous advertising campaigns to recruit new users that was defused only by regulatory agency action [144,145]. For decades Big Tobacco provided corporate sponsorship of various public events around the world, such as the Olympics, baseball and football games, and sporting events around the world. The fast food and beverage industries engage in similar marketing practices, sponsoring global events around the world. Big Tobacco shamelessly marketed their products to children (e.g., Joe Camel); while the food and beverage industries have followed suit (e.g., Ronald McDonald). Both have used deceptive business practices to maintain increased use of their product among "heavy users" [146,147].

8. Added Sugar Exerts Externalities

Substances that produce societal harms impact even the non-user. Second-hand smoke and drinking-driving provided strong arguments for tobacco and alcohol control, respectively. The above data demonstrate that the long-term healthcare, human, and economic costs of NCDs place the chronic effects of fructose overconsumption in the same category [148].

Sugared beverages alone kill 184,000 people per year globally [149]. The U.S. wastes $65 billion in work productivity and $150 billion in health care resources, and experiences a 50% increase in absenteeism and health insurance premiums, all to care for the co-morbidities of metabolic syndrome [150]. Currently, 75% of all health care dollars are spent on treating these diseases or resultant disabilities. Rising global NCD rates yield an annual mortality of 35 million people, with a disproportionate 80% of these deaths occurring in low- and middle-income countries, wasting precious medical resources [151]. Lastly, the past three Surgeons General and the Chairman of the Joint Chiefs of Staff have declared obesity a "threat to national security". The original Pentagon report from 2012 has been updated in 2018, and 33% of recruits are now deemed "Still Too Fat To Fight" [152]. Even among those recruited, 43% cannot be deployed into the field due to Stage 3 dental caries due to sugar consumption [153].

Population-wide sugar reduction would prevent premature death, save economies billions and improve quality of life for millions across the globe. Our UCSF group used advanced Markov modeling (using fatty liver disease as the sentinel disease) to demonstrate that reduction of added sugar consumption of just 20% (e.g., a tax) could reduce obesity, type 2 diabetes, heart disease, death rates, and medical expenditures within three years in the United States, and save $10 billion annually, while a 50% reduction (e.g., adhering to U.S. Dept. of Agriculture (USDA) guidelines) could save $31.8 billion annually [3]. On the productivity side, Morgan Stanley modeled global economic growth rates from 2015 to 2035 in low-sugar and high-sugar simulations [154], and showed that using a low-sugar case, economic growth would be maintained at 2.9%, while using a high-sugar case (e.g., the present), economic growth would slowly decline to 0.0%. Thus, the externalities of added sugar consumption are direct and affect everyone.

9. Food Industry Counters

9.1. Personal Responsibility

Education of the public through emphasis on "personal responsibility" over the last 30 years have not been effective in stemming the tide of obesity and metabolic syndrome. This should not be surprising, as educational efforts have been unsuccessful in reducing the consumption of other substances of abuse [9,155]. Add to this the fact that 74% of the items in the food supply are spiked with added sugar by the food industry [106]; thus it is virtually impossible for most individuals to disabuse sugar, and to be able to go "cold turkey" in order to reduce toxicity and dependence. This is especially true of the poor, who have limited access to healthy food, and are often limited in their purchases to high-sugar processed food on the Supplemental Nutrition Assistance Program (aka Food Stamps). The ostensible reason that the food industry has added more and more sugar to processed food is for "palatability". Indeed, when they do, we buy more; which reinforces the practice by increasing profits. Indeed, efforts to reduce the negative health impact of "junk food" by former Pepsi CEO Indra Nooyi by introducing a "good for you" category (to offset their "fun for you" category) have met with rancor by her own Board of Directors due to a $349 million reduction in profits [156].

The personal responsibility strategy was first deployed by tobacco companies in 1962 as a reason to keep on smoking [157]. This ideology requires four pre-requisites:

9.1.1. Knowledge

Information labelling is not easily understandable by the regular consumer buying food products in the supermarket. Many will trust and buy a product on the way it is promoted, rather than on its nutritional value. Until recently, the US Institute of Medicine, and in the UK and the rest of Europe for the past 15 years, guideline daily amounts on labels have suggested that daily consumption of up to 22 teaspoons of sugar is healthful [158].

9.1.2. Access

Over 70% of foods in the supermarket contain added sugar—it has become almost unavoidable. Processed sugary food and drinks have permeated workplaces, gyms, and schools. Several American hospitals (including UCSF), and the British National Health Service (NHS) have instituted a ban on sugary drinks sold in hospitals, in order to provide a role model for the public. Our UCSF group has documented the metabolic health benefits of a workplace ban on sugared beverages [159].

9.1.3. Affordability

One should be able to afford their choice, and society has to afford it too. Healthy food was twice as expensive as processed food in 2002, and its cost increased by the equivalent of US $0.22 per year over the next 10 years, compared with processed food, which increased by the equivalent of US $0.09 per year [160].

9.1.4. Non-Anarchy

The medical costs of chronic metabolic disease due to sugar consumption will cause a doubling of Medicare costs in the next decade [161], bankrupting health care systems around the world [162,163], and the NHS is under an ever-tighter squeeze, resulting in lengthier waiting times [164]. The argument that your actions cannot harm anyone else ignores the diet-related harm experienced by children who are especially vulnerable to poor diet at critical development stages.

Americans currently consume an average of 19.5 tsp/day of added sugar. The American Heart Association has recommended a reduction in added sugar consumption to 6 tsp/day for women and 9 tsp/day for men, a reduction by $2/3$ to $3/4$ in amount. Of these 22 tsp, $1/3$ can be found in beverages, and 1/6 in desserts. This means that fully $\frac{1}{2}$ of the added sugar in our diet is in foods that we did not know contained sugar, such as salad dressing, bread, tomato sauce, ketchup, and many other common food items. Thus, even if we removed all the soft drinks and desserts from our diet, we would still be over our "sugar limit", which has been set so high by the food industry. Thus, "personal responsibility' alone cannot be expected to confer any relief. Indeed, our food supply has been "adulterated" by the addition of added sugar by the food industry. Furthermore, there are 262 names for sugar, most of which are unknown to the population at large [165]. As the Nutrition Labeling and Education Act of 1990 [166] requires listing food ingredients by mass, the food industry can hide added sugar by using various forms of sugar and thus moving each form further down the label, so that the consumer does not know that the food they are purchasing is laden with added sugar [167]. Furthermore, while each disease within metabolic syndrome can be temporized, there is no pharmacologic "fix" for metabolic syndrome itself. Paracelsus said in 1537: "The dose determines the poison". Added sugar has an upper limit of 25–37.5 gm/day for adults and 12 gm/day for children; and we have been placed over our limit by the food industry.

The reduction of added sugar from the American diet must become the top priority to reverse the prevalence and severity of NCDs. Prevention strategies of necessity must occur through public health interventions to alter the food environment. But how? Food is a personal choice, most consider sugar as just "empty" calories, and if individuals want to consume their discretionary calories as sugar, why should they not be allowed to do so? Yet, tobacco and alcohol similarly pose significant societal threats due to their abuse, toxicity, ubiquity, and externalities (negative impact on society) [155,168], and they are regulated [169].

9.2. Is Added Sugar 'Food'?

The food industry will debate any argument for regulating added sugar with two talking points. First, they will point out that sugar is a primary component of fruit, and fruit has been shown to be preventive against NCDs [170]. In contradistinction, fruit juice has been shown to be correlated with these same diseases [76,171]. The reason is that the fiber prevents intestinal absorption, thus reducing the systemic burden of the sugar in whole fruit [172]. Second, the industry argues that dietary sugar is on the FDA's Generally Recognized as Safe (GRAS) list, which gives the food industry license to use any amount of sugar in any foods they wish. Fructose was grandfathered into the first GRAS list in 1958, as it was "natural" and had been used for generations without any obvious ill effects—although sugar was known to be associated with gout as early as the 17th century [173], and known to raise serum uric acid levels (the mechanism of gout) in 1967 [174]. It should be noted that inclusion on the GRAS list prior to 1 January 1958 was through either scientific procedures or experience based on common use in food (requiring a substantial history of consumption for food use by a significant number of consumers) and thought there is reasonable certainty that the substance is not harmful under the intended conditions of use (Food, Drugs, and Cosmetics Act (FDCA) 321(s), 21 CFR 170.30(c), 170.3(f)). However, in 1958 our consumption of added sugar averaged 2 ounces per day, and currently it averages 6.5 ounces per day. Thus, GRAS determinations in 1958 do not hold for today's food supply. The issue of GRAS outliving its intentions is seen for trans-fats and salt; both used by the processed food industry, both proven to be detrimental at doses above what were thought to be safe, and now both under scrutiny by the FDA (although not removed from the GRAS list).

Trans-fats used to be "food", but subsequent research showed they cause heart disease and other metabolic diseases. Nitrates used to be "food", yet research showed they cause colon cancer. Both were eventually removed from the GRAS list, and are now regulated as food additives. Ethanol has always been a food additive, and caffeine dosage above 0.02% (in cola drinks) is similarly regulated.

The question is, does added sugar legally qualify as food? It depends on how you define the word "food". The Food, Drug, and Cosmetics Act (FDCA, 1938) 321.201(f) defines the term "food" as: *(1) articles used for food or drink for man or other animals, (2) chewing gum, and (3) articles used for components of any such article.* The first rule of vocabulary is that you are not allowed to use the word in the definition. The Merriam-Webster Dictionary defines "food" as: *a material consisting essentially of* protein, carbohydrate, and fat used in the body of an organism to sustain growth, repair, and vital processes and to furnish energy. Fructose supplies energy, so that should make it a food. Or does it? Ethanol supplies energy (7 kcal/gm), but it is clearly not a food. There is no biochemical reaction in any eukaryote that requires it. When consumed chronically and in high dose, ethanol is toxic, unrelated to its calories or effects on weight. Not everyone who is exposed becomes addicted, but enough do to warrant public health intervention [175]. Clearly, ethanol is NOT a food, it is a food additive. Similarly, *added sugar is a food additive*—like ethanol, it is not essential for life, it is toxic in chronically high dosage, and a good percentage of the population is addicted. Indeed, the petitioning for removal of fructose from the GRAS list is being currently being entertained by public health non-governmental organizations (NGOs).

10. Possible Societal Interventions

In the last 30 years, there have been four global cultural tectonic shifts in behavior to ameliorate four public health problems: (a) smoking in public places; (b) drunk driving; (c) bicycle helmets and seat belts; (d) condoms in public bathrooms. In each case, public education was necessary but not sufficient, and some form of regulatory policy also had to be enacted to insure compliance. There are many lessons from alcohol and tobacco control policies that can be brought to bear on sugar and ultraprocessed food.

10.1. Public Education

One the most important things we have learned from tobacco and alcohol policy research is that public education, despite being the most popular and a necessary component of prevention, does not work alone [168,176]. Evidence from the U.S. suggests that government labels warning consumers about the health effects of excessive drinking have no effect on alcohol consumption, but might have had some limited effect on risky drinking patterns, such as drunk driving [177]. The most popular approaches–school-based health education, public information campaigns, product labeling, and government guidelines—do not work in isolation [178,179]. It should be noted that education *alone* has not solved any substance of abuse. Nonetheless, education softens the playing field, so that societal policy interventions can become acceptable and take hold.

We must take a look as to what works to reduce the consumption of addictive substances. Research on alcohol policy demonstrates that regulatory controls on the pricing, marketing, and distribution of alcohol are highly effective worldwide in reducing the negative impacts of alcohol consumption [10,168,176]. This strategy has also been effective with tobacco [180]. There are three ways to reduce availability: pricing strategies (e.g., taxation), restriction of access (e.g., blue laws), and interdiction (e.g., banning). No one thinks interdiction is a good idea—alcohol prohibition was tried, and was singularly unsuccessful.

10.2. Pricing Strategies-Taxation

Society accepts taxation because taxes affect only those who use those products. While tobacco and ethanol are significant burdens to society, sugar is by far and away the most expensive burden. The question is, what is the real goal? Making money for the state, or reduction in consumption? Because if you reduce consumption, you limit revenue generation. For a tax on a hedonic substance to work, it has to hurt. Most soda taxes are 10%, but an Oxford group modeled that a soda tax would have to be at least 20% to reduce general consumption [181].

The good news is that due to the emergence of the science around sugar and the inability of education to stop the diabetes pandemic, six American cities and 28 countries globally have enacted sugar taxes, and others are considering some form of legislation [182].

10.3. Pricing Strategies-Subsidies

Agricultural subsidies are payments and other kinds of support extended by the U.S. federal government to certain farmers and agribusinesses. They are a holdover from the original Farm Bill of

1933, when it was necessary to provide cheap food to a destitute population across the country. In the U.S., currently seven states are awarded 45% of the subsidies: Texas 9.6%; Iowa 8.4%; Illinois 6.9%; Minnesota 5.8%; Nebraska 5.7%; Kansas 5.5%; and North Dakota 5.3% [183]; and these are the states that that are the largest producers of corn, soybeans, wheat, and rice—the basics for ultraprocessed food production. There is no economist on the planet who believes in food subsidies, because they distort the market. They make available the wrong stuff while making the right stuff harder to afford. As long as commodities are cheap, real food will stay out of reach for much of the population.

What would happen if subsidies ended? The Giannini group at UC Berkeley modeled what food would actually cost; and the only two items that would increase in price are sugar and corn [184], which is just what we would want to happen. Not surprisingly, these are two of the major industries fighting to maintain the status quo. Still, people will argue, the overall price of food will go up. Well maybe it should, The U.S. spends the least percentage of GDP on food of all nations at 7%—that is because all the food is commodity crop-based and processed. The next two are the UK at 9% and Australia at 11%, the three fattest nations [185].

10.4. Restriction of Access-Workplace Bans

The workplace presents an educational moment and venue. At UCSF, all sugared beverage sales—soda and flavored coffee drinks—were banned from sale in the cafeterias, vanished from patients' meal trays, and disappeared from the menus of any vendors bringing food onto campus. We studied a subgroup of 214 employees who regularly drank sugared beverages before and one year after the ban was put in place [159]. They reported a daily intake of 35 ounces at baseline and 18 ounces at follow-up—a 17-ounce decrease, a cut by almost half. In addition, waist circumference reduced by 2.1 cm. Reductions in sugared beverage intake correlated with improvements in waist circumference, insulin sensitivity, and a pattern of reduction in blood lipids. Some employers may face challenges in implementing a workplace culture where SSB sales bans are perceived as paternalistic. Nevertheless, this proves the *Iron Law* does indeed work.

10.5. Restriction of Access-Stipends

The U.K. provides people with a monthly stipend—which can only be exchanged for real food [186]. This allows each person to use their stipends to vote on local food policy, and in so doing, promote local farmers and organic practices.

10.6. Combination Strategies-Differential Subsidization

Differential subsidization combines the "carrot and stick" approach—the inducement with the punishment [187]. Differential subsidization was employed in 1977 in the Nordic countries, including Sweden, Denmark and Norway, to curb the increasing number of alcoholics in their respective countries. The three countries collectively adopted two pieces of legislation: first, they nationalized the liquor stores resulting in the same products sold at the same amount everywhere; second, they taxed high-alcohol spirits, and then used the money from the tax to subsidize low-alcohol beer. In doing so, they were able to nudge the public away from hard spirits and toward the low-alcohol beer, thus, reducing alcohol consumption. In the process, hospitalizations decreased, car accidents reduced, cirrhosis of the liver declined, and economic productivity improved [188].

This could easily be used to cut sugared beverage consumption—tax soda, and use the revenue generated from the tax to subsidize water. The beverage makers will not care, because they are also selling the water. It is just a straight up exchange, nudging people to a healthier option with a zero-sum scheme. In so doing, you can "nudge" people into doing the right thing, and they won't complain—and most of the time, they will not even notice they have been nudged.

11. Conclusions

When it comes to public health, personal intervention (read: rehab) must be balanced with societal intervention (read: laws). For tobacco, alcohol, opioids, cholera, HIV, lead, pollution, and venereal disease, invoking "personal responsibility" and railing against the "nanny state" was ultimately unsuccessful, and both forms of intervention were ultimately deemed necessary. For added sugar and NCDs, we currently have nothing. The argument for societal intervention in NCDs has been lacking because the food industry has convinced the public that "a calorie is a calorie", that sugar are just "empty calories", and that "personal responsibility" is the answer. While public educational efforts are necessary to warn about the hazards of chronic excessive sugar consumption, they will not be sufficient, as has been seen for every other hedonic substance.

Added sugar, like tobacco, alcohol, cocaine, and opioids, meets public health criteria for societal intervention, i.e., regulation. The roadmap to successful intervention is complex, but we have templates based on how tobacco and alcohol regulation were enacted. As with tobacco and alcohol, the *Iron Law of Public Health* is in force, which states that reduction in availability results in reduction in consumption, which results in reduction in health harms [10]. Policies that target availability, affordability or acceptability (e.g., the Mexico sugar tax) are effective in curbing sugar consumption [111]. But similar to what occurred with the tobacco industry (e.g., *Merchants of Doubt*), the sugar industry, their legislative partners, and their political allies have utilized numerous instruments to deflect culpability and derail policy changes. Some involve influencing science, some involve influencing public opinion, and yet others influence legislatures directly [189]. These activities must be understood and countered before any specific and meaningful policy measures can be proffered.

In this article, I have provided evidence that: (1) sugar is addictive and toxic unrelated to calories; (2) sugar reduction confers health and societal benefits; (3) added sugar, and by inference ultraprocessed food, meets criteria for regulation; (4) sugar reduction is not only possible but required to save health and healthcare, and (5) societal interventions to reduce consumption of processed foods containing added sugar are achievable and necessary. Those interventions (administrative, legislative, judicial) will likely be geographically, politically, and culturally specific; and certain policy interventions will not work in certain venues.

Author Contributions: Along with informal consultations with those mentioned above, R.H.L. researched, designed, drafted, and authored this article. All authors have read and agreed to the published version of the manuscript.

Funding: This research received no external funding.

Acknowledgments: I wish to thank my fellow UCSF/Touro University research team members, especially Alejandro Gugliucci, Jean-Marc Schwarz, Kathy Mulligan, Sue Noworolski, Grace Jones, and Ayca Erkin-Cakmak. I need to thank my UCSF policy colleagues, Laura Schmidt, Claire Brindis, and Elissa Epel. Lastly, I thank my legal colleagues, David Faigman and Marsha Cohen at UC Hastings College of the Law, and Michael Roberts and Diana Winters at the UCLA Resnick Center for Food Policy and Obesity, who have also been instrumental in the policy analysis.

Conflicts of Interest: Lustig has never accepted money from the food industry, and has no disclosures with respect to this article. However, Dr. Lustig has authored five popular books as a public health service: *Fat Chance: Beating the Odds Against Sugar, Processed Food, Obesity, and Disease* (2013); *Sugar Has 56 Names: a Shopper's Guide* (2013); *The Fat Chance Cookbook* (2014); *The Hacking of the American Mind: The Science Behind the Corporate Takeover of our Bodies and Brains* (2017); and *Metabolical—the Lure and the Lies of Processed Food, Nutrition, and Modern Medicine* (2021). He is Chief Science Officer of the non-profit *Eat REAL* (US) and advisor to the non-profits *Action on Sugar* (UK) and the Center for Humane Technology (US). He is also Chief Medical Officer of the for-profit entities *BioLumen Technologies* (US) and *Foogal* (US), and consultant to *Simplex Health* (US).

References

1. Benziger, C.P.; Roth, G.A.; Moran, A.E. The Global Burden of Disease Study and the Preventable Burden of NCD. *Glob. Heart* **2016**, *11*, 393–397. [CrossRef] [PubMed]
2. Global Burden of Disease Causes of Death Collaborators. Global, regional, and national age-sex specific mortality for 264 causes of death, 1980–2016: A systematic analysis for the Global Burden of Disease Study 2016. *Lancet* **2017**, *390*, 1151–1210. [CrossRef]
3. Vreman, R.A.; Goodell, A.J.; Rodriguez, L.A.; Porco, T.C.; Lustig, R.H.; Kahn, J.G. Health and economic benefits of reducing sugar intake in the United States, including effects via non-alcoholic fatty liver disease: A microsimulation model. *BMJ Open* **2017**, *7*, e103543. [CrossRef] [PubMed]
4. Press, A. Medicare will Become Insolvent in 2026, U.S. Government Says. *Los Angeles Times*. 5 June 2018. Available online: https://www.latimes.com/nation/nationnow/la-na-pol-medicare-finances-20180605-story.html (accessed on 27 September 2020).
5. Yach, D.; Hawkes, C.; Gould, C.L.; Hofman, K.J. The global burden of chronic diseases: Overcoming impediments to prevention and control. *JAMA* **2004**, *291*, 2616–2622. [CrossRef]
6. U.N. General Assembly. Prevention and control of non-communicable diseases. In *U.N. General Assembly*; U.N. General Assembly: New York, NY, USA, 2010.
7. Johnston, L.D.; Miech, R.A.; O'Malley, P.M.; Bachman, J.G.; Schulenberg, J.E.; Patrick, M.E. *Monitoring the Future National Survey Results on Drug Use 1975–2018: Overview, Key Findings on Adolescent Drug Use*; University of Michigan: Ann Arbor, MI, USA, 2019.
8. Room, R. International control of alcohol: Alternative paths forward. *Drug Alcohol Rev.* **2006**, *25*, 581–595. [CrossRef]
9. Room, R.; Babor, T.; Rehm, J. Alcohol and public health. *Lancet* **2005**, *365*, 519–530. [CrossRef]
10. Room, R.; Schmidt, L.A.; Rehm, J.; Mäkela, P. International regulation of alcohol. *Br. Med. J.* **2008**, *337*, a2364. [CrossRef]
11. Lustig, R.H. Sickeningly sweet: Does sugar cause diabetes? Yes. *Can. J. Diabetes* **2016**, *40*, 282–287. [CrossRef]
12. Basu, S.; Yoffe, P.; Hills, N.; Lustig, R.H. The relationship of sugar to population-level diabetes prevalence: An econometric analysis of repeated cross-sectional data. *PLoS ONE* **2013**, *8*, e57873. [CrossRef] [PubMed]
13. Sepúlveda, J.; Murray, C. The state of global health in 2014. *Science* **2014**, *345*, 1275–1278. [CrossRef]
14. Chan, J.M.; Rimm, E.B.; Colditz, G.A.; Stampfer, M.J.; Willett, W.C. Obesity, fat distribution, and weight gain as risk factors for clinical diabetes in men. *Diabetes Care* **1994**, *17*, 961–969. [CrossRef]
15. McLaughlin, T.; Abbasi, F.; Cheal, K.; Chu, J.; Lamendola, C.; Reaven, G.M. Use of metabolic markers to identify overweight individuals who are insulin resistant. *Ann. Int. Med.* **2003**, *139*, 802–809. [CrossRef]
16. Chen, D.L.; Liess, C.; Poljak, A.; Xu, A.; Zhang, J.; Thoma, C.; Trenell, M.; Milner, B.; Jenkins, A.B.; Chisholm, D.J.; et al. Phenotypic characterization of insulin-resistant and insulin-sensitive obesity. *J. Clin. Endocrinol. Metab.* **2015**, *100*, 4082–4091. [CrossRef] [PubMed]
17. Abbasi, F.; Chu, J.W.; Lamendola, C.; McLaughlin, T.; Hayden, J.; Reaven, G.M.; Reaven, P.D. Discrimination between obesity and insulin resistance in the relationship with adiponectin. *Diabetes* **2004**, *53*, 585–590. [CrossRef]
18. Voulgari, C.; Tentolouris, N.; Dilaveris, P.; Tousoulis, D.; Katsilambros, N.; Stefanadis, C. Increased heart failure risk in normal-weight people with metabolic syndrome compared with metabolically healthy obese individuals. *J. Am. Coll. Cardiol.* **2011**, *58*, 1343–1350. [CrossRef]
19. Araújo, J.; Cai, J.; Stevens, J. Prevalence of Optimal Metabolic Health in American Adults: National Health and Nutrition Examination Survey 2009–2016. *Metab. Syndr. Relat. Disord.* **2019**, *17*, 46–52. [CrossRef] [PubMed]
20. Rosenbloom, A.L.; Guevara Aguirre, J.; Rosenfeld, R.G.; Fielder, P.J. The little women of Loja-growth hormone-receptor deficiency in an inbred population of southern Ecuador. *N. Engl. J. Med.* **1990**, *323*, 1367–1374. [CrossRef]
21. Menke, A.; Casagrande, S.; Geiss, L.; Cowie, C.C. Prevalence of and trends in diabetes among adults in the United States, 1988–2012. *JAMA* **2015**, *314*, 1052–1062. [CrossRef]
22. Wiegand, S.; Maikowski, U.; Blankenstein, O.; Biebermann, H.; Tarnow, P.; Gruters, A. Type 2 diabetes and impaired glucose tolerance in European children and adolescents with obesity—A problem that is no longer restricted to minority groups. *Eur. J. Endocrinol.* **2004**, *151*, 199–206. [CrossRef]

23. Biltoft, C.A.; Muir, A. The metabolic syndrome in children and adolescents: A clinician's guide. *Adolesc. Med. State Art Rev.* **2009**, *20*, 109–120.
24. Gibney, M.J. Ultra-Processed Foods: Definitions and Policy Issues. *Curr. Dev. Nutr.* **2019**, *3*, nzy077. [CrossRef]
25. Moubarac, J.C.; Parra, D.; Cannon, G.; Monteiro, C.A. Food classification systems based on food processing: Significance and implications for policies and actions. A systematic literature review and assessment. *Curr. Obes. Rep.* **2014**, *3*, 256–272. [CrossRef]
26. Juul, F.; Martinez-Steele, E.; Parekh, N.; Monteiro, C.A.; Chang, V.W. Ultra-processed food consumption and excess weight among US adults. *Br. J. Nutr.* **2018**, *120*, 90–100. [CrossRef]
27. Monteiro, C.A.; Moubarac, J.C.; Levy, R.B.; Canella, D.S.; Louzada, M.L.D.C.; Cannon, G. Household availability of ultra-processed foods and obesity in nineteen European countries. *Public Health Nutr.* **2018**, *21*, 18–26. [CrossRef]
28. Srour, B.; Fezeu, L.K.; Kesse-Guyot, E.; Allès, B.; Debras, C.; Druesne-Pecollo, N.; Chazelas, E.; Deschasaux, M.; Hercberg, S.; Galan, P.; et al. Ultraprocessed Food Consumption and Risk of Type 2 Diabetes Among Participants of the NutriNet-Santé Prospective Cohort. *JAMA Intern. Med.* **2020**, *180*, 283–291. [CrossRef]
29. Srour, B.; Fezeu, L.K.; Kesse-Guyot, E.; Allès, B.; Méjean, C.; Andrianasolo, R.M.; Chazelas, E.; Deschasaux, M.; Hercberg, S.; Galan, P.; et al. Ultra-processed food intake and risk of cardiovascular disease: Prospective cohort study (NutriNet-Santé). *BMJ* **2019**, *365*, l1451. [CrossRef]
30. Fiolet, T.; Srour, B.; Sellem, L.; Kesse-Guyot, E.; Allès, B.; Méjean, C.; Deschasaux, M.; Fassier, P.; Latino-Martel, P.; Beslay, M.; et al. Consumption of ultra-processed foods and cancer risk: Results from NutriNet-Santé prospective cohort. *BMJ* **2018**, *360*, k322. [CrossRef]
31. Popkin, B.M.; Adair, L.S.; Ng, S.W. Global nutrition transition and the pandemic of obesity in developing countries. *Nutr. Rev.* **2012**, *70*, 3–21. [CrossRef]
32. De Vogli, R.; Kouvonen, A.; Gimeno, D. The influence of market deregulation on fast food consumption and body mass index: A cross-national time series analysis. *Bull. World Health Organ.* **2014**, *92*, 99–107. [CrossRef] [PubMed]
33. GBD Diet Collaborators. Health effects of dietary risks in 195 countries, 1990–2017: A systematic analysis for the Global Burden of Disease Study 2017. *Lancet* **2019**, *393*, 1958–1972. [CrossRef]
34. Ziauddeen, H.; Farooqi, I.S.; Fletcher, P.C. Obesity and the brain: How convincing is the addiction model? *Nat. Rev. Neurosci.* **2012**, *13*, 279–286. [CrossRef]
35. Avena, N.M.; Gearhardt, A.N.; Gold, M.S.; Wang, G.J.; Potenza, M.N. Tossing the baby out with the bathwater after a brief rinse? The potential downside of dismissing food addiction based on limited data. *Nat. Rev. Neurosci.* **2012**, *13*, 514. [CrossRef]
36. Ziauddeen, H.; Farooqi, I.S.; Fletcher, P.C. Food addiction: Is there a baby in the bathwater? *Nat. Rev. Neurosci.* **2012**, *13*, 514. [CrossRef]
37. Moss, M. *Salt, Sugar, Fat: How the Food Giants Hooked Us*; Random House: New York, NY, USA, 2013.
38. Kessler, D.A. *The End of Overeating: Taking Control of the Insatiable American Appetite*; Rodale: New York, NY, USA, 2010.
39. Volkow, N.D.; Wise, R.A. How can drug addiction help us understand obesity? *Nat. Neurosci.* **2005**, *8*, 555–560. [CrossRef] [PubMed]
40. Fortuna, J.L. The obesity epidemic and food addiction: Clinical similarities to drug dependence. *J. Psychoact. Drugs* **2012**, *44*, 56–63. [CrossRef]
41. Wang, G.J.; Volkow, N.D.; Thanos, P.K.; Fowler, J.S. Similarity between obesity and drug addiction as assessed by neurofunctional imaging: A concept review. *J. Addict. Res.* **2004**, *23*, 39–53. [CrossRef] [PubMed]
42. Garber, A.K.; Lustig, R.H. Is fast food addictive? *Curr. Drug Abuse Rev.* **2011**, *4*, 146–162. [CrossRef]
43. Avena, N.M.; Bocarsly, M.E.; Hoebel, B.G.; Gold, M.S. Overlaps in the nosology of substance abuse and overeating: The translational implications of "food addiction". *Curr. Drug Abuse Rev.* **2011**, *4*, 133–139. [CrossRef]
44. Schulte, E.M.; Avena, N.M.; Gearhardt, A.N. Which foods may be addictive? The roles of processing, fat content, and glycemic load. *PLoS ONE* **2015**, *10*, e0117959. [CrossRef] [PubMed]
45. Richmond, R.L.; Roberto, C.A.; Gearhardt, A.N. The association of addictive-like eating with food intake in children. *Appetite* **2017**, *117*, 82–90. [CrossRef]

46. Hebebrand, J.; Albayrak, O.; Adan, R.; Antel, J.; Dieguez, C.; de Jong, J.; Leng, G.; Menzies, J.; Mercer, J.G.; Murphy, M.; et al. "Eating addiction", rather than "food addiction", better captures addictive-like eating behavior. *Neurosci. Biobehav. Rev.* **2014**, *47*, 295–300. [CrossRef]
47. Ruddock, H.K.; Christiansen, P.; Halford, J.C.G.; Hardman, C.A. The development and validation of the Addiction-like Eating Behaviour Scale. *Int. J. Obes.* **2017**, *41*, 1710–1717. [CrossRef]
48. NeuroFAST. NeuroFAST Consensus Opinion on Food Addiction. 2014. Available online: http://www.neurofast.eu/consensus (accessed on 27 September 2020).
49. Pesis, E. The role of the anaerobic metabolites, acetaldehyde and ethanol, in fruit ripening, enhancement of fruit quality and fruit deterioration. *Postharvest Biol. Technol.* **2005**, *37*, 1–19. [CrossRef]
50. Markus, C.R.; Rogers, P.J.; Brouns, F.; Schepers, R. Eating dependence and weight gain; no human evidence for a 'sugar-addiction' model of overweight. *Appetite* **2017**, *114*, 64–72. [CrossRef]
51. Mason, A.E.; Lustig, R.H.; Brown, R.R.; Acree, M.; Bacchetti, P.; Moran, P.J.; Dallman, M.; Laraia, B.; Adler, N.; Hecht, F.M.; et al. Acute responses to opioidergic blockade as a biomarker of hedonic eating among obese women enrolled in a mindfulness-based weight loss intervention trial. *Appetite* **2015**, *91*, 311–320. [CrossRef]
52. Mason, A.E.; Laraia, B.; Daubenmier, J.; Hecht, F.M.; Lustig, R.H.; Puterman, E.; Adler, N.; Dallman, M.; Kiernan, M.; Gearhardt, A.N.; et al. Putting the brakes on the "drive to eat": Pilot effects of naltrexone and reward-based eating on food cravings among obese women. *Eat Behav.* **2015**, *19*, 53–56. [CrossRef]
53. Mason, A.E.; Epel, E.S.; Aschbacher, K.; Lustig, R.H.; Acree, M.; Kristeller, J.; Cohn, M.; Dallman, M.; Moran, P.J.; Bacchetti, P.; et al. Reduced reward-driven eating accounts for the impact of a mindfulness-based diet and exercise intervention on weight loss: Data from the SHINE randomized controlled trial. *Appetite* **2016**, *100*, 86–93. [CrossRef]
54. Rudenga, K.J.; Small, D.M. Ventromedial prefrontal cortex response to concentrated sucrose reflects liking rather than sweet quality coding. *Chem. Senses* **2013**, *38*, 585–594. [CrossRef]
55. Mattes, R.D. The taste for salt in humans. *Am. J. Clin. Nutr.* **1997**, *65*, 692S–697S. [CrossRef]
56. Harris, G.; Booth, D.A. Infants' preference for salt in food: Its dependence upon recent dietary experience. *J. Reprod. Infant Psychol.* **1987**, *5*, 94–104. [CrossRef]
57. Dietary Guidelines Advisory Committee. *Report of the Dietary Guidelines Advisory Committee on the Dietary Guidelines for Americans, 2015*; Agricultural Research Division, U.S. Department of Agriculture: Washington, DC, USA, 2016. Available online: http://www.cnpp.usda.gov/DGAs2010-DGACReport.htm (accessed on 27 September 2020).
58. Kim, G.H.; Lee, H.M. Frequent consumption of certain fast foods may be associated with an enhanced preference for salt taste. *J. Hum. Nutr. Diet.* **2009**, *22*, 475–480. [CrossRef]
59. Cocores, J.A.; Gold, M.S. The salted food addiction hypothesis may explain overeating and the obesity epidemic. *Med. Hypotheses* **2009**, *73*, 892–899. [CrossRef]
60. Kochli, A.; Tenenbaum-Rakover, Y.; Leshem, M. Increased salt appetite in patients with congenital adrenal hyperplasia 21-hydroxylase deficiency. *Am. J. Physiol. Reg. Integr. Comp. Physiol.* **2005**, *288*, R1673–R1681. [CrossRef]
61. McCarron, D.A.; Geerling, J.C.; Kazaks, A.G.; Stern, J.S. Can dietary sodium intake be modified by public policy? *Clin. J. Am. Soc. Nephrol.* **2009**, *4*, 1878–1882. [CrossRef]
62. He, F.J.; Pombo-Rodrigues, S.; Macgregor, G.A. Salt reduction in England from 2003 to 2011: Its relationship to blood pressure, stroke and ischaemic heart disease mortality. *BMJ Open* **2014**, *4*, e004549. [CrossRef]
63. Blundell, J.E.; Stubbs, R.J.; Golding, C.; Croden, F.; Alam, R.; Whybrow, S.; Le Noury, J.; Lawton, C.L. Resistance and susceptibility to weight gain: Individual variability in response to a high-fat diet. *Physiol. Behav.* **2005**, *86*, 614–622. [CrossRef]
64. Drewnowski, A.; Greewood, M.R. Cream and sugar: Human preferences for high-fat foods. *Physiol. Behav.* **1983**, *30*, 629–633. [CrossRef]
65. Hu, T.; Mills, K.T.; Yao, L.; Demanelis, K.; Eloustaz, M.; Yancy, W.S.; Kelly, T.N.; He, J.; Bazzano, L.A. Effects of low-carbohydrate diets versus low-fat diets on metabolic risk factors: A meta-analysis of randomized controlled clinical trials. *Am. J. Epidemiol.* **2012**, *176* (Suppl. 7), S44–S54. [CrossRef]
66. Paoli, A.; Rubini, A.; Volek, J.S.; Grimaldi, K.A. Beyond weight loss: A review of the therapeutic uses of very-low-carbohydrate (ketogenic) diets. *Eur. J. Clin. Nutr.* **2013**, *67*, 789–796. [CrossRef]

67. Griffiths, R.R.; Chausmer, A.L. Caffeine as a model drug of dependence: Recent developments in understanding caffeine withdrawal, the caffeine dependence syndrome, and caffeine negative reinforcement. *Nihon Shinkei Seishin Yakurigaku Zasshi* **2000**, *20*, 223–231.
68. Bernstein, G.A.; Carroll, M.E.; Walters, D.N.; Crosby, R.D.; Perwien, A.R.; Benowitz, N.L. Caffeine withdrawal in normal school-age children. *J. Am. Acad. Child Adolesc. Psychiatry* **1998**, *37*, 858–865. [CrossRef]
69. Bernstein, G.A.; Carroll, M.E.; Thuras, P.D.; Cosgrove, K.P.; Roth, M.E. Caffeine dependence in teenagers. *Drug Alcohol Depend.* **2002**, *66*, 1–6. [CrossRef]
70. Couturier, E.G.; Laman, D.M.; van Duijn, M.A.; van Duijn, H. Influence of caffeine and caffeine withdrawal on headache and cerebral blood flow velocities. *Cephalalgia* **1997**, *17*, 188–190. [CrossRef]
71. Nawrot, P.; Jordan, S.; Eastwood, J.; Rotstein, J.; Hugenholtz, A.; Feeley, M. Effects of caffeine on human health. *Food Addit. Contam.* **2003**, *20*, 1–30. [CrossRef]
72. Huang, C.; Dumanovsky, T.; Silver, L.D.; Nonas, C.; Bassett, M.T. Calories from beverages purchased at 2 major coffee chains in New York City, 2007. *Prev. Chronic Dis.* **2009**, *6*, A118. [PubMed]
73. Griffiths, R.R.; Vernotica, E.M. Is caffeine a flavoring agent in cola soft drinks? *Arch. Fam. Med.* **2000**, *9*, 727–734. [CrossRef]
74. Dumanovsky, T.; Nonas, C.A.; Huang, C.Y.; Silver, L.D.; Bassett, M.T. What people buy from fast-food restaurants: Caloric content and menu item selection, New York City 2007. *Obesity* **2007**, *17*, 1369–1374. [CrossRef]
75. Vartanian, L.R.; Schwartz, M.B.; Brownell, K.D. Effects of soft drink consumption on nutrition and health: A systematic review and meta-analysis. *Am. J. Public Health* **2007**, *97*, 667–675. [CrossRef]
76. Imamura, F.; O'Connor, L.; Ye, Z.; Mursu, J.; Hayashino, Y.; Bhupathiraju, S.N.; Forouhi, N.G. Consumption of sugar sweetened beverages, artificially sweetened beverages, and fruit juice and incidence of type 2 diabetes: Systematic review, meta-analysis, and estimation of population attributable fraction. *BMJ* **2015**, *351*, h3576. [CrossRef]
77. Stevens, B.; Yamada, J.; Ohlsson, A.; Haliburton, S.; Shorkey, A. Sucrose for analgesia in newborn infants undergoing painful procedures. *Cochrane Database Syst. Rev.* **2016**, *7*, CD001069. [CrossRef]
78. Ifland, J.R.; Preuss, H.G.; Marcus, M.T.; Rourke, K.M.; Taylor, W.C.; Burau, K.; Jacobs, W.S.; Kadish, W.; Manso, G. Refined food addiction: A classic substance use disorder. *Med. Hypotheses* **2009**, *72*, 518–526. [CrossRef] [PubMed]
79. Corsica, J.A.; Spring, B.J. Carbohydrate craving: A double-blind, placebo-controlled test of the self-medication hypothesis. *Eat. Behav.* **2008**, *9*, 447–454. [CrossRef] [PubMed]
80. Benton, D. The plausibility of sugar addiction and its role in obesity and eating disorders. *Clin. Nutr.* **2010**, *29*, 288–303. [CrossRef]
81. Ventura, E.E.; Davis, J.N.; Goran, M.I. Sugar content of popular sweetened beverages based on objective laboratory analysis: Focus on fructose content. *Obesity* **2010**, *19*, 668–674. [CrossRef]
82. Dela Cruz, J.A.; Coke, T.; Bodnar, R.J. Simultaneous detection of c-Fos activation from mesolimbic and mesocortical dopamine reward sites following naive sugar and fat ingestion in rats. *J. Vis. Exp.* **2016**, *114*. [CrossRef]
83. Spangler, R.; Wittkowski, K.M.; Goddard, N.L.; Avena, N.M.; Hoebel, B.G.; Leibowitz, S.F. Opiate-like effects of sugar on gene expression in reward areas of the rat brain. *Mol. Brain Res.* **2004**, *124*, 134–142. [CrossRef]
84. Pelchat, M.L.; Johnson, A.; Chan, R.; Valdez, J.; Ragland, J.D. Images of desire: Food-craving activation during fMRI. *Neuroimage* **2004**, *23*, 1486–1493. [CrossRef] [PubMed]
85. Avena, N.M.; Rada, P.; Hoebel, B.G. Evidence for sugar addiction: Behavioral and neurochemical effects of intermittent, excessive sugar intake. *Neurosci. Biobehav. Rev.* **2008**, *32*, 20–39. [CrossRef] [PubMed]
86. Lenoir, M.; Serre, F.; Cantin, L.; Ahmed, S.H. Intense sweetness surpasses cocaine reward. *PLoS ONE* **2007**, *2*, e698. [CrossRef]
87. Lustig, R.H.; Mulligan, K.; Noworolski, S.M.; Gugliucci, A.; Erkin-Cakmak, A.; Wen, M.J.; Tai, V.W.; Schwarz, J.M. Isocaloric fructose restriction and metabolic improvement in children with obesity and metabolic syndrome. *Obesity* **2016**, *24*, 453–460. [CrossRef]
88. Gugliucci, A.; Lustig, R.H.; Caccavello, R.; Erkin-Cakmak, A.; Noworolski, S.M.; Tai, V.W.; Wen, M.J.; Mulligan, K.; Schwarz, J.M. Short-term isocaloric fructose restriction lowers apoC-III levels and yields less atherogenic lipoprotein profiles in children with obesity and metabolic syndrome. *Atherosclerosis* **2016**, *253*, 171–177. [CrossRef]

89. Schwarz, J.M.; Noworolski, S.M.; Erkin-Cakmak, A.; Korn, N.J.; Wen, M.J.; Tai, V.W.; Jones, G.M.; Palii, S.P.; Velasco-Alin, M.; Pan, K.; et al. Impact of dietary fructose restriction on liver fat, de novo lipogenesis, and insulin kinetics in children with obesity. *Gastroenterology* **2017**, *153*, 743–752. [CrossRef] [PubMed]
90. Teff, K.L.; Grudziak, J.; Townsend, R.R.; Dunn, T.N.; Grant, R.W.; Adams, S.H.; Keim, N.L.; Cummings, B.P.; Stanhope, K.L.; Havel, P.J. Endocrine and metabolic effects of consuming fructose- and glucose-sweetened beverages with meals in obese men and women: Influence of insulin resistance on plasma triglyceride responses. *J. Clin. Endocrinol. Metab.* **2009**, *94*, 1562–1569. [CrossRef]
91. Banks, W.A.; Coon, A.B.; Robinson, S.M.; Moinuddin, A.; Shultz, J.M.; Nakaoke, R.; Morley, J.E. Triglycerides induce leptin resistance at the blood-brain barrier. *Diabetes* **2004**, *53*, 1253–1260. [CrossRef]
92. Hommel, J.D.; Trinko, R.; Sears, R.M.; Georgescu, D.; Liu, Z.W.; Gao, X.B.; Thurmon, J.J.; Marinelli, M.; DiLeone, R.J. Leptin receptor signaling in midbrain dopamine neurons regulates feeding. *Neuron* **2006**, *51*, 801–810. [CrossRef]
93. Jastreboff, A.M.; Sinha, R.; Lacadie, C.; Small, D.M.; Sherwin, R.S.; Potenza, M.N. Neural correlates of stress- and food cue-induced food craving in obesity: Association with insulin levels. *Diabetes Care* **2013**, *36*, 394–402. [CrossRef] [PubMed]
94. Hill, J.W.; Williams, K.W.; Ye, C.; Luo, J.; Balthasar, N.; Coppari, R.; Cowley, M.A.; Cantley, L.C.; Lowell, B.B.; Elmquist, J.K. Acute effects of leptin require PI3K signaling in hypothalamic proopiomelanocortin neurons in mice. *J. Clin. Investig.* **2008**, *118*, 1796–1805. [CrossRef] [PubMed]
95. Teff, K.L.; Elliott, S.S.; Tschop, M.; Kieffer, T.J.; Rader, D.; Heiman, M.; Townsend, R.R.; Keim, N.L.; D'Alessio, D.; Havel, P.J. Dietary fructose reduces circulating insulin and leptin, attenuates postprandial suppression of ghrelin, and increases triglycerides in women. *J. Clin. Endocrinol. Metab.* **2004**, *89*, 2963–2972. [CrossRef]
96. Lindqvist, A.; Baelemans, A.; Erlanson-Albertsson, C. Effects of sucrose, glucose and fructose on peripheral and central appetite signals. *Regul. Pept.* **2008**, *150*, 26–32. [CrossRef]
97. Rorabaugh, J.M.; Stratford, J.M.; Zahniser, N.R. Differences in bingeing behavior and cocaine reward following intermittent access to sucrose, glucose or fructose solutions. *Neuroscience* **2015**, *301*, 213–220. [CrossRef]
98. Purnell, J.Q.; Klopfenstein, B.A.; Stevens, A.A.; Havel, P.J.; Adams, S.H.; Dunn, T.N.; Krisky, C.; Rooney, W.D. Brain functional magnetic resonance imaging response to glucose and fructose infusions in humans. *Diabetes Obes. Metab.* **2011**, *13*, 229–234. [CrossRef]
99. Page, K.A.; Chan, O.; Arora, J.; Belfort-Deaguiar, R.; Dzuira, J.; Roehmholdt, B.; Cline, G.W.; Naik, S.; Sinha, R.; Constable, R.T.; et al. Effects of fructose vs glucose on regional cerebral blood flow in brain regions involved with appetite and reward pathways. *JAMA* **2013**, *309*, 63–70. [CrossRef]
100. Wölnerhanssen, B.K.; Meyer-Gerspach, A.C.; Schmidt, A.; Zimak, N.; Peterli, R.; Beglinger, C.; Borgwardt, S. Dissociable behavioral, physiological and neural effects of acute glucose and fructose ingestion: A pilot study. *PLoS ONE* **2015**, *10*, e0130280. [CrossRef]
101. Jastreboff, A.M.; Sinha, R.; Arora, J.; Giannini, C.; Kuba, T.J.; Malik, S.; Van Name, M.A.; Santoro, N.; Savoye, M.; Duran, E.J.; et al. Altered brain response to drinking glucose and fructose in obese adolescents. *Diabetes* **2016**, *65*, 1929–1939. [CrossRef]
102. Stice, E.; Burger, K.S.; Yokum, S. Relative ability of fat and sugar tastes to activate reward, gustatory, and somatosensory regions. *Am. J. Clin. Nutr.* **2013**, *98*, 1377–1384. [CrossRef]
103. American Psychiatric Association. *Diagnostic and Statistical Manual of Mental Disorders: DSM-5*; American Psychiatric Association: Washington, DC, USA, 2013.
104. Gordon, E.L.; Ariel-Donges, A.H.; Bauman, V.; Merlo, L.J. What Is the Evidence for "Food Addiction?" A Systematic Review. *Nutrients* **2018**, *10*, 477. [CrossRef]
105. Lustig, R.H. Fructose: It's alcohol without the "buzz". *Adv. Nutr.* **2013**, *4*, 226–235. [CrossRef] [PubMed]
106. Ng, S.W.; Slining, M.M.; Popkin, B.M. Use of caloric and noncaloric sweeteners in US consumer packaged foods, 2005–2009. *J. Acad. Nutr. Diet.* **2012**, *112*, 1828–1834. [CrossRef] [PubMed]
107. Andreyeva, T.; Long, M.W.; Brownell, K.D. The impact of food prices on consumption: A systematic review of research on the price elasticity of demand for food. *Am. J. Public Health* **2010**, *100*, 216–222. [CrossRef]
108. Wayne, G.F.; Carpenter, C.M. Tobacco industry manipulation of nicotine dosing. *Handb. Exp. Pharmacol.* **2009**, *192*, 457–485.

109. Segal, T. Profit Margin for Food and Beverage Sector. Available online: https://www.investopedia.com/ask/answers/071015/what-profit-margin-usual-company-food-and-beverage-sector.asp (accessed on 27 September 2020).
110. Chayka, K. Why coffee shortages won't change the price of your Frappucino. *Pacific Standard*, 30 July 2014.
111. Colchero, M.A.; Rivera-Dommarco, J.; Popkin, B.M.; Ng, S.W. In Mexico, evidence of sustained consumer response two years after implementing a sugar-sweetened beverage tax. *Health Aff.* **2017**, *36*, 564–571. [CrossRef]
112. Lustig, R.H. Fructose: Metabolic, hedonic, and societal parallels with ethanol. *J. Am. Diet. Assoc.* **2010**, *110*, 1307–1321. [CrossRef]
113. Onishi, Y.; Honda, M.; Ogihara, T.; Sakoda, H.; Anai, M.; Fujishiro, M.; Ono, H.; Shojima, N.; Fukushima, Y.; Inukai, K.; et al. Ethanol feeding induces insulin resistance with enhanced PI 3-kinase activation. *Biochem. Biophys. Res. Commun.* **2003**, *303*, 788–794. [CrossRef]
114. Softic, S.; Cohen, D.E.; Kahn, C.R. Role of dietary fructose and hepatic de novo lipogenesis in fatty liver disease. *Dig. Dis. Sci.* **2016**, *61*, 1282–1293. [CrossRef]
115. Stanhope, K.L.; Schwarz, J.M.; Havel, P.J. Adverse metabolic effects of dietary fructose: Results from recent epidemiological, clinical, and mechanistic studies. *Curr. Opin. Lipidol.* **2013**, *24*, 198–206. [CrossRef]
116. Lim, J.S.; Mietus-Snyder, M.; Valente, A.; Schwarz, J.M.; Lustig, R.H. The role of fructose in the pathogenesis of NAFLD and the metabolic syndrome. *Nat. Rev. Gastroenterol. Hepatol.* **2010**, *7*, 251–264. [CrossRef]
117. Dills, W.L. Protein fructosylation: Fructose and the Maillard reaction. *Am. J. Clin. Nutr.* **1993**, *58*, 779S–787S. [CrossRef] [PubMed]
118. Bremer, A.A.; Mietus-Snyder, M.L.; Lustig, R.H. Toward a unifying hypothesis of metabolic syndrome. *Pediatrics* **2012**, *129*, 557–570. [CrossRef]
119. Mortera, R.R.; Bains, Y.; Gugliucci, A. Fructose at the crossroads of the metabolic syndrome and obesity epidemics. *Front. Biosci.* **2019**, *24*, 186–211.
120. Rodríguez-Mortera, R.; Luevano-Contreras, C.; Solorio-Meza, S.; Caccavello, R.; Bains, Y.; Garay-Sevilla, M.E.; Gugliucci, A. Higher D-lactate levels are associated with higher prevalence of small dense low-density lipoprotein in obese adolescents. *Clin. Chem. Lab. Med.* **2018**, *56*, 1100–1108. [CrossRef]
121. Erkin-Cakmak, A.; Bains, Y.; Caccavello, R.; Noworolski, S.M.; Schwarz, J.M.; Mulligan, K.; Lustig, R.H.; Gugliucci, A. Isocaloric Fructose Restriction Reduces Serum d-Lactate Concentration in Children With Obesity and Metabolic Syndrome. *J. Clin. Endocrinol. Metab.* **2019**, *104*, 3003–3011. [CrossRef] [PubMed]
122. van Buul, V.J.; Tappy, L.; Brouns, F.J. Misconceptions about fructose-containing sugars and their role in the obesity epidemic. *Nutr. Res. Rev.* **2014**, *27*, 119–130. [CrossRef]
123. Mozaffarian, D.; Hao, T.; Rimm, E.B.; Willett, W.C.; Hu, F.B. Changes in diet and lifestyle and long-term weight gain in women and men. *N. Engl. J. Med.* **2011**, *364*, 2392–2404. [CrossRef]
124. Te Morenga, L.; Mallard, S.; Mann, J. Dietary sugars and body weight: Systematic review and meta-analyses of randomised controlled trials and cohort studies. *BMJ* **2013**, *346*, e7492. [CrossRef]
125. Bentley, R.A.; Ruck, D.J.; Fouts, H.N. U.S. obesity as delayed effect of excess sugar. *Econ. Hum. Biol.* **2020**, *36*, 100818. [CrossRef]
126. Gulati, S.; Misra, A. Sugar intake, obesity, and diabetes in India. *Nutrients* **2014**, *6*, 5955–5974. [CrossRef]
127. Deshpande, G.; Mapanga, R.F.; Essop, M.F. Frequent sugar-sweetened beverage consumption and the onset of cardiometabolic diseases: Cause for concern? *J. Endocr. Soc.* **2017**, *1*, 1372–1385. [CrossRef] [PubMed]
128. Malik, V.S.; Popkin, B.M.; Bray, G.A.; Despres, J.P.; Hu, F.B. Sugar-sweetened beverages, obesity, type 2 diabetes mellitus, and cardiovascular disease risk. *Circulation* **2010**, *121*, 1356–1364. [CrossRef]
129. Bray, G.A. Energy and fructose from beverages sweetened with sugar or high-fructose corn syrup pose a health risk for some people. *Adv. Nutr.* **2013**, *4*, 220–225. [CrossRef]
130. Ruff, J.S.; Suchy, A.K.; Hugentobler, S.A.; Sosa, M.M.; Schwartz, B.L.; Morrison, L.C.; Gieng, S.H.; Shigenaga, M.K.; Potts, W.K. Human-relevant levels of added sugar consumption increase female mortality and lower male fitness in mice. *Nat. Commun.* **2013**, *4*, 2245. [CrossRef] [PubMed]
131. Bremer, A.A.; Stanhope, K.L.; Graham, J.L.; Cummings, B.P.; Wang, W.; Saville, B.R.; Havel, P.J. Fructose-fed rhesus monkeys: A nonhuman primate model of insulin resistance, metabolic syndrome, and type 2 diabetes. *Clin. Transl. Sci.* **2011**, *4*, 243–252. [CrossRef]
132. EPIC-Interact Consortium. Consumption of sweet beverages and type 2 diabetes incidence in European adults: Results from EPIC-InterAct. *Diabetologia* **2013**, *56*, 1520–1530. [CrossRef]

133. Rodriguez, L.A.; Madsen, K.A.; Cotterman, C.; Lustig, R.H. Added sugar intake and metabolic syndrome in US adolescents: Cross-sectional analysis of NHANES 2005–2012. *Public Health Nutr.* **2016**, *19*, 2424–2434. [CrossRef]
134. Castro, V. Pure, white and deadly ... expensive: A bitter sweetness in health care expenditure. *Health Econ.* **2017**, *26*, 1644–1666. [CrossRef]
135. Barker, F.G. What is medical evidence? *Clin. Neurosurg.* **2009**, *56*, 24–33.
136. Stanhope, K.L.; Schwarz, J.M.; Keim, N.L.; Griffen, S.C.; Bremer, A.A.; Graham, J.L.; Hatcher, B.; Cox, C.L.; Dyachenko, A.; Zhang, W.; et al. Consuming fructose-, not glucose-sweetened beverages increases visceral adiposity and lipids and decreases insulin sensitivity in overweight/obese humans. *J. Clin. Investig.* **2009**, *119*, 1322–1334. [CrossRef]
137. Maersk, M.; Belza, A.; Stødkilde-Jørgensen, H.; Ringgaard, S.; Chabanova, E.; Thomsen, H.; Pedersen, S.B.; Astrup, A.; Richelsen, B. Sucrose-sweetened beverages increase fat storage in the liver, muscle, and visceral fat depot: A 6-mo randomized intervention study. *Am. J. Clin. Nutr.* **2012**, *95*, 283–289. [CrossRef]
138. Bray, G.A. How bad is fructose? *Am. J. Clin. Nutr.* **2007**, *86*, 895–896. [CrossRef]
139. Vos, M.B.; Kimmons, J.E.; Gillespie, C.; Welsh, J.; Blanck, H.M. Dietary fructose consumption among US children and adults: The Third National Health and Nutrition Examination Survey. *Medscape J. Med.* **2008**, *10*, 160.
140. Popkin, B.M.; Hawkes, C. Sweetening of the global diet, particularly beverages: Patterns, trends, and policy responses. *Lancet Diabetes Endccrinol.* **2016**, *4*, 174–186. [CrossRef]
141. Kuchler, F.; Stewart, H. *Price Trends Are Similar for Fruits, Vegetables, and Snack Foods*; U.S. Department of Agriculture: Washington, DC, USA, 2008. Available online: https://www.ers.usda.gov/webdocs/publications/45951/12368_err55.pdf?v=7164.8 (accessed on 27 September 2020).
142. Food and Nutrition Board, Institute of Medicine. *Food Marketing to Children and Youth: Threat or Opportunity?* National Academies Press: Washington, DC, USA, 2006; Available online: https://www.nap.edu/catalog/11514/food-marketing-to-children-and-youth-threat-or-opportunity (accessed on 27 September 2020).
143. Moodie, R.; Stuckler, D.; Monteiro, C.; Sheron, N.; Neal, B.; Thamarangsi, T.; Lincoln, P.; Casswell, S.; Lancet NCD Action Group. Profits and pandemics: Prevention of harmful effects of tobacco, alcohol, and ultra-processed food and drink industries. *Lancet* **2013**, *381*, 670–679. [CrossRef]
144. *Altria Group Inc. v. Good. 555 U.S. 70*; 2008; pp. 70–71. Available online: https://en.wikipedia.org/wiki/Altria_Group,_Inc._v._Good (accessed on 27 September 2020).
145. *FTC v. Sugar Information, Inc.*; 1972; Volume 81, F.T.C. 711; Available online: https://en.wikipedia.org/wiki/Altria_Group,_Inc._v._Good (accessed on 27 September 2020).
146. *Small v. Lorillard Tobacco Co. 94 N.Y.2d 43, 894*; 1999; pp. 894–895. Available online: https://en.wikipedia.org/wiki/Altria_Group,_Inc._v._Good (accessed on 27 September 2020).
147. *Pelman ex rel. Pelman v. McDonald's Corp. 396 F.3d 508*; 2005; pp. 508–509. Available online: https://en.wikipedia.org/wiki/Altria_Group,_Inc._v._Good (accessed on 27 September 2020).
148. Jarl, J.; Johansson, P.; Eriksson, A.; Eriksson, M.; Gerdtham, U.G.; Hemström, O.; Selin, K.H.; Lenke, L.; Ramstedt, M.; Room, R. The societal cost of alcohol consumption: An estimation of the economic and human cost including health effects in Sweden, 2002. *Eur. J. Health Econ.* **2008**, *9*, 351–360. [CrossRef] [PubMed]
149. Singh, G.M.; Micha, R.; Khatibzadeh, S.; Lim, S.; Ezzati, M.; Mozaffarian, D.; Global Burden of Diseases Nutrition and Chronic Diseases Expert Group (NutriCoDE). Estimated global, regional, and national disease burdens related to sugar-sweetened beverage consumption in 2010. *Circulation* **2015**, *132*, 639–666. [CrossRef]
150. Finkelstein, E.A.; DiBonaventura, M.; Burgess, S.M.; Hale, B.C. The costs of obesity in the workplace. *J. Occup. Environ. Med.* **2010**, *52*, 971–976. [CrossRef]
151. Strong, K.; Mathers, C.; Leeder, S.; Beaglehole, R. Preventing chronic diseases: How many lives can we save? *Lancet* **2005**, *366*, 1578–1582. [CrossRef]
152. Christeson, W.; Taggart, A.D.; Messner-Zidell, S.; Kiernan, M.; Cusick, J.; Day, R. Still too Fat to Fight. 2018. Available online: https://en.wikipedia.org/wiki/Altria_Group,_Inc._v._Good (accessed on 27 September 2020).
153. Mongeau, S.W. USAF Dental readiness classifications and caries-risk assessment. *Mil. Med.* **2008**, *173*, 42–47. [CrossRef]
154. Morgan Stanley Research. The Bittersweet Aftertaste of Sugar. 2015. Available online: http://static.latribune.fr/463077/etude-morgan-stanley-impact-diabete-sur-l-economie-mondiale.pdf (accessed on 27 September 2020).

155. Engelhard, C.L.; Garson, A.; Dorn, S. *Reducing Obesity: Policy Strategies from the Tobacco Wars*; Urban Institute: Washington, DC, USA, 2009.
156. Seabrook, J. Snacks for a fat planet. *New Yorker*, 16 May 2011.
157. Proctor, R.N. *Golden Holocaust: Origins of the Cigarette Catastrophe and the Case for Abolition*; University of California Press: Berkeley, CA, USA, 2011.
158. Pomeranz, J.L. The bittersweet truth about sugar labeling regulations: They are achievable and overdue. *Am. J. Public Health* **2012**, *102*, e14–e20. [CrossRef]
159. Epel, E.S.; Hartman, A.; Jacobs, L.M.; Leung, C.; Cohn, M.A.; Jensen, L.; Ishkanian, L.; Wojcicki, J.; Mason, A.E.; Lustig, R.H.; et al. Association of a workplace sales ban on sugar-sweetened beverages with employee consumption of sugar sweetened beverages and health. *JAMA Int. Med.* **2020**, *180*, 1–8. [CrossRef]
160. Jones, N.R.; Conklin, A.I.; Suhrcke, M.; Monsivais, P. The growing price gap between more and less healthy foods: Analysis of a novel longitudinal UK dataset. *PLoS ONE* **2014**, *9*, e109343. [CrossRef]
161. Cubanski, J.; Neuman, T. *The Facts on Medicare Spending and Financing*; Henry, J., Ed.; Kaiser Family Foundation: Washington, DC, USA, 2017; Available online: https://www.kff.org/medicare/issue-brief/the-facts-on-medicare-spending-and-financing/ (accessed on 27 September 2020).
162. Credit Suisse Research Institute. *Sugar: Consumption at a Crossroads*; Credit Suisse Research Institute: New York, NY, USA, 2013; Available online: http://wphna.org/wp-content/uploads/2014/01/13-09_Credit_Suisse_Sugar_crossroads.pdf (accessed on 27 September 2020).
163. Global Burden of Metabolic Risk Factors for Chronic Diseases Collaboration. Cardiovascular disease, chronic kidney disease, and diabetes mortality burden of cardiometabolic risk factors from 1980 to 2010: A comparative risk assessment. *Lancet Diabetes Endocrinol.* **2014**, *2*, 634–647. [CrossRef]
164. Triggle, N. NHS Ranked 'Number One' Health System. Available online: http://www.bbc.com/news/health-40608253 (accessed on 27 September 2020).
165. Hypoglycemia Support Foundation. Added Sugar Repository. Available online: https://hypoglycemia.org/added-sugar-repository/ (accessed on 27 September 2020).
166. U.S. Congress. Nutrition Labeling and Education Act. In *Public Law 101–535*; U.S. Congress: Washington, DC, USA, 1990. Available online: http://thomas.loc.gov/cgi-bin/bdquery/z?d101:H.R.3562 (accessed on 27 September 2020).
167. Lustig, R.H. Defusing the healthcare time bomb. *San Francisco Chronicle*. 6 January 2013. Available online: http://www.sfgate.com/opinion/article/Defusing-the-health-care-time-bomb-4168827.php (accessed on 27 September 2020).
168. Babor, T.; Caetano, R.; Casswell, S.; Edwards, G.; Giesbrecht, N.; Graham, K.; Grube, J.; Gruenewald, P.; Hill, L.; Holder, H.; et al. *Alcohol: No Ordinary Commodity—Research and Public Policy*; Oxford University Press: Oxford, UK, 2003.
169. Lustig, R.H.; Schmidt, L.A.; Brindis, C.D. The toxic truth about sugar. *Nature* **2012**, *487*, 27–29. [CrossRef] [PubMed]
170. Gan, Y.; Tong, X.; Li, L.; Cao, S.; Yin, X.; Gao, C.; Herath, C.; Li, W.; Jin, Z.; Chen, Y.; et al. Consumption of fruit and vegetable and risk of coronary heart disease: A meta-analysis of prospective cohort studies. *Int. J. Cardiol.* **2015**, *183*, 129–137. [CrossRef]
171. Schulze, M.B.; Manson, J.E.; Ludwig, D.S.; Colditz, G.A.; Stampfer, M.J.; Willett, W.C.; Hu, F.B. Sugar-sweetened beverages, weight gain, and incidence of type 2 diabetes in young and middle-aged women. *JAMA* **2004**, *292*, 927–934. [CrossRef]
172. Reynolds, A.; Mann, J.; Cummings, J.; Winter, N.; Mete, E.; Te Morenga, L. Carbohydrate quality and human health: A series of systematic reviews and meta-analyses. *Lancet* **2019**, *393*, 434–445. [CrossRef]
173. Mintz, S. *Sweetness and Power, The Place of Sugar in Modern History*; Penguin: New York, NY, USA, 1985.
174. Perheentupa, J.; Raivio, K. Fructose-induced hyperuricaemia. *Lancet* **1967**, *2*, 528–531. [CrossRef]
175. Tupala, E.; Tiihonen, J. Dopamine and alcoholism: Neurobiological basis of ethanol abuse. *Prog. Neuropsychopharmacol. Biol. Psychiatry* **2004**, *28*, 1221–1247. [CrossRef] [PubMed]
176. Edwards, G.; Anderson, P.; Babor, T.F.; Casswell, S.; Ferrence, R.; Giesbrecht, N.; Godfrey, C.; Holder, H.D.; Lemmens, P.H.; Mäkelä, K.; et al. Retail price influences on alcohol consumption, and taxation on alcohol as a prevention strategy. In *Alcohol Policy and the Public Good*; Edwards, G., Ed.; Oxford University Press: New York, NY, USA, 1994; pp. 109–213.

177. Greenfield, T.K.; Graves, K.L.; Kaskutas, L.A. Alcohol warning labels for prevention: National survey results. *Alcohol Health Res. World* **1993**, *17*, 67–75.
178. Walls, H.L.; Peeters, A.; Proietto, J.; McNeil, J.J. Public health campaigns and obesity—A critique. *BMC Public Health* **2011**, *11*, 136. [CrossRef]
179. Gonzalez-Suarez, C.; Worley, A.; Grimmer-Somers, K.; Dones, V. School-based interventions on childhood obesity: A meta-analysis. *Am. J. Prev. Med.* **2009**, *37*, 418–427. [CrossRef]
180. Siegel, R.L.; Miller, K.D.; Iemal, A. Cancer statistics, 2020. *CA* **2020**, *70*, 7–30. [CrossRef] [PubMed]
181. Briggs, A.D.M.; Mytton, O.T.; Kehlbacher, A.; Tiffin, R.; Elhussein, A.; Rayner, M.; Jebb, S.A.; Blakely, T.; Scarborough, P. Health impact assessment of the UK soft drinks industry levy: A comparative risk assessment modelling study. *Lancet Public Health* **2016**, *2*, e15–e22. [CrossRef]
182. Lee, Y.; Mozaffarian, D.; Sy, S.; Liu, J.; Wilde, P.E.; Marklund, M.; Abrahams-Gessel, S.; Gaziano, T.A.; Micha, R. Health Impact and Cost-Effectiveness of Volume, Tiered, and Absolute Sugar Content Sugar-Sweetened Beverage Tax Policies in the United States: A Microsimulation Study. *Circulation* **2020**, *142*, 523–534. [CrossRef]
183. Amadeo, K. Farm Subsidies with Pros, Cons, and Impact How Farm Subsidies Affect You. Available online: https://www.thebalance.com/farm-subsidies-4173885 (accessed on 4 July 2019).
184. Alston, J.M.; Sumner, D.A.; Vosti, S.A. *Farm Subsidies and Obesity in the United States*; University of California: Berkeley, CA, USA, 2007; Available online: http://giannini.ucop.edu/media/are-update/files/articles/v11n2_1.pdf (accessed on 27 September 2020).
185. Menzel, P. Hungry Planet: What the World Eats—In pictures. *The Guardian*. 6 May 2019. Available online: https://www.theguardian.com/lifeandstyle/gallery/2013/may/06/hungry-planet-what-world-eats (accessed on 27 September 2020).
186. Crossley, D. 10 Reasons to Take "Our Future in the Land" Seriously. Available online: https://www.foodethicscouncil.org/10-reasons-to-take-our-future-in-the-land-seriously/ (accessed on 27 September 2020).
187. Schmidt, L.A.; Patel, A.; Brindis, C.D.; Lustig, R.H. Towards evidence-based policies for reduction of dietary sugars: Lessons from the alcohol experience. In *Dietary Sugars and Health*; Goran, M.I., Tappy, L., Le, K.A., Eds.; Taylor and Francis: Milton Park, UK, 2014; pp. 371–390.
188. Room, R. *The Effects of Nordic Alcohol Policies: What Happens to Drinking and Harm When Alcohol Controls Change?* Nordic Council for Alcohol and Drug Research: Helsinki, Finland, 2002.
189. Lima, J.M.; Galea, S. Corporate practices and health: A framework and mechanisms. *Glob. Health* **2018**, *14*, 21. [CrossRef]

Publisher's Note: MDPI stays neutral with regard to jurisdictional claims in published maps and institutional affiliations.

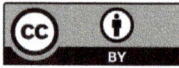

© 2020 by the author. Licensee MDPI, Basel, Switzerland. This article is an open access article distributed under the terms and conditions of the Creative Commons Attribution (CC BY) license (http://creativecommons.org/licenses/by/4.0/).

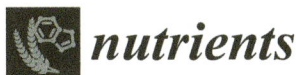

Review

Food Addiction and Psychosocial Adversity: Biological Embedding, Contextual Factors, and Public Health Implications

David A. Wiss [1], Nicole Avena [2,3] and Mark Gold [4,*]

1. Fielding School of Public Health, University of California Los Angeles, Los Angeles, CA 90095, USA; dwiss@ucla.edu
2. Department of Neuroscience, Icahn School of Medicine at Mount Sinai, New York, NY 10029, USA; nicoleavena@gmail.com
3. Department of Psychology, Princeton University, Princeton, NJ 08540, USA
4. School of Medicine, Washington University in St. Louis, St. Louis, MO 63130, USA
* Correspondence: drmarkgold@gmail.com; Tel.: +1-904-955-7079

Received: 18 September 2020; Accepted: 13 November 2020; Published: 16 November 2020

Abstract: The role of stress, trauma, and adversity particularly early in life has been identified as a contributing factor in both drug and food addictions. While links between traumatic stress and substance use disorders are well documented, the pathways to food addiction and obesity are less established. This review focuses on psychosocial and neurobiological factors that may increase risk for addiction-like behaviors and ultimately increase BMI over the lifespan. Early childhood and adolescent adversity can induce long-lasting alterations in the glucocorticoid and dopamine systems that lead to increased addiction vulnerability later in life. Allostatic load, the hypothalamic-pituitary-adrenal axis, and emerging data on epigenetics in the context of biological embedding are highlighted. A conceptual model for food addiction is proposed, which integrates data on the biological embedding of adversity as well as upstream psychological, social, and environmental factors. Dietary restraint as a feature of disordered eating is discussed as an important contextual factor related to food addiction. Discussion of various public health and policy considerations are based on the concept that improved knowledge of biopsychosocial mechanisms contributing to food addiction may decrease stigma associated with obesity and disordered eating behavior.

Keywords: food addiction; eating disorder; obesity; stress; trauma; early life adversity; adverse childhood experience; dopamine; epigenetics; biopsychosocial

1. Background

The quest to discover the precise mechanisms of hedonic overeating began decades ago. While many theories have been proposed, none have been widely accepted, and the obesity epidemic continues to grow. The *Nutrition Transition* theory describes a global trend toward consumption of processed foods that are low in fiber and high in added sugars and fats [1]. The changing global food landscape in the past four decades have increased access to convenient "snack" foods and decreased time spent preparing foods at home [2]. Several lines of research have explored the idea that highly palatable foods can alter brain reward pathways. For example, a landmark study showed that dopamine (DA) receptors were significantly lower in individuals with obesity [3]. Soon after, investigators documented overlapping neuroimaging characteristics in humans with obesity and those with substance use disorders (SUDs), showing reductions in DA-D2 receptors [4]. It was then suggested that individuals may overeat to compensate for DA-D2 receptor dysfunction [5]. To date, it is not clear whether these neurochemical associations are a cause of addiction-like overeating or a consequence [6]. However, similar to other addictions, changes that occur in obesity show that food reinforcement adapts, strongly implicating biological underpinnings. Given the limited success in reversing the obesity trends, a better understanding of the various biopsychosocial mechanisms may help inform public health efforts.

Bart Hoebel pioneered the concept of food addiction (FA) research using animal models, showing evidence of bingeing, withdrawal, craving, and concomitant changes in dopaminergic and opioidergic systems in response to overeating sugar [7–14]. In rodent studies, early life adversity (ELA) has been shown to induce alterations in DA neuronal activity and synaptic function [15], impacting reward-directed behavior and partially accounting for individual variation along the mesolimbic DA projection [16]. More recently it has been shown that chronic stress dysregulates the reward system, promotes addiction-like eating, and contributes to the development of obesity [17]. Furthermore, palatable diets buffer against the negative impact of social stressors in juvenile rats [18]. Interestingly, environmental enrichment (larger space with conspecifics and novel objects) reduced sugar seeking and consumption [19]. Other rodent studies documented early and persistent alterations in amygdala circuitry and function following exposure to ELA, which were not diminished when the stressor was removed [20]. This suggests that ELA is not always redeemable by subsequent experience. At present, there is a gap in our understanding of how various forms of stress, trauma, and adversity link to addiction-like eating in real-world settings, particularly when viewed in social context, as well as over the lifespan.

In humans, various forms of ELA are associated with illicit drug use later in life [21–23]. In addition, there are established links between ELA and obesity [21,24], however, the exact mechanisms are not understood. A recent systematic review on childhood obesity implicated stress as a midstream factor that can lead to "junk food" self-medication and subtle addiction, in order to alleviate uncomfortable emotional states [25]. In a nationally representative sample of young adults (n = 10,813) exposure to multiple types of child maltreatment predicted excessive sugary beverage consumption [26]. In a Brazilian sample (n = 7639) FA was independently associated with early life physical and sexual abuse [27]. A positron emission tomography (PET) study also found that long-term exposure to adversity is associated with reduced striatal DA synthesis capacity [28]. Functional magnetic resonance imaging (fMRI) studies have linked ELA to blunted subjective responses to reward-predicting cues [29], and to altered connectivity in the extended reward network, leading to increased vulnerability to FA and obesity later in life [30]. While there are sufficient data that describes life course associations between ELA and adult weight outcomes [24], the actual biological mechanisms are less understood, which is a primary focus of this review. Another aim is to integrate psychologically relevant contextual factors such as weight stigma and pathological dieting.

The purpose of this review is to focus on literature from FA as well as obesity in the context of exposure to trauma, stress, and adversity, in an effort to answer three questions: (1) is FA a biologically plausible explanation for a life course association between ELA and obesity? (2) how might other relevant psychological, social, and environmental factors contribute to FA and to obesity? (see Figure 1) and finally, (3) what does it mean for public health? For simplicity, we have conceptually merged stress/trauma/adversity (STA) at several points throughout, particularly when reviewed outside of the context of early life, however we acknowledge these are not identical concepts. We also acknowledge that FA does not always lead to obesity, and that obesity can occur in the absence of FA. Additionally, ELA is used synonymously with adverse childhood experience (ACE) to describe exposures in the first 18 years of life. This review draws from literature across multiple disciplines in order to consider both individual and population health perspectives, and to describe contextual factors related to the neurobiology of FA. It is important to translate obesity science into a relevant social context, in order to identify achievable intervention targets which may have a meaningful impact upstream.

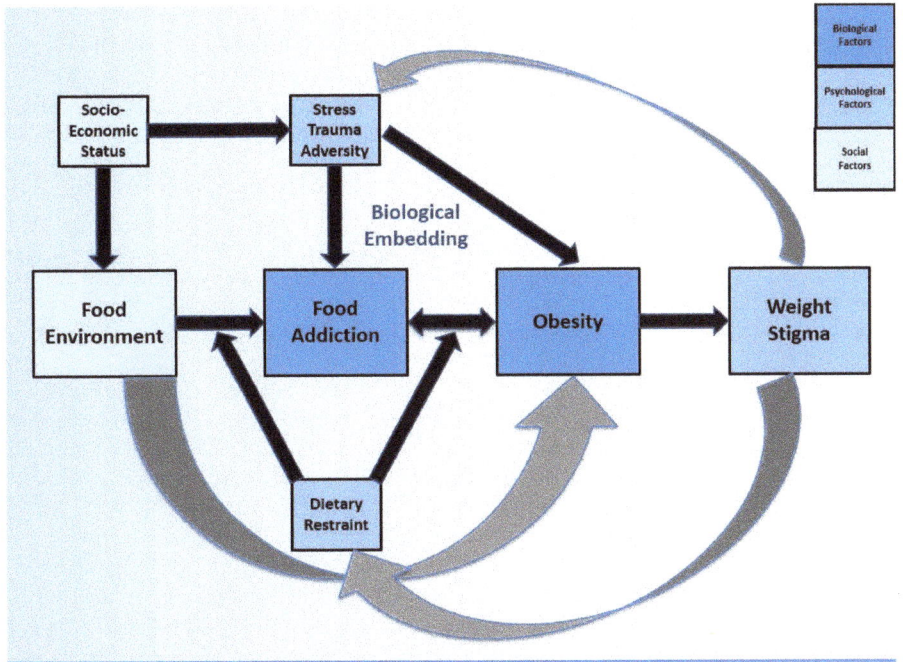

Figure 1. Food addiction and obesity following exposure to stress, trauma, and adversity: A biopsychosocial perspective of contextual factors.

1.1. The Biopsychosocial Model & Other Foundational Theories

Social and biological processes overlap and are inextricably linked. However, research methods are often incapable of capturing all features of an observed phenomenon, such as the various drivers of obesity (see Figure 1). Another example is how addiction neuroscience overlooks key social factors such as exclusion and marginalization which would make these findings more clinically relevant [31]. Biopsychosocial models were originally proposed by Engel as a new way to understand health and disease, by considering influence from various domains [32]. Biopsychosocial obesity research has found that lower educational attainment is associated with higher BMI, after adjusting for biological (energy intake and expenditure), psychological (decisional balance) and social (support) factors [33]. A biopsychosocial approach to childhood obesity should consider the (1) biology of the child (2) family environment and immediate psychosocial influences and (3) wider environmental, social, and cultural influences [34]. This creates opportunity for collaboration across multiple academic and clinically-focused disciplines. The current review employs a biopsychosocial perspective on FA, considering obesity as one possible outcome. This manuscript also incorporates Krieger's *Ecosocial Theory* which emphasizes the social production of disease over biomedical individualism, describing "embodiment" as the biological incorporation of social and ecological circumstances into everyday life [35]. A *Life Course Perspective* is used to link ELA to adult health [36–38]. Finally, a *Developmental Psychology* perspective views human development as relational, pertaining to dynamics (e.g., community features) which require individuals to be contextually situated into multidirectional and reciprocating ecological systems [39–41].

1.2. Food Addiction & Eating Disorders

With the validation of the *Yale Food Addiction Scale* (YFAS) in 2009 [42] and the updated YFAS 2.0 in 2016 [43], FA in humans has been operationalized across hundreds of studies. At the present time, FA has not been recognized as an official eating disorder (ED) in the Diagnostic and Statistical Manual (DSM) of Mental Disorders. Unique aspects of addictions include the importance of the substance, withdrawal, and tolerance, whereas unique aspects of EDs include restraint/rules, and shape/weight concerns [44]. It is well-established that dietary restraint/restriction can lead to rebound bingeing [45] yet it remains unclear if this is a cause or consequence of FA symptoms (discussed in Section 5.1). Thus, disordered eating characterized by dietary restraint provides important context for FA data. It has been recently suggested that the presence of dieting behavior must be carefully evaluated in order to separate the FA "signal" from the "noise" [46]. For example, ED research has identified significant overlap between FA and bulimia nervosa (BN), with FA symptoms improving when BN symptoms remit [47]. FA prevalence is the highest in BN [48] compared with other EDs, suggesting that FA treatment models should consider symptom contribution from dietary restraint and other compensatory behaviors. It has been proposed that FA is a transdiagnostic disorder associated with neurobiological vulnerability in certain people, who are more susceptible to using food as a coping mechanism [49]. It has also been shown that FA predicts a worse treatment outcome in patients with binge eating disorder (BED) [50].

Among those with an ED diagnosis, Brewerton (2017) proposed that the presence of FA be conceptualized as a meaningful correlate of post-traumatic stress disorder (PTSD) severity and symptoms [51]. For example, data from the Nurses' Health Study II has shown that severe physical and sexual abuse are associated with a 90% increase in FA risk [52]. The same dataset also suggested that symptoms of PTSD are associated with an increased prevalence of FA [53]. In a sample of 301 overweight and obese women, the association between FA and childhood trauma remained significant after adjusting for potential confounders such as socioeconomic status (SES) [54]. In a sample of bariatric surgery seeking patients (n = 1586), elevated ACE scores correlated with an increased likelihood of screening positive for FA [55]. A recent meta-analysis showed that multiple ACEs increased the odds of adult obesity by 46% (95% CI: 28–64%) [24] but several unmeasured confounders likely influence this estimate, such as the presence of EDs and SUDs, which frequently cluster, co-occur, and lead to weight fluctuations [56,57]. Therefore, risk estimates between childhood adversity and adult obesity would likely be higher after adjusting for these diagnoses often associated with dietary restriction and weight control, however this has not been formally tested. While data linking ELA to EDs are robust, only recently has it been shown that FA symptoms can mediate this pathway, as well as exacerbate ED symptoms significantly across all forms of childhood maltreatment [58]. Although EDs are not directly featured in Figure 1, the constructs of dietary restraint and weight stigma are used to contextualize important associations between EDs and FA. Notwithstanding, there are likely paths from ELA to obesity that are better captured by more classic ED pathology (e.g., BED) rather than FA, which are not directly featured by the model.

2. Food Addiction Neuroscience & Social Context

A frequent criticism of FA data in clinical settings is that the measure itself does not account for restrained eating [46] (discussed in Section 5.1). Another criticism is that it remains unclear how to intervene once FA has been detected. A recent systematic review of mostly pilot and feasibility studies concluded that currently there are no empirically supported psychosocial interventions for FA [59]. The authors recommend that clinicians assess for comorbid ED, and if present, provide evidence-based treatments (e.g., cognitive behavioral therapy) for those conditions. There is growing support for the FA construct in studies using the YFAS as well as neuroimaging studies on obesity that do not use "food addiction" terminology, with several examples provided below. It is worth noting that many authors reject the FA term in favor of other language such as eating addiction [60], or with additional qualifiers such as refined or processed food addiction [61,62], and even food use disorder [63]. Figure 1 proposes that FA is one driver of obesity, although there are several others, including some not captured by the model (discussed further in Section 2.1).

Neurobiological overlaps between obesity and addiction have been described within the mesolimbic pathway between the ventral tegmental area (VTA) and the ventral striatum, with further projection to limbic (amygdala and hippocampus) and cortical regions (prefrontal cortex [PFC] and cingulate gyrus) [64]. Recent data suggests that among 110 healthy lean adults, exposure to a Western-style diet for one week led to rapid declines in hippocampal-dependent learning and memory, as well as appetitive control [65]. Research has shown that obesity (similar to SUD) is associated with deficits in executive functioning, an umbrella term encompassing the higher-order cognitive processes that help people take goal-directed action [66]. In a sample of women with obesity (n = 36), FA severity has been associated with impaired decision-making, compared to controls [67]. Resting-state fMRI data has shown decreased functional connectivity in the frontal gyrus in adults with obesity (n = 20) compared to controls [68]. A large cross-sectional study of children ages 9–11 (n = 2700) showed that increased BMI is associated with a reduced mean cortical thickness as well as lower executive functioning [69]. A follow-up report from the same study (n = 3190) suggested that BMI is associated with PFC development as well as diminished working memory [70]. Interestingly, a nationally representative sample of US adults (n = 4769 mean age 29) found that obesity is associated with poor working memory in women, but not men [71]. While tempting to consider that biological sex differences explain these findings, social context would suggest that the experience of weight stigma (discussed in Section 5.2), which is higher in women than men [72] may be a contributing factor. Recent data on school-age children (n = 176) suggests that weight-related stereotype threat (fear of confirming a negative stereotype) may explain working memory deficits more so than excess body weight [73].

Among patients with obesity (n = 224), FA is more closely correlated with psychological factors (depressive symptoms, quality of life) than with metabolic parameters (BMI, fat percentage, waist circumference) [74]. In a small sample of adult community members (n = 52), individuals with FA had significantly higher scores on depressive symptoms, emotion dysregulation, emotional eating, demand characteristics, motives, impulsivity, and family history of mental health problems and addiction [75]. Impulsivity can be defined as decision-making with limited forethought (rash-spontaneous behavior), having strong associations with FA [76–79]. Impulsivity hinders inhibitory control and is associated with increased intake of food [80] and drugs [81], often heightened in response to novel stimuli [82]. Delay discounting (preference for "smaller sooner" rather than "larger later" rewards) is closely associated with impulsivity and has been correlated with YFAS scores [83]. These authors believe it to be a predisposing factor rather than a consequence, although bidirectionality is likely. It has been suggested that impulsivity-related domains such as lower self-control, higher reward sensitivity, and negative affect help explain some similarities between addiction and obesity [84]. While impulsivity has heritable components linked to the mesocorticolimbic system [85] as well as serotonin-related candidate genes (e.g., HTR2A) [86], the potential for these traits to be influenced by epigenetic modification following psychosocial adversity will be explored in Section 3.1.

2.1. Food Environment as a Driver of Food Addiction & Obesity

The proposed pathways in Figure 1 suggest that FA may partially mediate the relationship between the food environment and obesity. Other pathways also exist. For example, census tract data have been used to show that wealthier neighborhoods (using median income) have better access (physical availability) to markets with healthier foods compared to poor neighborhoods [87]. Considering the importance of the built environment, neighborhood features (e.g., crime) that discourage outdoor physical activity are consistently linked to higher BMIs [88]. Recognizing that built, socioeconomic, and social characteristics co-occur [89], several investigators have advocated for a better understanding of theory-driven mediators and moderators in the relationship between neighborhood context and obesity [90,91]. Given the link between STA and FA, unsafe environments associated with lower SES neighborhoods are likely to impact BMI through increases in reward-based eating. It has been established that diet quality tends to follow a SES gradient [92]. It has also been shown that parental fruit/vegetable consumption is linked to adolescent fruit/vegetable consumption [93], suggesting that the home food environment is important. Not eating dinner as a family has also been linked with increased BMI in kindergarten age children, regardless of SES [94]. It has been proposed that the maltreatment-obesity association is spurious, driven by confounding through the home food environment. However, after testing, researchers have found limited confounding influence [95] which supports arguments in favor of biological mechanisms.

Innovative methods that assess food environments include examining the (1) ratio of fast-food to full-service restaurants (2) ratio of bars/pubs to liquor stores and (3) presence of markets [96]. Multilevel models typically adjust for individual factors (education, hours of walking per week) as well as neighborhood factors (deprivation, walkability score). Perhaps the combination of food environment features matters more than individual components [96]. While several studies have described neighborhood "food swamps" (high density of high-calorie junk food) as predictive of obesity [97], few studies have looked at the potential roles of psychosocial pathways (mental health and wellbeing) [98]. A recent systematic review found that overall psychological resources (i.e., stress) had more consistent evidence of mediation than external neighborhood in the relationship between SES and BMI [91]. One study (n = 1112 adults) showed that paths from neighborhood characteristics to BMI could be partially explained by psychological distress and measures of inflammation [99] (discussed in Section 3). Taken together, FA is one potential pathway linking the food environment to obesity, however there is a "backdoor path" [100] through SES to STA, as well as a pathway that may not include FA (i.e., through the built environment). Comprehensive biopsychosocial frameworks cannot be tested or explained by any single study. There is conceptual support for the theory that the external environment (quick, cheap, highly palatable foods) is an upstream driver of EDs however this not been thoroughly investigated (discussed in Section 6.1). Figure 1 represents a synthesis of literature reviewed so far, as well as a roadmap for subsequent sections.

2.2. Socioeconomic Status

Given the inverse relationship between SES and BMI [101,102], obesity can also be viewed as a social phenomenon. This negative relationship has been shown in numerous countries outside of the US (e.g., Netherlands, Turkey, Morocco, South Asia) [103]. Hot-spot analysis in the US shows that higher BMI clusters are more likely in socioeconomically disadvantaged minority neighborhoods [104]. Meanwhile, large datasets (n = 43,864) have shown that obesity risk is decreased when positive contextual factors (maternal mental health, school safety, and child resilience) are present [105]. A large population-based cohort from the UK (n = 18,733) found that home-based deprivation was more closely associated with changes in child BMI than school-based deprivation [106]. On the other hand, some authors believe that the root cause of ACEs are largely based in the community, originating from an accumulation of contextual risk factors beyond a child's control, including family history, failed attachment, safety/security, and neighborhood risks [107]. While models of addiction and obesity are incomplete without psychosocial context, current research methods cannot adequately contextualize risk. Hence, literature from multiple disciplines was used to synthesize our conceptual model, which could be expanded with additional constructs such as resilience.

To illustrate further, a recent study showed that individuals with higher ACE scores were more likely to report not finishing high school, unemployment, and living below the poverty level [108]. Sustained activation and loss of capacity to respond to chronic stress might lead to a higher risk of illness and disease among people in lower SES categories [109]. It has been recognized that the processes which mediate the relationship between ELA and adult obesity might differ between men and women [110–112]. For example, a recent systematic review found that perceived stress from structural racism and weight stigma among black women creates negative emotions which predict emotional eating [113]. These stressors may then increase metabolic disturbance. Obesity itself can be a stressful state due to high prevalence of weight stigma [114] (discussed in Section 5.2), as highlighted by the feedback loop in Figure 1. Obesity may be driving changes in stress biology rather than stress biology driving obesity [115]. Next, we consider the impact of ELA (as well as STA more broadly) from a life course perspective, describing precise (as well as candidate) mechanisms by which social factors impact health, seen primarily through recent SUD and obesity research.

3. Biological Embedding of Stress, Trauma, & Adversity

The fetal and infant origins of adult disease was proposed by Barker in 1990 [116]. This focus on the biological basis of disease gave rise to concepts such as allostatic load (AL), defined as the "cost of chronic exposure to fluctuating or heightened neural or neuroendocrine response resulting from repeated or chronic environmental challenge" [117]. This can be operationalized using a range of biomarkers that indicate inflammation and long-term "weathering." A simpler definition of AL is the price of adaption that leads to disease states over time. It has been suggested that frequent activation of the stress response and the failure to shut off allostatic activity creates "wear and tear" [118]. A landmark study showed that higher AL scores were associated with poorer cognitive and physical functioning, increasing the risk of cardiovascular diseases independent of sociodemographic risk factors [119]. Higher levels of AL (indexed by measures of blood pressure, C-reactive protein, fibrinogen, cholesterol ratio, triglycerides, and cortisol) have been observed in higher weight individuals [120]. This research suggested that these cumulatively elevated biomarkers link to decreased inhibitory control, highlighting the potential for disordered eating to become very difficult to overcome, similar to drug addiction.

It has been suggested that inflammatory mediators act on cortico-amygdala (threat) and cortico-basal ganglia (reward) circuits in a manner which predisposes individuals to "self-medicating" behaviors such as drug use, smoking, and the excess consumption of highly palatable foods [121]. Such behaviors further propagate inflammation and create a self-sustaining feedback loop. The "neuroimmune network hypothesis" proposes that ELA amplifies the communication between the brain and the immune system, promoting low grade peripheral inflammation [122]. The "glucocorticoid cascade hypothesis" posits that stress hormones impair brain function which further increases cortisol levels [123]. Adolescents exposed to childhood adversity have larger pituitary gland volume, associated with lower cortisol awakening response [124]. These authors propose that attenuation of hypothalamic-pituitary-adrenal (HPA) axis function may derive from stress-induced chronic hyperactivation during childhood. Heightened susceptibility may be due to differences in corticotrophin-releasing hormone (CRH) within the HPA axis, responsible for the output of cortisol [125]. Individual differences in inflammatory reactivity might explain why people have differing susceptibility to the consequences of stress, which may include neuroinflammation from stress-induced pro-inflammatory cytokines [126]. A recent cohort study of nine- and ten-year-old children showed that pro-inflammatory diets (i.e., high in saturated fats) increase neuroinflammation in reward-related brain regions, which in turn lead to further unhealthy eating and obesity [127].

A meta-analysis of 1781 people documented significantly decreased hippocampal volumes following ELA, with weaker evidence of increased amygdala volumes [128]. Alterations in corticolimbic circuitry following exposure to trauma make adolescents (n = 64) less able to relax and more vulnerable to risky behavior [129]. Other observable neural changes following ELA include (1) structural variation in gray and white matter (2) functional variation in brain activity and functional connectivity and (3) altered neurotransmitter metabolism [130]. In line with what has been observed in rodent studies [131], these effects might not be restricted to one's own lifespan but may also be transmitted to offspring [132]. It is well established that paternal drug exposure has long-lasting consequences including altered drug sensitivity in subsequent generations [133] but only recently has intergenerational transmission of trauma consistent with epigenetic explanations been described [134]. In animal models, the effects of maternal care on developing DA pathways and reward-directed behavior may account for individual differences in the mesolimbic DA system [16]. In social context, addictions may promote compromised parenting increasing the possibility that suboptimal care may be provided to the next generation. There is a timely need for longitudinal studies that capture the precise biological mechanisms that link ELA to addictions over time, as well as their consequences.

3.1. Epigenetic Mechanisms of Biological Embedding

Epigenetics is the study of how the environment regulates the genome, best described as changes in gene function without changes in gene sequence. DNA methylation is an enzymatically-catalyzed modification of DNA and is one plausible mechanism through which early life exposures (low SES, nutritional patterns) become biologically embedded [135]. Methylation changes are apparent even years after the exposure but can be reversible in some cases. Epigenetic processes may be a key mediator between social environments during childhood and disease risk throughout life. Both DNA methylation and demethylation mechanisms are likely recruited during early life unfavorable experiences [136]. Other forms of epigenetic modification include histone modification and noncoding ribonucleic acids [137].

A milestone study confirmed what had been previously shown in animal models: human parental care impacts epigenetic regulation of hippocampal glucocorticoid receptor gene (NR3C1) expression [138]. Such epigenetic marks that persist into adulthood may influence vulnerability for psychopathology through its impact on HPA axis function. However, it is difficult to determine if DNA methylation changes are the immediate results of ELA or a consequence of the phenotypes associated with such adversity [139]. Notwithstanding, NR3C1 has been linked to prenatal stress [140] and is the most studied gene to date related to abuse and neglect [141]. Other genes involved in HPA axis regulation such as corticotrophin-releasing factor (CRF) have been investigated [142]. It is not implausible that developmental programming of the HPA axis and subsequent regulation of the stress response might impact addiction susceptibility, thereby increasing intake of substances known to activate reward pathways, including highly palatable food.

Epigenetic control of the expression of opioid receptor genes (mu-, delta-, and kappa-) has been reviewed in the context of SUDs [143]. While methylation at the mu-opioid receptor (MOR) gene is most strongly associated with drug addiction [144] as well as incentive motivation for processed food [145,146], decreased methylation at the kappa-opioid receptor (KOR) in the anterior insula has been shown in child abuse [147] (discussed further in Section 4.1). In this study of postmortem brain structures, the investigators were unable to detect a change in MOR expression, suggesting different epigenetic signatures associated with addictions and ELA. It is worth noting that different drugs have impacts at different brain regions and many include histone modifications in the nucleus accumbens (NAc) [148]. Other potentially relevant epigenetic modifications include the serotonin transporters [149–151] and proopiomelanocortin (POMC) [152]. Additional research is needed to determine how various epigenetic modifications associate with various forms of disordered eating, including FA.

In a sample of 206 women with bulimic symptomatology, there was evidence of increased methylation of the DA-D2 gene promoter, compared to controls [153]. Taq1A polymorphisms at the D2 receptor has been well-studied and known to influence impulsive behavior [154]. Recent data shows that DNA methylation in obesity-related genes may relate to obesity risk in adolescents [155]. Increased obesity susceptibility genes (e.g., FTO) have been found in the insula and substantia nigra (brain regions involved in addiction and reward) [156]. It has been shown that the methylation status on DA signaling genes (SLC18A1 and SLC6A3) might underlie epigenetic mechanisms contributing to carbohydrate and calorie consumption, as well as fat deposition [157]. Recently authors have linked specific dietary components with the gut microbiome in an effort to determine epigenetic factors on offspring susceptibility to obesity [158]. Expression levels of candidate genes implicated in glucose and energy homeostasis (e.g., HDAC7 and IGF2BP2) could be epigenetically regulated by gut bacterial populations [159]. The link between epigenetic marks and gut microbes appear to be mediated by host-microbial metabolites acting as substrates and cofactors for key epigenetic enzymes in the host [160]. More research linking epigenetics to the microbiome is timely and warranted, particularly in the context of dysfunctional eating behavior (including both under- and overeating).

4. Stress & Obesity

While a PTSD diagnosis is associated with an altered stress response, chronic stress can exist in the absence of PTSD, and has been the focus of several investigations related to eating behavior. Multiple pathways have been described which link stress to obesity, including (1) interference with cognitive processes (executive function, self-regulation) (2) behavior (eating, physical activity, sleep) (3) physiological changes (HPA axis, reward processing, gut microbiome) and (4) production of biochemical hormones and peptides (leptin, ghrelin, neuropeptide Y) [114]. At a basic level, stress may lead to food consumption in the absence of hunger. It is established that poor executive functioning is associated with consumption of palatable food, leading to inflammation and metabolic changes promoting weight gain [161–163]. Other pathways which have been identified include the autonomic nervous system (cardiovascular functioning), the epigenome (intergenerational transmission), and the metabolome (profile of metabolites in body) [164]. The vagus nerve (part of the autonomic nervous system) has been identified as an important physiological stress pathway linked to gut microbiota [165]. With rising interest in the gut-brain axis, novel pathways which include FA are being explored [166]. FA can be considered as a partial mediator in the stress-obesity pathway, likely resulting from one or many of the biologically embedded pathways described herein.

To illustrate further, individual differences in neural response to food cues under stress have been observed in human neuroimaging studies [167], lending support to differential susceptibility. It is well established that amygdala function is moderated by stress-induced glucocorticoid (GC) release [20], and a less efficient HPA axis negative feedback loop may represent a deficiency in emotion and stress regulation [168]. Highly palatable foods stimulate stress hormones that alter the limbic system (emotions) and striatal (motivational) pathways, promoting further food craving and excessive intake [169]. Rewarding foods upregulate CRF in the amygdala and related limbic striatal pathways. The most direct physiological pathway is dominated by cortisol, which stimulates fat storage and changes dietary behavior through increased reward sensitivity (DA and opioid systems) and increased appetite (arcuate nucleus in the hypothalamus) [165]. Future research should attempt to clarify the biological embedding of chronic stress both in the absence and presence of diagnosed PTSD, specifically impacting reward-related pathways associated with consumption behavior. Additionally, more research is needed on biopsychosocial factors of resilience in the context of both FA and obesity.

4.1. Stress & Addictions

Given the established links between stress and obesity, these links can be used to conceptualize relationships between stress and FA. The phenomenon of stress-induced reinstatement of drug-seeking is generalizable to other substances, including food [170]. To illustrate, the DA and GC systems are both highly involved in substance addictions, and ELA may induce long-lasting alterations in these systems. One of the most profound effects of stress is the activation of the HPA axis with release of CRF from the paraventricular nucleus. Human studies have shown stress exposure increases alcohol craving [171]. Both chronic stress and long-standing alcohol use promote PFC dysfunction [172]. Changes in CRF activity that result from chronic alcohol exposure within the extended amygdala network is thought to be key factor in withdrawal symptoms [173]. It has been proposed that repeated altered activity in the DA system and sustained activation of the CRF system leads to AL and negative emotional states [174]. The central thesis in Koob's allostatic view of stress and addiction is that stress leads to changes in brain CRF that have a direct impact on addiction [175]. Withdrawal can produce elevated levels of GCs and increase release of CRF in the central nucleus of the amygdala [175].

It has also been suggested that increased CRF alters serotonin release in the brain which facilitates DA in the accumbens [176]. Prolonged exposure to stress can lead to irregular changes in GC receptor density (epigenetics) which may increase the reinforcing effects of alcohol and drugs [177,178].

Interestingly, a higher salivary cortisol level in response to stress has been associated with higher drop-out rates in treatment [179]. It has also been suggested that variability in stress-related genes may contribute to the ability of certain individuals to remain abstinent from heroin, possibly due to higher stress resilience [180]. Importantly, not only does STA increase addiction behaviors, some authors have suggested this association also exists in the opposite direction [181,182]. With illicit drugs, their procurement and use can predispose individuals to traumatic stress [183,184]. In animal models, chronic opioid pretreatment is able to robustly augment associative fear learning [185]. These changes were not observed when opioids were given after the traumatic event, and potentiation lasted beyond discontinuation of drug exposure. This concept has been thoroughly described as part of the withdrawal process in widely accepted addiction models [186–188]. However, more research is needed to understand how long-term exposure to highly palatable foods may alter one's long-term response to stressful life experiences, and how this dynamic can play out in reciprocal and bidirectional ways, for example in the presence of weight stigma and dietary restraint (and cumulatively over time).

A recent review of preclinical data suggests three mechanisms by which DA and GCs interact: (1) GCs upregulate tyrosine hydroxylase (rate-limiting enzyme in DA synthesis) (2) GCs down-regulate monoamine oxidase (enzyme responsible for DA removal) and (3) GCs are hypothesized to decrease DA uptake subsequently increasing synaptic DA [189]. Clearly stress enhances substance abuse-related effects at multiple points along the mesolimbic projection. The KOR system plays an important role in behavioral stress responses and has been implicated in stress-induced maladaptive responses [190]. While MOR activation produces euphoria, KOR is generally aversive and may contribute to negative affect states in withdrawal. According to some authors, it is possible that a stress-induced increase in KOR function promotes drug seeking by reducing DA transmission [190]. Meanwhile, reduced MOR has been observed in comorbid binge eating disorder and obesity [191] and across SUDs [144] which strongly suggest neurochemical overlap in these conditions, and which can persist despite weight loss or periods of drug abstinence. Any change in stress neurobiology is likely to influence reward. Based on observed deficits in the ventral striatum, reward responsiveness and processing may be a primary mediator of the effects of ELA [192]. Taken together, FA is a biologically plausible explanation for the life course association between ELA and obesity, however important contextual factors from the psychological domain deserve further consideration.

5. Psychological Correlates of Food Addiction & Obesity

Thus far we have highlighted several social and environmental factors associated with STA and addiction-like eating. We have reviewed emerging data on the biological embedding of adversity, which may increase an individual's susceptibility to FA, and potentially lead to obesity over time. Based on the overlap between FA and EDs as well as SUDs, we have recommended including these variables into statistical models which investigate weight outcomes. Finally, we have proposed a comprehensive conceptual framework to further contextualize these relationships by including two psychological (as well as socially constructed) correlates of FA, EDs, and obesity: dietary restraint and weight stigma.

5.1. Dietary Restraint

Restrained eating is generally defined as a cognitive effort to eat less in order to lose weight [193], which has been viewed both as the problem and solution to obesity [194]. More recently it has become clear that theories of weight loss based on low-calorie dieting are failing, likely due to neurochemical, endocrine, and gastrointestinal factors which are not adequately captured by simple models of energy balance. While the concept of dietary restraint has been linked to some positive outcomes (e.g., weight management, prevention efforts) [195], it is included in our model as a risk factor for eating pathology, often associated with EDs (sometimes referred to as restriction). A classic study conducted by Ancel Keys in the 1940s examined the link between starvation and changes in human biology and behavior [196]. The study showed that significant (intentional) weight loss produced the onset of binge eating in 30% of participants (n = 36). Many of the individuals who were reduced to 50% of their baseline caloric intake for extended periods of time (months) began collecting recipes and cookbooks. The finding that caloric restriction leads to preoccupation with food has been widely cited in the ED literature. Meanwhile, it is less clear if deliberate efforts to eat differently (focusing on dietary quality rather than quantity) should be classified as pathological restraint. Extreme diets intended for health reasons which impair daily function have been described as "orthorexia nervosa" which appears to be growing problem [197]. Research linking FA recovery to orthorexia is timely and warranted.

A dieting intervention on 121 females which included monitoring and restricting showed that monitoring increases perceived stress, while restricting increases the cortisol output [198]. Dieting is stressful, which may explain why engaging in dieting behaviors aimed at losing weight can actually have the opposite effect. Future iterations of Figure 1 may include an arrow directly from dietary restraint to STA, whereas in the current model there is only a backdoor path through weight stigma. A twin study from Finland (n = 4129) showed that dieters are prone to future weight gain independent of genetic factors [199]. A recent fMRI study showed that "successful" restrained eaters had stronger activation in the middle frontal gyrus and cerebellum (associated with executive function and inhibition) suggesting that food temptations may trigger processes of positive inhibition in some, but not others [200]. It is likely that altered neurochemistry from SUD and/or ELA/STA will impact the degree of success with dietary restraint. More research is needed on the impact of trauma on various eating behaviors, including restriction. It will prove important to better define dietary restraint in the context of FA recovery.

There is considerable debate on how to approach FA from a nutritional standpoint, including incorporating FA data into the traditional ED landscape [201]. Meule has stated that "dietary restraint does not have to be dysfunctional as long as flexible elements are added" [202]. Based on available data linking FA and EDs (Section 1.2), it is proposed that restrained eating moderates the link between food environment and FA, as well as the link between FA and obesity (Figure 1). In other words, individuals engaging in dietary restraint are predicted to display higher levels of FA severity. Future research should examine the directionality as well as cumulative interplay of this relationship. Furthermore, it is proposed that individuals who meet criteria for FA and engage in dietary restraint may experience different effects on their weight status, depending on whether or not the restraint is successful, unsuccessful, pathological, or part of a restrictive ED. These theories need to be tested in both observational and experimental studies in an effort to better develop the emerging field of behavioral health nutrition. Recently, an 8-step process has been proposed to help clinicians discern FA from dietary restraint in order to inform inclusive vs. exclusive nutrition strategies [46]. The key discerning factors include the presence of SUD, PTSD, and ELA, which, if all present, can provide more confidence in the strength of an FA signal, particularly in the absence of dieting behaviors.

5.2. Weight Stigma

Weight stigma has been described as a "vicious cycle" where weight stigma begets weight gain [203]. Similar to dieting, the experience of stigmatization increases cortisol, which may drive food consumption by sensitizing the reward system [203]. In addition to increased cortisol, weight stigma also increases oxidative stress [204] providing further evidence of biological embedding. In a large sample of adolescents (n = 115,180), perceiving one's body as overweight increases risk of suicidality [205]. Conceptually, weight stigma is similar to other forms of STA, which we consider as midstream drivers of eating behavior and subsequent weight outcomes, both through biological and psychosocial pathways. While unproven, it is possible that body dissatisfaction and self-stigma drives avoidance behaviors (e.g., weight loss to avoid adiposity) which is similar to the avoidance experience in PTSD. This may be one reason why efforts to lose weight can be persistent (or even relentless) for so many, despite the fact that weight loss efforts have been unsuccessful (or unsustainable) in the past.

In a large national sample (n = 5129), weight discrimination was associated with overeating (specifically convenience foods) and less regular meal timing [206]. Individuals who are the target of weight stigma have been shown to decrease self-control and perceived capacity for weight management [207]. In a large sample of adolescents (n = 1497), FA and psychological distress mediated the association between weight-related self-stigma and binge eating [208]. It is worth acknowledging differences between externalized (others) and internalized (self) weight bias. It has also been shown that some people will experience longer term distress from weight stigma than others [209]. Perceptions and/or experiences of weight bias in primary care settings have been shown to negatively influence patient engagement with health care services [210]. In summary, weight stigma has emerged as an important component of obesity context, with strong arguments in favor of adopting weight-inclusive health policy [211]. While the FA explanation for weight control has been shown to decrease weight stigma among groups [212,213] it has been suggested that FA can increase internalized weight stigma among individuals [214]. More research is needed on the role of weight stigma driving dietary restraint, both as a cause and consequence of addiction-like eating.

6. What Does It Mean for Public Health?

Research on biological programming attempts to identify the most critical and sensitive periods that underlie the developmental origins of later childhood and adult disease [215]. It has been suggested that the timing of adversity explains more variability in DNA methylation than the accumulation or recency of exposure [216]. It has also been observed that different dimensions of adversity have distinct influences on neurodevelopment [217]. The exact mechanisms which link human DNA methylation with psychological disorders have not been elucidated [151]. What we do know is that the cumulative effects of STA can impact neural function with significant implications for substance-seeking behaviors. All addictions share a common neurobiology and have known relationships to STA in both directions. Sugar, salt, and fat added to foods make them more palatable and reinforce "drug-like" behavior with loss of control, continued use despite consequences, binge episodes, and other similarities with traditional drugs of abuse. It is clear that obesity causes changes in opioid and DA signaling which alter reward processing [218]. Given the established links between ELA and the propensity for behavioral health disorders including SUD, ED, and FA, prevention efforts might have a meaningful impact upstream. Addressing clusters of disorders with shared underpinnings jointly may be more fruitful than a one-disorder-at-a-time approach [122].

A recent study of New Orleans children showed that neighborhood stress exerts a direct influence on obesity, after adjusting for diet and activity [219]. Such findings support the need to improve social conditions rather than efforts to address obesity at the individual level. It will be important to identify positive contextual factors such as neighborhood and school safety, as well as resilience [105] and develop community-based programs that promote these protective factors. Resiliency-building programs that reduce delay discounting may decrease addictive behaviors [220]. Meanwhile, socioeconomic differences in the quality of early life create "cumulative disadvantage" that contribute to gradients in health status [37]. SES indicators are upstream determinants of health while biological factors are more proximate determinants [221]. Neighborhood disadvantage creates social context which may become biologically embedded [222]. The impact of low SES can become embedded into inflammatory processes, the HPA axis, and neural function/structure, all of which are epigenetically controlled [135]. It is not unreasonable to assume that normalizing/improving HPA axis function may be beneficial in the treatment and relapse of addiction-related disorders. Given that epigenetic patterns are sculpted during early life [137], reducing stressors appears crucial to the long-term management of FA.

A "systems thinking" multilevel approach will be critical to reverse obesity trends. For example, trauma-informed treatment and stress management curriculum should be made available in underserved communities, starting with schools [107]. Mobilizing cross-sector interdisciplinary partnerships to connect ELA to later life health outcomes will be critical. It has been stated that "fostering increased societal awareness about toxic stress exposures that are often hidden, stigmatized, and attached to shame needs to occur across generations" [223]. Greater awareness of the biological mechanisms discussed herein are likely to reduce weight stigma, which is a known barrier for individual help-seeking behaviors in those with obesity [224] as well as SUDs [225]. Feelings of rejection associated with weight stigma and disordered eating are additional stressors which may further perpetuate a negative cycle [114,168]. A recent study showed that the FA model explanation for obesity resulted in lower stigma than the traditional "diet and exercise" explanation that attributes obesity to personal responsibility [213]. Given that weight stigma is a psychosocial contributor to maladaptive eating behavior, interventions targeting stigma (at the individual and societal levels) are warranted.

6.1. Food Policy

This paper has reviewed evidence to suggest that improving the early childhood environment might impact obesity risk and therefore should be a public health priority. Meanwhile, if reward-related neuroadaptations associated with addiction persist over time, addressing only the underlying factors may fail to create lasting changes in eating behavior, suggesting that policies targeting the food environment will also be important. Given that the food environment in the US promotes easy access to foods with addictive potential [226] it is not unreasonable to hypothesize that highly palatable foods leave a biological imprint which may perpetuate FA symptoms across the lifespan and into subsequent generations, as has been shown in animal models [131]. Western-style diets rapidly impair appetitive control, compared to those on their habitual diet [65]. Combined with heightened susceptibility to STA stemming from ELA, efforts to address the obesity epidemic may be futile without strategic multilevel interventions targeting corporate responsibility (i.e., "Big Food") [227].

There is mounting evidence of the harmful effects of processed foods in contemporary diets. A recent trial comparing the caloric intake of those on ultra-processed foods (containing minimal whole foods) compared to unprocessed/whole foods for two weeks found ad libitum intake was increased by approximately 500 kcal/day on the ultra-processed diet [228]. Not surprisingly, people gained weight on the ultra-processed diet and lost weight on the unprocessed. Cross-sectional data (NHANES 2005–2014) has shown that higher consumption of ultra-processed foods is associated with excess weight and is more pronounced in females [229]. A study from Spain showed that four or more servings per day of ultra-processed foods is associated with a 62% increased hazard for all-cause mortality, where each additional serving increased all-cause mortality by 18% [230]. It remains unclear if the negative health effects are due to the direct impact of the processed foods, or the displacement of nutrient-dense high-fiber foods protective against oxidative stress and associated inflammation.

Public health interventions to increase access to healthy foods in lower SES communities have been unsuccessful in reducing obesity, therefore new approaches are needed. Identifying certain foods to be addictive may encourage collective efforts to avoid them [231] and is associated with support for policies to curb their use [232] similar to how public health officials addressed Big Tobacco. Only recently have researchers and policy makers begun to explore targeting the food environment in universal ED prevention efforts [233]. It has been suggested that "processed food addiction is the result of an intentional epidemic of addiction not an incidental by-product of Western environments" [62]. The term "processed food addiction" implicates the food industry rather than the individual. There is a critical need for increased awareness of FA and the role played by multinational food corporations in promoting processed foods with addictive qualities [214]. Evidence suggests that aggressive marketing of these foods to children, adolescents, and young adults disproportionately affects vulnerable groups [234–238]. While it is highly unlikely that food companies will re-formulate their products based on self-regulation, it also unrealistic to expect food-addicted individuals to regularly avoid food-related temptations. Policy support should include warning labels, industry reductions on sugar, and product bans (e.g., energy drinks) [232] while legal tools include advertising restrictions and class-action litigation [239]. Several authors have recommended policies restricting fast food advertising to adolescents [240,241]. Based on growing evidence for FA, this may be indicated.

7. Conclusions

The biological underpinnings of addictions strongly imply a role for ELA in the development of FA and obesity. Importantly, ELA can alter the physiological response to various forms of psychosocial STA across multiple body systems, which can have a cumulative impact on health behaviors over the lifespan. FA research which began in animal models has since been described in human neuroimaging studies which capture neurobiological and behavioral overlap between FA and SUDs. A biopsychosocial perspective on FA considers biomarkers such as inflammatory markers and other measures of AL, the HPA axis including the output of cortisol, epigenetic mechanisms including those that influence the HPA axis, and various structural, functional, and morphological brain changes, following exposure to ELA and STA. In order to contextualize risk, a biopsychosocial model considers the upstream drivers and fundamental causes of health disparities, such as SES and environmental (e.g., neighborhood) factors that impact food access and food choices. Furthermore, obesity frameworks should incorporate weight stigma as an important cause and consequence of the epidemic, suggested herein as a form of STA that can also become biological embedded. Finally, the role of dietary restraint has been included as an important psychological factor that should be accounted for when conceptualizing FA and obesity, particularly given the strong relationship between ELA and EDs, as recently reviewed elsewhere [46].

Stress proliferates over the life course and across generations, widening health disparities between advantaged and disadvantaged groups [242]. This might explain why public health nutrition interventions in low SES communities have had limited success. Consumption of highly palatable foods to "self-medicate" the long-term biological impact of chronic stress may be a critical factor in understanding the obesity crisis. This is particularly true for marginalized groups with less access (e.g., affordability) to unprocessed foods. Higher SES groups are more likely to have success in reducing addiction-like eating compared to lower SES groups who are constrained by access and resources. Public health interventions should account for the growing inequities in health outcomes. Biopsychosocial approaches that consider the cumulative interplay between social and biological factors are helpful when conceptualizing multiple systems driving substance-related disorders, whether it be alcohol, drugs, nicotine, or food [243]. A biopsychosocial model may contribute to conceptual and methodological advances in our understanding and treatment of obesity. Meanwhile, separating constructs into biological, psychological, and social factors (as in Figure 1) can be contraindicated by ecological models that emphasize the dynamic reciprocity between these levels. However, our conceptual model has discerned between these factors in order to encourage further contextual analysis of FA.

Based on the biological plausibility of FA as a consequence of psychosocial STA, potential solutions to the obesity epidemic may include: (1) improve social conditions in order to reduce exposure to ELA, as well develop community-based programs for early intervention (2) decrease weight stigma based on FA data implying that body weight is not simply a "choice" (3) mind-body approaches (e.g., yoga, meditation) designed to improve the human stress response and (4) policy proposals aimed at the food industry to reduce exposure to highly palatable foods. More information is needed about the role of nutrition in the reversibility of unfavorable gene expression. More research is needed to investigate whether long-term dietary changes such as abstaining from highly palatable foods is even feasible. If so, will this improve the microbiome and stimulate/reverse epigenetic change and/or lead to altered reward pathways in the brain? At a minimum, it is reasonable to predict that reducing exposure to addiction-like eating can improve executive functioning. Since dietary restraint is a known risk factor for the development of EDs, drastic individual nutrition changes should be implemented in consultation with a qualified professional such as a registered dietitian nutritionist, particularly when there is underlying trauma and/or SUD. Treatment models should be trauma-informed and include staff trainings.

FA and SUD share multiple predisposing factors including ELA which can become biologically embedded. These findings may link social determinants to specific health outcomes and elucidate pathway effects of risk across the life course. Epigenetic processes may be a key mediator between social environments during childhood and disease risk in adulthood. Mediating mechanisms such as

AL, the HPA axis, DNA methylation, and altered reward sensitivity (i.e., dopamine systems) have scientific merit, however the fundamental causes of health inequalities present in society should not be overlooked. Low SES and neighborhood disadvantage remain important drivers of ELA, particularly within the context of the obesity epidemic. The cumulative effects of STA that impact neural function and heighten threat vigilance have significant implications for substance-seeking behaviors, including eating. The FA construct has gained credibility from animal and human studies reviewed herein, which may help reduce stigma associated with addiction-like behaviors, including obesity. More research is needed to understand the differential impact of inflammatory signaling markers on the brain, including assessment of blood brain barrier integrity. The study of neuroinflammation is likely to add explanatory power to our conceptual model and guide future research questions.

If the DSM accepts FA, it will lead to better treatment and eventually public health efforts to improve the national food environment and global nutrition landscape. More resources should be allocated for nutrition education during pregnancy and lactation, particularly in underserved communities where stress and adversity are high, and the food environment is suboptimal. Applying the FA framework has the potential to influence the way people view food, and to ultimately decrease addiction in future generations. FA treatment does not always require specific "food abstinence" but it does warrant reduced exposure and harm reduction strategies. Given the strong evidence that neurobiological responses to food differ among people, personalized precision nutrition interventions are warranted. In order for these strategies to be successful, cultural shifts around food norms will be necessary. Furthermore, FA is both an individual and collective health problem, and should be addressed at the societal level with broad policy interventions. We propose that unregulated promotion of addictive foods by the food industry are major contributors of obesity, particularly in the face of disadvantage and distress. Government interdiction may be required to reduce the epidemic of obesity and the growing problem of food addiction. Multidisciplinary efforts using trauma-informed integrated biopsychosocial frameworks will be necessary to reverse obesity trends.

Author Contributions: Conceptual model, literature review, and first draft preparation (D.A.W.). Draft revisions (N.A. & M.G.). All authors have read and agreed to the published version of the manuscript.

Funding: This research received no external funding.

Conflicts of Interest: The authors declare no conflict of interest.

References

1. Popkin, B.M. Nutritional Patterns and Transitions. *Popul. Dev. Rev.* **1993**, *19*, 138–157. [CrossRef]
2. Hall, K.D. Did the Food Environment Cause the Obesity Epidemic? *Obesity* **2018**, *26*, 11–13. [CrossRef] [PubMed]
3. Wang, G.-J.; Volkow, N.D.; Logan, J.; Pappas, N.R.; Wong, C.T.; Zhu, W.; Netusll, N.; Fowler, J.S. Brain dopamine and obesity. *Lancet* **2001**, *357*, 354–357. [CrossRef]
4. Volkow, N.D.; Wise, R.A. How can drug addiction help us understand obesity? *Nat. Neurosci.* **2005**, *8*, 555–560. [CrossRef] [PubMed]
5. Stice, E.; Spoor, S.; Bohon, C.; Small, D. Relation Between Obesity and Blunted Striatal Response to Food Is Moderated by TaqIA A1 Allele. *Science* **2008**, *322*, 449–452. [CrossRef]
6. Saules, K.K.; Carr, M.M.; Herb, K.M. Overeating, Overweight, and Substance Use: What Is the Connection? *Curr. Addict. Rep.* **2018**, *5*, 232–242. [CrossRef]
7. Gold, M.S. From bedside to bench and back again: A 30-year saga. *Physiol. Behav.* **2011**, *104*, 157–161. [CrossRef]
8. Avena, N.M.; Hoebel, B.G. A diet promoting sugar dependency causes behavioral cross-sensitization to a low dose of amphetamine. *Neuroscience* **2003**, *122*, 17–20. [CrossRef]
9. Hoebel, B.G.; Avena, N.M.; Rada, P. Accumbens dopamine-acetylcholine balance in approach and avoidance. *Curr. Opin. Pharmacol.* **2007**, *7*, 617–627. [CrossRef]
10. Hoebel, B.G. Brain neurotransmitters in food and drug reward. *Am. J. Clin. Nutr.* **1985**, *42*, 1133–1150. [CrossRef] [PubMed]

11. Rada, P.; Avena, N.M.; Hoebel, B.G. Daily bingeing on sugar repeatedly releases dopamine in the accumbens shell. *Neuroscience* **2005**, *134*, 737–744. [CrossRef] [PubMed]
12. Avena, N.M.; Rada, P.; Hoebel, B.G. Underweight rats have enhanced dopamine release and blunted acetylcholine response in the nucleus accumbens while bingeing on sucrose. *Neuroscience* **2008**, *156*, 865–871. [CrossRef] [PubMed]
13. Avena, N.M.; Rada, P.; Hoebel, B.G. Evidence for sugar addiction: Behavioral and neurochemical effects of intermittent, excessive sugar intake. *Neurosci. Biobehav. Rev.* **2008**, *32*, 20–39. [CrossRef] [PubMed]
14. Wiss, D.A.; Avena, N.; Rada, P. Sugar Addiction: From Evolution to Revolution. *Front. Psychiatry* **2018**, *9*, 545. [CrossRef]
15. Kim, S.; Kwok, S.; Mayes, L.C.; Potenza, M.N.; Rutherford, H.J.; Strathearn, L. Early adverse experience and substance addiction: Dopamine, oxytocin, and glucocorticoid pathways. *Ann. N. Y. Acad. Sci.* **2017**, *1394*, 74–91. [CrossRef]
16. Peña, C.; Neugut, Y.D.; Calarco, C.A.; Champagne, F.A. Effects of maternal care on the development of midbrain dopamine pathways and reward-directed behavior in female offspring. *Eur. J. Neurosci.* **2014**, *39*, 946–956. [CrossRef]
17. Wei, N.-L.; Quan, Z.-F.; Zhao, T.; Yu, X.-D.; Xie, Q.; Zeng, J.; Ma, F.-K.; Wang, F.; Tang, Q.-S.; Wu, H.; et al. Chronic stress increases susceptibility to food addiction by increasing the levels of DR2 and MOR in the nucleus accumbens. *Neuropsychiatr. Dis. Treat.* **2019**, *15*, 1211–1229. [CrossRef]
18. MacKay, J.C.; Kent, P.; James, J.S.; Cayer, C.; Merali, Z. Ability of palatable food consumption to buffer against the short- and long-term behavioral consequences of social defeat exposure during juvenility in rats. *Physiol. Behav.* **2017**, *177*, 113–121. [CrossRef]
19. Grimm, J.W.; Hyde, J.; Glueck, E.; North, K.; Ginder, D.; Jiganti, K.; Hopkins, M.; Sauter, F.; MacDougall, D.; Hovander, D. Examining persistence of acute environmental enrichment-induced anti-sucrose craving effects in rats. *Appetite* **2019**, *139*, 50–58. [CrossRef]
20. Cohen, M.; Jing, D.; Yang, R.R.; Tottenham, N.; Lee, F.S.; Casey, B. Early-life stress has persistent effects on amygdala function and development in mice and humans. *Proc. Natl. Acad. Sci. USA* **2013**, *110*, 18274–18278. [CrossRef]
21. Felitti, V.J.; Anda, R.F.; Nordenberg, D.; Williamson, D.F.; Spitz, A.M.; Edwards, V.; Koss, M.P.; Marks, J.S. Relationship of Childhood Abuse and Household Dysfunction to Many of the Leading Causes of Death in Adults The Adverse Childhood Experiences (ACE) Study. *Am. J. Prev. Med.* **1998**, *14*, 245–258. [CrossRef]
22. Levis, S.C.; Bentzley, B.S.; Molet, J.; Bolton, J.L.; Perrone, C.R.; Baram, T.Z.; Mahler, S.V. On the early life origins of vulnerability to opioid addiction. *Mol. Psychiatr.* **2019**, 1–8. [CrossRef] [PubMed]
23. Al'Absi, M. The influence of stress and early life adversity on addiction: Psychobiological mechanisms of risk and resilience. *Int. Rev. Neurobiol.* **2020**, *152*, 71–100. [CrossRef] [PubMed]
24. Wiss, D.A.; Brewerton, T.D. Adverse Childhood Experiences and Adult Obesity: A Systematic Review of Plausible Mechanisms and Meta-Analysis of Cross-Sectional Studies. *Physiol. Behav.* **2020**, *223*, 112964. [CrossRef]
25. Hemmingsson, E. Early Childhood Obesity Risk Factors: Socioeconomic Adversity, Family Dysfunction, Offspring Distress, and Junk Food Self-Medication. *Curr. Obes. Rep.* **2018**, *7*, 204–209. [CrossRef]
26. Cammack, A.L.; Gazmararian, J.A.; Suglia, S.F. History of child maltreatment and excessive dietary and screen time behaviors in young adults: Results from a nationally representative study. *Prev. Med.* **2020**, *139*, 106176. [CrossRef]
27. Nunes-Neto, P.R.; Köhler, C.A.; Schuch, F.B.; Solmi, M.; Quevedo, J.; Maes, M.; Murru, A.; Vieta, E.; McIntyre, R.S.; McElroy, S.L.; et al. Food addiction: Prevalence, psychopathological correlates and associations with quality of life in a large sample. *J. Psychiatr. Res.* **2018**, *96*, 145–152. [CrossRef]
28. Bloomfield, M.A.; McCutcheon, R.A.; Kempton, M.; Freeman, T.P.; Howes, O. The effects of psychosocial stress on dopaminergic function and the acute stress response. *Elife* **2019**, *8*, e46797. [CrossRef]
29. Dillon, D.G.; Holmes, A.J.; Birk, J.L.; Brooks, N.; Lyons-Ruth, K.; Pizzagalli, D.A. Childhood Adversity Is Associated with Left Basal Ganglia Dysfunction During Reward Anticipation in Adulthood. *Biol. Psychiat.* **2009**, *66*, 206–213. [CrossRef]
30. Osadchiy, V.; Mayer, E.A.; Bhatt, R.; Labus, J.S.; Gao, L.; Kilpatrick, L.A.; Liu, C.; Tillisch, K.; Naliboff, B.; Chang, L.; et al. History of early life adversity is associated with increased food addiction and sex-specific alterations in reward network connectivity in obesity. *Obes. Sci. Pract.* **2019**, *5*, 416–436. [CrossRef]

31. Heilig, M.; Epstein, D.H.; Nader, M.A.; Shaham, Y. Time to connect: Bringing social context into addiction neuroscience. *Nat. Rev. Neurosci.* **2016**, *17*, 592–599. [CrossRef] [PubMed]
32. Engel, G.L. The need for a new medical model: A challenge for biomedicine. *Science* **1977**, *196*, 129–136. [CrossRef] [PubMed]
33. Baughman, K.; Logue, E.; Sutton, K.; Capers, C.; Jarjoura, D.; Smucker, W. Biopsychosocial characteristics of overweight and obese primary care patients: Do psychosocial and behavior factors mediate sociodemographic effects? *Prev. Med.* **2003**, *37*, 129–137. [CrossRef]
34. Qu, Y.; Galván, A.; Fuligni, A.J.; Telzer, E.H. A Biopsychosocial Approach to Examine Mexican American Adolescents' Academic Achievement and Substance Use. *RSF Russell Sage Found. J. Sci.* **2018**, *4*, 84–97. [CrossRef]
35. Krieger, N. Theories for social epidemiology in the 21st century: An ecosocial perspective. *Int. J. Epidemiol.* **2001**, *30*, 668–677. [CrossRef] [PubMed]
36. Elder, G.H., Jr. The Life Course as Developmental Theory. *Child. Dev.* **1998**, *69*, 1–12. [CrossRef]
37. Hertzman, C. The biological embedding of early experience and its effects on health in adulthood. *Ann. N. Y. Acad. Sci.* **1999**, *896*, 85–95. [CrossRef]
38. Ben-Shlomo, Y.; Kuh, D. A life course approach to chronic disease epidemiology: Conceptual models, empirical challenges and interdisciplinary perspectives. *Int. J. Epidemiol.* **2002**, *31*, 285–293. [CrossRef]
39. Lerner, R.M. The Place of Learning within the Human Development System: A Developmental Contextual Perspective. *Hum. Dev.* **1995**, *38*, 361–366. [CrossRef]
40. Overton, W.F.; Lerner, R.M. Fundamental Concepts and Methods in Developmental Science: A Relational Perspective. *Res. Hum. Dev.* **2014**, *11*, 63–73. [CrossRef]
41. Lerner, R.M.; Johnson, S.K.; Buckingham, M.H. Relational Developmental Systems-Based Theories and the Study of Children and Families: Lerner and Spanier (1978) Revisited. *J. Fam. Theor. Rev.* **2015**, *7*, 83–104. [CrossRef]
42. Gearhardt, A.N.; Corbin, W.R.; Brownell, K.D. Preliminary validation of the Yale Food Addiction Scale. *Appetite* **2009**, *52*, 430–436. [CrossRef] [PubMed]
43. Gearhardt, A.N.; Corbin, W.R.; Brownell, K.D. Development of the Yale Food Addiction Scale Version 2.0. *Psychol. Addict. Behav.* **2016**, *30*, 113–121. [CrossRef] [PubMed]
44. Schulte, E.M.; Grilo, C.M.; Gearhardt, A.N. Shared and unique mechanisms underlying binge eating disorder and addictive disorders. *Clin. Psychol. Rev.* **2016**, *44*, 125–139. [CrossRef] [PubMed]
45. Racine, S.E.; Burt, A.S.; Iacono, W.G.; McGue, M.; Klump, K.L. Dietary restraint moderates genetic risk for binge eating. *J. Abnorm. Psychol.* **2011**, *120*, 119–128. [CrossRef] [PubMed]
46. Wiss, D.; Brewerton, T. Separating the Signal from the Noise: How Psychiatric Diagnoses Can Help Discern Food Addiction from Dietary Restraint. *Nutrients* **2020**, *12*, 2937. [CrossRef]
47. Meule, A.; von Rezori, V.; Blechert, J. Food Addiction and Bulimia Nervosa. *Eur. Eat. Disord. Rev.* **2014**, *22*, 331–337. [CrossRef]
48. Meule, A.; Gearhardt, A.N. Ten Years of the Yale Food Addiction Scale: A Review of Version 2.0. *Curr. Addict. Rep.* **2019**, *6*, 218–228. [CrossRef]
49. Fernandez-Aranda, F.; Karwautz, A.; Treasure, J. Food addiction: A transdiagnostic construct of increasing interest. *Eur. Eat. Disord. Rev.* **2018**, *26*, 536–540. [CrossRef]
50. Romero, X.; Agüera, Z.; Granero, R.; Sánchez, I.; Riesco, N.; Jiménez-Murcia, S.; Gisbert-Rodriguez, M.; Sánchez-González, J.; Casalé, G.; Baenas, I.; et al. Is food addiction a predictor of treatment outcome among patients with eating disorder? *Eur Eat. Disord Rev.* **2019**, *27*, 700–711. [CrossRef]
51. Brewerton, T.D. Food addiction as a proxy for eating disorder and obesity severity, trauma history, PTSD symptoms, and comorbidity. *Eat. Weight. Disord. Stud. Anorex. Bulim. Obes.* **2017**, *22*, 241–247. [CrossRef] [PubMed]
52. Mason, S.M.; Flint, A.J.; Field, A.E.; Austin, B.S.; Rich-Edwards, J.W. Abuse victimization in childhood or adolescence and risk of food addiction in adult women. *Obesity* **2013**, *21*, E775–E781. [CrossRef] [PubMed]
53. Mason, S.M.; Flint, A.J.; Roberts, A.L.; Agnew-Blais, J.; Koenen, K.C.; Rich-Edwards, J.W. Posttraumatic Stress Disorder Symptoms and Food Addiction in Women by Timing and Type of Trauma Exposure. *JAMA Psychiatry* **2014**, *71*, 1271–1278. [CrossRef] [PubMed]

54. Imperatori, C.; Innamorati, M.; Lamis, D.A.; Farina, B.; Pompili, M.; Contardi, A.; Fabbricatore, M. Childhood trauma in obese and overweight women with food addiction and clinical-level of binge eating. *Child. Abus. Negl.* **2016**, *58*, 180–190. [CrossRef]
55. Holgerson, A.A.; Clark, M.M.; Ames, G.E.; Collazo-Clavell, M.L.; Kellogg, T.A.; Graszer, K.M.; Kalsy, S.A.; Grothe, K. Association of Adverse Childhood Experiences and Food Addiction to Bariatric Surgery Completion and Weight Loss Outcome. *Obes. Surg.* **2018**, *28*, 3386–3392. [CrossRef]
56. Warren, C.S.; Lindsay, A.R.; White, E.K.; Claudat, K.; Velasquez, S.C. Weight-related concerns related to drug use for women in substance abuse treatment: Prevalence and relationships with eating pathology. *J. Subst. Abus. Treat.* **2013**, *44*, 494–501. [CrossRef]
57. Wiss, D.A.; Waterhous, T.S. Nutrition Therapy for Eating Disorders, Substance Use Disorders, and Addictions. In *Eating Disorders, Addictions and Substance Use Disorders, Research, Clinical and Treatment Perspectives*; Springer: Berlin/Heidelberg, Germany, 2014; pp. 509–532. ISBN 9783642453779.
58. Khalil, R.B.; Sleilaty, G.; Richa, S.; Seneque, M.; Iceta, S.; Rodgers, R.; Alacreu-Crespo, A.; Maimoun, L.; Lefebvre, P.; Renard, E.; et al. The Impact of Retrospective Childhood Maltreatment on Eating Disorders as Mediated by Food Addiction: A Cross-Sectional Study. *Nutrients* **2020**, *12*, 2969. [CrossRef]
59. Cassin, S.E.; Sijercic, I.; Montemarano, V. Psychosocial Interventions for Food Addiction: A Systematic Review. *Curr. Addict. Rep.* **2020**, *7*, 9–19. [CrossRef]
60. Hebebrand, J.; Albayrak, Ö.; Adan, R.; Antel, J.; Dieguez, C.; de Jong, J.; Leng, G.; Menzies, J.; Mercer, J.G.; Murphy, M.; et al. "Eating addiction", rather than "food addiction", better captures addictive-like eating behavior. *Neurosci. Biobehav. Rev.* **2014**, *47*, 295–306. [CrossRef]
61. Ifland, J.R.; Preuss, H.G.; Marcus, M.T.; Rourke, K.M.; Taylor, W.C.; Burau, K.; Jacobs, W.S.; Kadish, W.; Manso, G. Refined food addiction: A classic substance use disorder. *Med. Hypotheses* **2009**, *72*, 518–526. [CrossRef]
62. Ifland, J.; Preuss, H.G.; Marcus, M.T.; Rourke, K.M.; Taylor, W.; Wright, T.H. Clearing the Confusion around Processed Food Addiction. *J. Am. Coll. Nutr.* **2015**, *34*, 240–243. [CrossRef] [PubMed]
63. Nolan, L.J. Is it time to consider the "food use disorder?" *Appetite* **2017**, *115*, 16–18. [CrossRef] [PubMed]
64. Volkow, N.D.; Wang, G.-J.; Tomasi, D.; Baler, R.D. Obesity and addiction: Neurobiological overlaps. *Obes. Rev.* **2013**, *14*, 2–18. [CrossRef] [PubMed]
65. Stevenson, R.J.; Francis, H.M.; Attuquayefio, T.; Gupta, D.; Yeomans, M.R.; Oaten, M.J.; Davidson, T. Hippocampal-dependent appetitive control is impaired by experimental exposure to a Western-style diet. *R. Soc. Open Sci.* **2020**, *7*, 191338. [CrossRef]
66. Dohle, S.; Diel, K.; Hofmann, W. Executive functions and the self-regulation of eating behavior: A review. *Appetite* **2018**, *124*, 4–9. [CrossRef]
67. Steward, T.; Mestre-Bach, G.; Vintró-Alcaraz, C.; Lozano-Madrid, M.; Agüera, Z.; Fernández-Formoso, J.A.; Granero, R.; Jiménez-Murcia, S.; Vilarrasa, N.; García-Ruiz-de-Gordejuela, A.; et al. Food addiction and impaired executive functions in women with obesity. *Eur. Eat. Disord. Rev.* **2018**, *26*, 574–584. [CrossRef]
68. Chao, S.-H.; Liao, Y.-T.; Chen, V.C.-H.; Li, C.-J.; McIntyre, R.S.; Lee, Y.; Weng, J.-C. Correlation between brain circuit segregation and obesity. *Behav. Brain Res.* **2018**, *337*, 218–227. [CrossRef]
69. Ronan, L.; Alexander-Bloch, A.; Fletcher, P.C. Childhood Obesity, Cortical Structure, and Executive Function in Healthy Children. *Cereb. Cortex* **2019**, *30*, 2519–2528. [CrossRef]
70. Laurent, J.S.; Watts, R.; Adise, S.; Allgaier, N.; Chaarani, B.; Garavan, H.; Potter, A.; Mackey, S. Associations Among Body Mass Index, Cortical Thickness, and Executive Function in Children. *JAMA Pediatr.* **2020**, *174*, 170. [CrossRef]
71. Yang, Y.; Shields, G.S.; Wu, Q.; Liu, Y.; Guo, C. Obesity is associated with poor working memory in women, not men: Findings from a nationally representative dataset of U.S. adults. *Eat. Behav.* **2019**, *35*, 101338. [CrossRef]
72. Sattler, K.M.; Deane, F.P.; Tapsell, L.; Kelly, P.J. Gender differences in the relationship of weight-based stigmatisation with motivation to exercise and physical activity in overweight individuals. *Health Psychol. Open* **2018**, *5*, 205510291875969. [CrossRef] [PubMed]
73. Guardabassi, V.; Tomasetto, C. Weight status or weight stigma? Obesity stereotypes—Not excess weight—Reduce working memory in school-aged children. *J. Exp. Child. Psychol.* **2019**, *189*, 104706. [CrossRef] [PubMed]

74. Kiyici, S.; Koca, N.; Sigirli, D.; Aslan, B.B.; Guclu, M.; Kisakol, G. Food Addiction Correlates with Psychosocial Functioning More Than Metabolic Parameters in Patients with Obesity. *Metab. Syndr. Relat. Disord.* **2020**, *18*, 161–167. [CrossRef] [PubMed]
75. Wenzel, K.R.; Weinstock, J.; McGrath, A.B. The Clinical Significance of Food Addiction. *J. Addict. Med.* **2020**, *14*, e153–e159. [CrossRef] [PubMed]
76. VanderBroek-Stice, L.; Stojek, M.K.; Beach, S.; vanDellen, M.R.; MacKillop, J. Multidimensional assessment of impulsivity in relation to obesity and food addiction. *Appetite* **2017**, *112*, 59–68. [CrossRef]
77. Wolz, I.; Granero, R.; Fernández-Aranda, F. A comprehensive model of food addiction in patients with binge-eating symptomatology: The essential role of negative urgency. *Compr. Psychiatry* **2017**, *74*, 118–124. [CrossRef]
78. Meule, A.; de Zwaan, M.; Müller, A. Attentional and motor impulsivity interactively predict 'food addiction' in obese individuals. *Compr. Psychiatry* **2017**, *72*, 83–87. [CrossRef]
79. Maxwell, A.L.; Gardiner, E.; Loxton, N.J. Investigating the relationship between reward sensitivity, impulsivity, and food addiction: A systematic review. *Eur. Eat. Disord. Rev. J. Eat. Disord. Assoc.* **2020**, *28*, 368–384. [CrossRef]
80. Nederkoorn, C.; Guerrieri, R.; Havermans, R.; Roefs, A.; Jansen, A. The interactive effect of hunger and impulsivity on food intake and purchase in a virtual supermarket. *Int. J. Obes.* **2009**, *33*, 905–912. [CrossRef]
81. Trifilieff, P.; Martinez, D. Imaging addiction: D2 receptors and dopamine signaling in the striatum as biomarkers for impulsivity. *Neuropharmacology* **2014**, *76*, 498–509. [CrossRef]
82. Savage, S.W.; Zald, D.H.; Cowan, R.L.; Volkow, N.D.; Marks-Shulman, P.A.; Kessler, R.M.; Abumrad, N.N.; Dunn, J.P. Regulation of novelty seeking by midbrain dopamine D2/D3 signaling and ghrelin is altered in obesity. *Obesity* **2014**, *22*, 1452–1457. [CrossRef] [PubMed]
83. Kekic, M.; McClelland, J.; Bartholdy, S.; Chamali, R.; Campbell, I.C.; Schmidt, U. Bad Things Come to Those Who Do Not Wait: Temporal Discounting Is Associated with Compulsive Overeating, Eating Disorder Psychopathology and Food Addiction. *Front. Psychiatry* **2019**, *10*, 978. [CrossRef] [PubMed]
84. Michaud, A.; Vainik, U.; Garcia-Garcia, I.; Dagher, A. Overlapping Neural Endophenotypes in Addiction and Obesity. *Front. Endocrinol.* **2017**, *8*, 127. [CrossRef] [PubMed]
85. Moloney, G.M.; van Oeffelen, W.E.P.A.; Ryan, F.J.; van de Wouw, M.; Cowan, C.; Claesson, M.J.; Schellekens, H.; Dinan, T.G.; Cryan, J.F. Differential gene expression in the mesocorticolimbic system of innately high- and low-impulsive rats. *Behav. Brain Res.* **2019**, *364*, 193–204. [CrossRef] [PubMed]
86. Gray, J.C.; MacKillop, J.; Weafer, J.; Hernandez, K.M.; Gao, J.; Palmer, A.A.; Wit, H. de Genetic analysis of impulsive personality traits: Examination of a priori candidates and genome-wide variation. *Psychiatry Res.* **2018**, *259*, 398–404. [CrossRef]
87. Morland, K.; Wing, S.; Roux, A.; Poole, C. Neighborhood characteristics associated with the location of food stores and food service places. *Am. J. Prev. Med.* **2002**, *22*, 23–29. [CrossRef]
88. Black, J.L.; Macinko, J. Neighborhoods and obesity. *Nutr. Rev.* **2008**, *66*, 2–20. [CrossRef]
89. Carroll-Scott, A.; Gilstad-Hayden, K.; Rosenthal, L.; Peters, S.M.; McCaslin, C.; Joyce, R.; Ickovics, J.R. Disentangling neighborhood contextual associations with child body mass index, diet, and physical activity: The role of built, socioeconomic, and social environments. *Soc. Sci. Med.* **2013**, *95*, 106–114. [CrossRef]
90. Kim, Y.; Cubbin, C.; Oh, S. A systematic review of neighbourhood economic context on child obesity and obesity-related behaviours. *Obes. Rev.* **2019**, *20*, 420–431. [CrossRef]
91. Claassen, M.; Klein, O.; Bratanova, B.; Claes, N.; Corneille, O. A systematic review of psychosocial explanations for the relationship between socioeconomic status and body mass index. *Appetite* **2019**, *132*, 208–221. [CrossRef]
92. Darmon, N.; Drewnowski, A. Does social class predict diet quality? *Am. J. Clin. Nutr.* **2008**, *87*, 1107–1117. [CrossRef] [PubMed]
93. Fleary, S.A.; Ettienne, R. The relationship between food parenting practices, parental diet and their adolescents' diet. *Appetite* **2019**, *135*, 79–85. [CrossRef] [PubMed]
94. Williams, A.S.; Ge, B.; Petroski, G.; Kruse, R.L.; McElroy, J.A.; Koopman, R.J. Socioeconomic Status and Other Factors Associated with Childhood Obesity. *J. Am. Board Fam. Med.* **2018**, *31*, 514–521. [CrossRef] [PubMed]
95. Mason, S.; Santaularia, N.; Berge, J.; Larson, N.; Neumark-Sztainer, D. Is the childhood home food environment a confounder of the association between child maltreatment exposure and adult body mass index? *Prev. Med.* **2018**, *110*, 86–92. [CrossRef] [PubMed]

96. Walker, B.B.; Shashank, A.; Gasevic, D.; Schuurman, N.; Poirier, P.; Teo, K.; Rangarajan, S.; Yusuf, S.; Lear, S.A. The Local Food Environment and Obesity: Evidence from Three Cities. *Obesity* **2019**, *28*, 40–45. [CrossRef]
97. Cooksey-Stowers, K.; Schwartz, M.B.; Brownell, K.D. Food Swamps Predict Obesity Rates Better Than Food Deserts in the United States. *Int. J. Environ. Res. Public Health* **2017**, *14*, 1366. [CrossRef]
98. Drewnowski, A.; Buszkiewicz, J.; Aggarwal, A.; Rose, C.; Gupta, S.; Bradshaw, A. Obesity and the Built Environment: A Reappraisal. *Obesity* **2019**, *28*, 22–30. [CrossRef]
99. Chirinos, D.A.; Garcini, L.M.; Seiler, A.; Murdock, K.W.; Peek, K.; Stowe, R.P.; Fagundes, C. Psychological and Biological Pathways Linking Perceived Neighborhood Characteristics and Body Mass Index. *Ann. Behav. Med.* **2018**, *53*, 827–838. [CrossRef]
100. Greenland, S.; Pearl, J.; Robins, J.M. Causal Diagrams for Epidemiologic Research. *Epidemiology* **1999**, *10*, 37–48. [CrossRef]
101. Sobal, J.; Stunkard, A.J. Socioeconomic Status and Obesity: A Review of the Literature. *Psychol. Bull.* **1989**, *105*, 260–275. [CrossRef]
102. McLaren, L. Socioeconomic Status and Obesity. *Epidemiol Rev.* **2007**, *29*, 29–48. [CrossRef] [PubMed]
103. De Wilde, J.; Eilander, M.; Middelkoop, B. Effect of neighbourhood socioeconomic status on overweight and obesity in children 2–15 years of different ethnic groups. *Eur. J. Public Health* **2019**, *29*, 796–801. [CrossRef] [PubMed]
104. Chen, M.; Creger, T.; Howard, V.; Judd, S.E.; Harrington, K.F.; Fontaine, K.R. Association of community food environment and obesity among US adults: A geographical information system analysis. *J. Epidemiol. Community Health* **2018**, *73*, 148–155. [CrossRef] [PubMed]
105. Lynch, B.A.; Rutten, L.J.; Wilson, P.M.; Kumar, S.; Phelan, S.; Jacobson, R.M.; Fan, C.; Agunwamba, A. The impact of positive contextual factors on the association between adverse family experiences and obesity in a National Survey of Children. *Prev. Med.* **2018**, *116*, 81–86. [CrossRef] [PubMed]
106. Twaits, A.; Alwan, N.A. The association between area-based deprivation and change in body-mass index over time in primary school children: A population-based cohort study in Hampshire, UK. *Int. J. Obes.* **2019**, *44*, 628–636. [CrossRef]
107. Ford, D.E. The Community and Public Well-being Model: A New Framework and Graduate Curriculum for Addressing Adverse Childhood Experiences. *Acad. Pediatrics* **2017**, *17*, S9–S11. [CrossRef]
108. Metzler, M.; Merrick, M.T.; Klevens, J.; Ports, K.A.; Ford, D.C. Adverse childhood experiences and life opportunities: Shifting the narrative. *Child. Youth Serv. Rev.* **2017**, *72*, 141–149. [CrossRef]
109. Kristenson, M.; Eriksen, H.R.; Sluiter, J.K.; Starke, D.; Ursin, H. Psychobiological mechanisms of socioeconomic differences in health. *Soc. Sci. Med.* **2004**, *58*, 1511–1522. [CrossRef]
110. Gunstad, J.; Paul, R.H.; Spitznagel, M.; Cohen, R.A.; Williams, L.M.; Kohn, M.; Gordon, E. Exposure to early life trauma is associated with adult obesity. *Psychiatry Res.* **2006**, *142*, 31–37. [CrossRef]
111. Friedman, E.M.; Montez, J.K.; Sheehan, C.M.; Guenewald, T.L.; Seeman, T.E. Childhood Adversities and Adult Cardiometabolic Health: Does the Quantity, Timing, and Type of Adversity Matter? *J. Aging Health* **2015**, *27*, 1311–1338. [CrossRef]
112. Mhamdi, S.E.; Lemieux, A.; Abroug, H.; Salah, A.B.; Bouanene, I.; Salem, K.B.; al'Absi, M. Childhood exposure to violence is associated with risk for mental disorders and adult's weight status: A community-based study in Tunisia. *J. Public Health* **2018**, *41*, 502–510. [CrossRef] [PubMed]
113. Pickett, S.; Burchenal, C.A.; Haber, L.; Batten, K.; Phillips, E. Understanding and effectively addressing disparities in obesity: A systematic review of the psychological determinants of emotional eating behaviours among Black women. *Obes. Rev.* **2020**, *21*, e13010. [CrossRef] [PubMed]
114. Tomiyama, A. Stress and Obesity. *Annu. Rev. Psychol.* **2019**, *70*, 703–718. [CrossRef] [PubMed]
115. Doom, J.R.; Lumeng, J.C.; Sturza, J.; Kaciroti, N.; Vazquez, D.M.; Miller, A.L. Longitudinal associations between overweight/obesity and stress biology in low-income children. *Int. J. Obes.* **2019**, *44*, 646–655. [CrossRef] [PubMed]
116. Barker, D. The fetal and infant origins of adult disease. *Br. Med. J.* **1990**, *301*, 1111. [CrossRef]
117. McEwen, B.S.; Stellar, E. Stress and the Individual: Mechanisms Leading to Disease. *Arch. Intern. Med.* **1993**, *153*, 2093–2101. [CrossRef]
118. McEwen, B.S. Stress, Adaption, and Disease. *Ann. N. Y. Acad. Sci.* **1998**, *840*, 33–44. [CrossRef]
119. Seeman, T.; Singer, B.; Rowe, J.; Horwitz, R.; McEwen, B. Price of adaptation—Allostatic load and its health consequences. MacArthur studies of successful aging. *Arch. Intern. Med.* **1997**, *157*, 2259–2268. [CrossRef]

120. Ottino-González, J.; Jurado, M.A.; García-García, I.; Caldú, X.; Prats-Soteras, X.; Tor, E.; Sender-Palacios, M.J.; Garolera, M. Allostatic load and executive functions in overweight adults. *Psychoneuroendocrinology* **2019**, *106*, 165–170. [CrossRef]
121. Nusslock, R.; Miller, G.E. Early-Life Adversity and Physical and Emotional Health Across the Lifespan: A Neuroimmune Network Hypothesis. *Biol. Psychiatry* **2016**, *80*, 23–32. [CrossRef]
122. Hostinar, C.E.; Nusslock, R.; Miller, G.E. Future Directions in the Study of Early-Life Stress and Physical and Emotional Health: Implications of the Neuroimmune Network Hypothesis. *J. Clin. Child. Adolesc. Psychol.* **2018**, *47*, 142–156. [CrossRef] [PubMed]
123. Sapolsky, R.; Krey, L.; McEwen, B. The neuroendocrinology of stress and aging: The glucocorticoid cascade hypothesis. *Endocr. Rev.* **1986**, *7*, 284–301. [CrossRef] [PubMed]
124. Kaess, M.; Whittle, S.; O'Brien-Simpson, L.; Allen, N.B.; Simmons, J.G. Childhood maltreatment, pituitary volume and adolescent hypothalamic-pituitary-adrenal axis—Evidence for a maltreatment-related attenuation. *Psychoneuroendocrinology* **2018**, *98*, 39–45. [CrossRef] [PubMed]
125. Boyce, T.W. Differential Susceptibility of the Developing Brain to Contextual Adversity and Stress. *Neuropsychopharmacology* **2015**, *41*, 142–162. [CrossRef] [PubMed]
126. Finnell, J.E.; Wood, S.K. Putative Inflammatory Sensitive Mechanisms Underlying Risk or Resilience to Social Stress. *Front. Behav. Neurosci.* **2018**, *12*, 240. [CrossRef] [PubMed]
127. Rapuano, K.M.; Laurent, J.S.; Hagler, D.J.; Hatton, S.N.; Thompson, W.K.; Jernigan, T.L.; Dale, A.M.; Casey, B.J.; Watts, R. Nucleus accumbens cytoarchitecture predicts weight gain in children. *Proc. Natl. Acad. Sci. USA* **2020**, *117*, 26977–26984. [CrossRef] [PubMed]
128. Calem, M.; Bromis, K.; McGuire, P.; Morgan, C.; Kempton, M.J. Meta-analysis of associations between childhood adversity and hippocampus and amygdala volume in non-clinical and general population samples. *Neuroimage Clin.* **2017**, *14*, 471–479. [CrossRef]
129. Elsey, J.; Coates, A.; Lacadie, C.M.; McCrory, E.J.; Sinha, R.; Mayes, L.C.; Potenza, M.N. Childhood Trauma and Neural Responses to Personalized Stress, Favorite-Food and Neutral-Relaxing Cues in Adolescents. *Neuropsychopharmacology* **2015**, *40*, 1580–1589. [CrossRef]
130. Berens, A.E.; Jensen, S.K.; Nelson, C.A. Biological embedding of childhood adversity: From physiological mechanisms to clinical implications. *BMC Med.* **2017**, *15*, 135. [CrossRef] [PubMed]
131. Wiss, D.A.; Criscitelli, K.; Gold, M.; Avena, N. Preclinical evidence for the addiction potential of highly palatable foods: Current developments related to maternal influence. *Appetite* **2017**, *115*, 19–27. [CrossRef] [PubMed]
132. Buss, C.; Entringer, S.; Moog, N.K.; Toepfer, P.; Fair, D.A.; Simhan, H.N.; Heim, C.M.; Wadhwa, P.D. Intergenerational Transmission of Maternal Childhood Maltreatment Exposure: Implications for Fetal Brain Development. *J. Am. Acad. Child. Adolesc. Psychiatry* **2017**, *56*, 373–382. [CrossRef]
133. Nieto, S.J.; Kosten, T.A. Who's your daddy? Behavioral and epigenetic consequences of paternal drug exposure. *Int. J. Dev. Neurosci.* **2019**, *78*, 109–121. [CrossRef]
134. Costa, D.L.; Yetter, N.; DeSomer, H. Intergenerational transmission of paternal trauma among US Civil War ex-POWs. *Proc. Natl. Acad. Sci. USA* **2018**, *115*, 11215–11220. [CrossRef] [PubMed]
135. Demetriou, C.A.; Veldhoven, K.; Relton, C.; Stringhini, S.; Kyriacou, K.; Vineis, P. Biological embedding of early-life exposures and disease risk in humans: A role for DNA methylation. *Eur. J. Clin. Investig.* **2015**, *45*, 303–332. [CrossRef] [PubMed]
136. Lutz, P.-E.; Turecki, G. DNA methylation and childhood maltreatment: From animal models to human studies. *Neuroscience* **2014**, *264*, 142–156. [CrossRef]
137. McGowan, P.O.; Szyf, M. The epigenetics of social adversity in early life: Implications for mental health outcomes. *Neurobiol. Dis.* **2010**, *39*, 66–72. [CrossRef] [PubMed]
138. McGowan, P.O.; Sasaki, A.; D'Alessio, A.C.; Dymov, S.; Labonté, B.; Szyf, M.; Turecki, G.; Meaney, M.J. Epigenetic regulation of the glucocorticoid receptor in human brain associates with childhood abuse. *Nat. Neurosci.* **2009**, *12*, 342–348. [CrossRef]
139. Szyf, M. DNA Methylation, Behavior and Early Life Adversity. *J. Genet. Genom.* **2013**, *40*, 331–338. [CrossRef]
140. Palma-Gudiel, H.; Córdova-Palomera, A.; Eixarch, E.; Deuschle, M.; Fañanás, L. Maternal psychosocial stress during pregnancy alters the epigenetic signature of the glucocorticoid receptor gene promoter in their offspring: A meta-analysis. *Epigenetics* **2015**, *10*, 893–902. [CrossRef]

141. Mitchell, C.; Schneper, L.M.; Notterman, D.A. DNA methylation, early life environment, and health outcomes. *Pediatric Res.* **2015**, *79*, 212–219. [CrossRef]
142. Bakusic, J.; Schaufeli, W.; Claes, S.; Godderis, L. Stress, burnout and depression: A systematic review on DNA methylation mechanisms. *J. Psychosom. Res.* **2017**, *92*, 34–44. [CrossRef] [PubMed]
143. Wei, L.-N. Epigenetic control of the expression of opioid receptor genes. *Epigenetics* **2008**, *3*, 119–121. [CrossRef] [PubMed]
144. Belzeaux, R.; Lalanne, L.; Kieffer, B.L.; Lutz, P.-E. Focusing on the Opioid System for Addiction Biomarker Discovery. *Trends Mol. Med.* **2018**, *24*, 206–220. [CrossRef] [PubMed]
145. Giuliano, C.; Cottone, P. The role of the opioid system in binge eating disorder. *CNS Spectr.* **2015**, *20*, 537–545. [CrossRef] [PubMed]
146. Pucci, M.; Bonaventura, M.; Vezzoli, V.; Zaplatic, E.; Massimini, M.; Mai, S.; Sartorio, A.; Scacchi, M.; Persani, L.; Maccarrone, M.; et al. Preclinical and Clinical Evidence for a Distinct Regulation of Mu Opioid and Type 1 Cannabinoid Receptor Genes Expression in Obesity. *Front. Genet.* **2019**, *10*, 523. [CrossRef]
147. Lutz, P.-E.; Gross, J.A.; Dhir, S.K.; Maussion, G.; Yang, J.; Bramoulle, A.; Meaney, M.J.; Turecki, G. Epigenetic Regulation of the Kappa Opioid Receptor by Child Abuse. *Biol. Psychiatry* **2018**, *84*, 751–761. [CrossRef] [PubMed]
148. Walker, D.M.; Nestler, E.J. Neuroepigenetics and addiction. *Sci. Direct* **2018**, *148*, 747–765. [CrossRef]
149. Denhardt, D.T. Effect of stress on human biology: Epigenetics, adaptation, inheritance, and social significance. *J. Cell. Physiol.* **2018**, *233*, 1975–1984. [CrossRef]
150. Seo, D.; Patrick, C.J.; Kennealy, P.J. Role of serotonin and dopamine system interactions in the neurobiology of impulsive aggression and its comorbidity with other clinical disorders. *Aggress. Violent Behav.* **2008**, *13*, 383–395. [CrossRef]
151. Kader, F.; Ghai, M.; Maharaj, L. The effects of DNA methylation on human psychology. *Behav Brain Res.* **2018**, *346*, 47–65. [CrossRef]
152. Candler, T.; Kühnen, P.; Prentice, A.M.; Silver, M. Epigenetic regulation of POMC; implications for nutritional programming, obesity and metabolic disease. *Front. Neuroendocrinol.* **2019**, *54*, 100773. [CrossRef] [PubMed]
153. Groleau, P.; Joober, R.; Israel, M.; Zeramdini, N.; DeGuzman, R.; Steiger, H. Methylation of the dopamine D2 receptor (DRD2) gene promoter in women with a bulimia-spectrum disorder: Associations with borderline personality disorder and exposure to childhood abuse. *J. Psychiatr. Res.* **2014**, *48*, 121–127. [CrossRef] [PubMed]
154. Jentsch, D.J.; Ashenhurst, J.R.; Cervantes, C.M.; Groman, S.M.; James, A.S.; Pennington, Z.T. Dissecting impulsivity and its relationships to drug addictions. *Ann. N. Y. Acad. Sci.* **2014**, *1327*, 1–26. [CrossRef] [PubMed]
155. He, F.; Berg, A.; Kawasawa, Y.; Bixler, E.O.; Fernandez-Mendoza, J.; Whitsel, E.A.; Liao, D. Association between DNA methylation in obesity-related genes and body mass index percentile in adolescents. *Sci. Rep.* **2019**, *9*, 1–8. [CrossRef] [PubMed]
156. Ndiaye, F.K.; Huyvaert, M.; Ortalli, A.; Canouil, M.; Lecoeur, C.; Verbanck, M.; Lobbens, S.; Khamis, A.; Marselli, L.; Marchetti, P.; et al. The expression of genes in top obesity-associated loci is enriched in insula and substantia nigra brain regions involved in addiction and reward. *Int. J. Obes.* **2020**, *44*, 539–543. [CrossRef] [PubMed]
157. Ramos-Lopez, O.; Riezu-Boj, J.I.; Milagro, F.I.; Martinez, A.J.; Project, M. Dopamine gene methylation patterns are associated with obesity markers and carbohydrate intake. *Brain Behav.* **2018**, *8*, e01017. [CrossRef] [PubMed]
158. Li, Y. Epigenetic Mechanisms Link Maternal Diets and Gut Microbiome to Obesity in the Offspring. *Front. Genet.* **2018**, *9*, 342. [CrossRef]
159. Ramos-Molina, B.; Sánchez-Alcoholado, L.; Cabrera-Mulero, A.; Lopez-Dominguez, R.; Carmona-Saez, P.; Garcia-Fuentes, E.; Moreno-Indias, I.; Tinahones, F.J. Gut Microbiota Composition Is Associated with the Global DNA Methylation Pattern in Obesity. *Front. Genet.* **2019**, *10*, 613. [CrossRef]
160. Miro-Blanch, J.; Yanes, O. Epigenetic Regulation at the Interplay Between Gut Microbiota and Host Metabolism. *Front. Genet.* **2019**, *10*, 638. [CrossRef]
161. Miller, A.L.; Lee, H.J.; Lumeng, J.C. Obesity-associated biomarkers and executive function in children. *Pediatr Res.* **2015**, *77*, 143–147. [CrossRef]

162. Favieri, F.; Forte, G.; Casagrande, M. The Executive Functions in Overweight and Obesity: A Systematic Review of Neuropsychological Cross-Sectional and Longitudinal Studies. *Front. Psychol* **2019**, *10*, 2126. [CrossRef] [PubMed]
163. Bourassa, K.; Sbarra, D.A. Body mass and cognitive decline are indirectly associated via inflammation among aging adults. *Brain Behav Immun* **2017**, *60*, 63–70. [CrossRef] [PubMed]
164. Miller, A.L.; Lumeng, J.C. Pathways of Association from Stress to Obesity in Early Childhood. *Obesity* **2016**. [CrossRef] [PubMed]
165. Michels, N. Biological underpinnings from psychosocial stress towards appetite and obesity during youth: Research implications towards metagenomics, epigenomics and metabolomics. *Nutr. Res. Rev.* **2019**, 282–293. [CrossRef]
166. Gupta, A.; Osadchiy, V.; Mayer, E.A. Brain–gut–microbiome interactions in obesity and food addiction. *Nat. Rev. Gastroentero* **2020**, 1–18. [CrossRef]
167. Wonderlich, J.A.; Breithaupt, L.; Thompson, J.C.; Crosby, R.D.; Engel, S.G.; Fischer, S. The impact of neural responses to food cues following stress on trajectories of negative and positive affect and binge eating in daily life. *J. Psychiatr. Res.* **2018**, *102*, 14–22. [CrossRef]
168. Chami, R.; Monteleone, A.; Treasure, J.; Monteleone, P. Stress hormones and eating disorders. *Mol. Cell. Endocrinol.* **2019**, *497*, 110349. [CrossRef]
169. Sinha, R. Role of addiction and stress neurobiology on food intake and obesity. *Biol. Psychol.* **2018**, *131*, 5–13. [CrossRef]
170. Mantsch, J.R.; Baker, D.A.; Funk, D.; Lê, A.D.; Shaham, Y. Stress-Induced Reinstatement of Drug Seeking: 20 Years of Progress. *Neuropsychopharmacol* **2016**, *41*, 335–356. [CrossRef]
171. McCaul, M.E.; Wand, G.S.; Weerts, E.M.; Xu, X. A paradigm for examining stress effects on alcohol-motivated behaviors in participants with alcohol use disorder. *Addict. Biol.* **2017**, *23*, 836–845. [CrossRef]
172. Blaine, S.K. Alcohol, stress, and glucocorticoids: From risk to dependence and relapse in alcohol use disorders. *Neuropharmacology* **2017**, *122*, 115–126. [CrossRef] [PubMed]
173. Becker, H.C. Influence of stress associated with chronic alcohol exposure on drinking. *Neuropharmacology* **2018**, *122*. [CrossRef] [PubMed]
174. George, O.; Moal, M.; Koob, G.F. Allostasis and addiction: Role of the dopamine and corticotropin-releasing factor systems. *Physiol. Behav.* **2012**, *106*, 58–64. [CrossRef] [PubMed]
175. Koob, G.F.; Schulkin, J. Addiction and Stress: An Allostatic View. *Neurosci. Biobehav. Rev.* **2019**, *106*, 245–262. [CrossRef] [PubMed]
176. Forster, G.L.; Anderson, E.M.; Scholl, J.L.; Lukkes, J.L.; Watt, M.J. Negative consequences of early-life adversity on substance use as mediated by corticotropin-releasing factor modulation of serotonin activity. *Neurobiol. Stress* **2018**, *9*, 29–39. [CrossRef] [PubMed]
177. Moustafa, A.A.; Parkes, D.; Fitzgerald, L.; Underhill, D.; Garami, J.; Levy-Gigi, E.; Stramecki, F.; Valikhani, A.; Frydecka, D.; Misiak, B. The relationship between childhood trauma, early-life stress, and alcohol and drug use, abuse, and addiction: An integrative review. *Curr. Psychol.* **2018**, 1–6. [CrossRef]
178. Kreek, M.; Nielsen, D.A.; Butelman, E.R.; LaForge, S.K. Genetic influences on impulsivity, risk taking, stress responsivity and vulnerability to drug abuse and addiction. *Nat. Neurosci.* **2005**, *8*, 1450–1457. [CrossRef]
179. Daughters, S.B.; Richards, J.M.; Gorka, S.M.; Sinha, R. HPA axis response to psychological stress and treatment retention in residential substance abuse treatment: A prospective study. *Drug Alcohol Depend.* **2009**, *105*, 202–208. [CrossRef]
180. Levran, O.; Peles, E.; Randesi, M.; da Rosa, J.; Shen, P.-H.; Rotrosen, J.; Adelson, M.; Kreek, M. Genetic variations in genes of the stress response pathway are associated with prolonged abstinence from heroin. *Pharmacogenomics* **2018**, *19*, 333–341. [CrossRef]
181. Jacques, A.; Chaaya, N.; Beecher, K.; Ali, S.A.; Belmer, A.; Bartlett, S. The impact of sugar consumption on stress driven, emotional and addictive behaviors. *Neurosci. Biobehav. Rev.* **2019**, *103*, 178–199. [CrossRef]
182. Evans, C.; Cahill, C. Neurobiology of opioid dependence in creating addiction vulnerability. *F1000Research* **2016**, *5*. [CrossRef]
183. Brady, K.T.; Dansky, B.S.; Sonne, S.C.; Saladin, M.E. Posttraumatic Stress Disorder and Cocaine Dependence: Order of Onset. *Am. J. Addict.* **1998**, *7*, 128–135. [CrossRef] [PubMed]
184. Cottler, L.B.; Compton, W.M.; Mager, D.; Spitznagel, E.L.; Janca, A. Posttraumatic stress disorder among substance users from the general population. *Am. J. Psychiatry* **1992**, *149*, 664–670. [CrossRef] [PubMed]

185. Pennington, Z.T.; Trott, J.M.; Rajbhandari, A.K.; Li, K.; Walwyn, W.M.; Evans, C.J.; Fanselow, M.S. Chronic opioid pretreatment potentiates the sensitization of fear learning by trauma. *Neuropsychopharmacol* **2019**, *45*, 482–490. [CrossRef] [PubMed]
186. Longo, D.L.; Volkow, N.D.; Koob, G.F.; McLellan, T.A. Neurobiologic Advances from the Brain Disease Model of Addiction. *N. Engl. J. Med.* **2016**, *374*, 363–371. [CrossRef]
187. Koob, G.F.; Volkow, N.D. Neurobiology of addiction: A neurocircuitry analysis. *Lancet Psychiatry* **2016**, *3*, 760–773. [CrossRef]
188. Volkow, N.D.; Koob, G. Brain disease model of addiction: Why is it so controversial? *Lancet Psychiatry* **2015**, *2*, 677–679. [CrossRef]
189. Mukhara, D.; Banks, M.L.; Neigh, G.N. Stress as a Risk Factor for Substance Use Disorders: A Mini-Review of Molecular Mediators. *Front. Behav. Neurosci.* **2018**, *12*, 309. [CrossRef]
190. Karkhanis, A.; Holleran, K.M.; Jones, S.R. International Review of Neurobiology. *Int. Rev. Neurobiol.* **2017**, *136*, 53–88. [CrossRef]
191. Joutsa, J.; Karlsson, H.K.; Majuri, J.; Nuutila, P.; Helin, S.; Kaasinen, V.; Nummenmaa, L. Binge eating disorder and morbid obesity are associated with lowered mu-opioid receptor availability in the brain. *Psychiatry Res. Neuroimaging* **2018**, *276*, 41–45. [CrossRef]
192. Novick, A.M.; Levandowski, M.L.; Laumann, L.; Philip, N.S.; Price, L.H.; Tyrka, A.R. The effects of early life stress on reward processing. *J. Psychiatr. Res.* **2018**, *101*, 80–103. [CrossRef] [PubMed]
193. Meule, A. Chapter 16 An Addiction Perspective on Eating Disorders and Obesity. *Eat. Disord. Obes. Child. Adolesc.* **2019**, 99–104. [CrossRef]
194. Monnier, L.; Schlienger, J.-L.; Colette, C.; Bonnet, F. The obesity treatment dilemma: Why dieting is both the answer and the problem? A mechanistic overview. *Diabetes Metab.* **2020**. [CrossRef] [PubMed]
195. Schaumberg, K.; Anderson, D.A.; Anderson, L.M.; Reilly, E.E.; Gorrell, S. Dietary restraint: What's the harm? A review of the relationship between dietary restraint, weight trajectory and the development of eating pathology. *Clin. Obes.* **2016**, *6*, 89–100. [CrossRef]
196. Keys, A.; Brožek, J.; Henschel, A.; Mickelsen, O.; Taylor, H.L. *The Biology of Human Starvation, Vols. 1 & 2*; University of Minnesota Press: Minneapolis, MN, USA, 1950.
197. Dunn, T.M.; Bratman, S. On orthorexia nervosa: A review of the literature and proposed diagnostic criteria. *Eat. Behav.* **2016**, *21*, 11–17. [CrossRef]
198. Tomiyama, A.J.; Mann, T.; Vinas, D.; Hunger, J.M.; Dejager, J.; Taylor, S.E. Low calorie dieting increases cortisol. *Psychosom Med.* **2010**, *72*, 357. [CrossRef]
199. Pietiläinen, K.H.; Saarni, S.E.; Kaprio, J.; Rissanen, A. Does dieting make you fat? A twin study. *Int. J. Obes.* **2011**, *36*, 456–464. [CrossRef]
200. Su, Y.; Bi, T.; Gong, G.; Jiang, Q.; Chen, H. Why Do Most Restrained Eaters Fail in Losing Weight?: Evidence from an fMRI Study. *Psychol. Res. Behav Manag.* **2019**, *12*, 1127–1136. [CrossRef]
201. Wiss, D.A.; Brewerton, T.D. Incorporating food addiction into disordered eating: The disordered eating food addiction nutrition guide (DEFANG). *Eat. Weight Disord. Stud. Anorex. Bulim. Obes.* **2017**, *22*, 49–59. [CrossRef]
202. Meule, A. A Critical Examination of the Practical Implications Derived from the Food Addiction Concept. *Curr. Obes. Rep.* **2019**, *8*, 11–17. [CrossRef]
203. Tomiyama, A.J. Weight stigma is stressful. A review of evidence for the Cyclic Obesity/Weight-Based Stigma model. *Appetite* **2014**, *82*, 8–15. [CrossRef] [PubMed]
204. Tomiyama, A.J.; Epel, E.S.; McClatchey, T.M.; Poelke, G.; Kemeny, M.E.; McCoy, S.K.; Daubenmier, J. Associations of Weight Stigma with Cortisol and Oxidative Stress Independent of Adiposity. *Health Psychol.* **2014**, *33*, 862–867. [CrossRef] [PubMed]
205. Daly, M.; Robinson, E.; Sutin, A.R. Perceived overweight and suicidality among US adolescents from 1999 to 2017. *Int. J. Obes.* **2020**, *44*, 2075–2079. [CrossRef] [PubMed]
206. Sutin, A.; Robinson, E.; Daly, M.; Terracciano, A. Weight discrimination and unhealthy eating-related behaviors. *Appetite* **2016**, *102*, 83–89. [CrossRef]
207. Major, B.; Rathbone, J.A.; Blodorn, A.; Hunger, J.M. The Countervailing Effects of Weight Stigma on Weight-Loss Motivation and Perceived Capacity for Weight Control. *Personal. Soc. Psychol. Bull.* **2020**, 146167220903184. [CrossRef]

208. Ahorsu, D.K.; Lin, C.-Y.; Imani, V.; Griffiths, M.D.; Su, J.-A.; Latner, J.D.; Marshall, R.D.; Pakpour, A.H. A prospective study on the link between weight-related self-stigma and binge eating: Role of food addiction and psychological distress. *Int. J. Eat. Disord.* **2020**, *53*, 442–450. [CrossRef]
209. Pudney, E.V.; Himmelstein, M.S.; Puhl, R.M.; Foster, G.D. Distressed or not distressed? A mixed methods examination of reactions to weight stigma and implications for emotional wellbeing and internalized weight bias. *Soc. Sci. Med.* **2020**, *249*, 112854. [CrossRef]
210. Alberga, A.S.; Edache, I.Y.; Forhan, M.; Russell-Mayhew, S. Weight bias and health care utilization: A scoping review. *Prim. Heal. Care Res. Dev.* **2019**, *20*, e116. [CrossRef]
211. Hunger, J.M.; Smith, J.P.; Tomiyama, A.J. An Evidence-Based Rationale for Adopting Weight-Inclusive Health Policy. *Soc. Issues Policy Rev.* **2020**, *14*, 73–107. [CrossRef]
212. Latner, J.D.; Puhl, R.M.; Murakami, J.M.; O'Brien, K.S. Food addiction as a causal model of obesity. Effects on stigma, blame, and perceived psychopathology. *Appetite* **2014**, *77*, 79–84. [CrossRef]
213. O'Brien, K.S.; Puhl, R.M.; Latner, J.D.; Lynott, D.; Reid, J.D.; Vakhitova, Z.; Hunter, J.A.; Scarf, D.; Jeanes, R.; Bouguettaya, A.; et al. The Effect of a Food Addiction Explanation Model for Weight Control and Obesity on Weight Stigma. *Nutrients* **2020**, *12*, 294. [CrossRef] [PubMed]
214. Cassin, S.E.; Buchman, D.Z.; Leung, S.E.; Kantarovich, K.; Hawa, A.; Carter, A.; Sockalingam, S. Ethical, Stigma, and Policy Implications of Food Addiction: A Scoping Review. *Nutrients* **2019**, *11*, 710. [CrossRef]
215. Rubin, L.P. Maternal and Pediatric Health and Disease: Integrating Biopsychosocial Models and Epigenetics. *Pediatric Res.* **2015**, *79*, 127–135. [CrossRef] [PubMed]
216. Dunn, E.C.; Soare, T.W.; Zhu, Y.; Simpkin, A.J.; Suderman, M.J.; Klengel, T.; Smith, A.; Ressler, K.; Relton, C.L. Sensitive periods for the effect of childhood adversity on DNA methylation: Results from a prospective, longitudinal study. *Biol. Psychiatry* **2019**, *85*, 838–849. [CrossRef] [PubMed]
217. Gabard-Durnam, L.J.; McLaughlin, K.A. Do Sensitive Periods Exist for Exposure to Adversity? *Biol. Psychiatry* **2019**, *85*, 789–791. [CrossRef]
218. Matikainen-Ankney, B.A.; Kravitz, A.V. Persistent effects of obesity: A neuroplasticity hypothesis. *Ann. N. Y. Acad. Sci.* **2018**, *1428*, 221–239. [CrossRef]
219. Theall, K.P.; Chaparro, P.M.; Denstel, K.; Bilfield, A.; Drury, S.S. Childhood obesity and the associated roles of neighborhood and biologic stress. *Prev. Med. Rep.* **2019**, *14*, 100849. [CrossRef]
220. Rung, J.M.; Peck, S.; Hinnenkamp, J.E.; Preston, E.; Madden, G.J. Changing Delay Discounting and Impulsive Choice: Implications for Addictions, Prevention, and Human Health. *Perspect. Behav Sci.* **2019**, *42*, 397–417. [CrossRef]
221. Bortz, W.M. Biological basis of determinants of health. *Am. J. Public Health* **2005**, *95*, 389–392. [CrossRef]
222. Lei, M.-K.; Beach, S.R.; Simons, R.L. Biological embedding of neighborhood disadvantage and collective efficacy: Influences on chronic illness via accelerated cardiometabolic age. *Dev. Psychopathol.* **2018**, *30*, 1797–1815. [CrossRef]
223. Dube, S.R. Continuing conversations about adverse childhood experiences (ACEs) screening: A public health perspective. *Child. Abus. Neglect.* **2018**, *85*, 180–184. [CrossRef] [PubMed]
224. Tomiyama, A.J.; Carr, D.; Granberg, E.M.; Major, B.; Robinson, E.; Sutin, A.R.; Brewis, A. How and why weight stigma drives the obesity 'epidemic' and harms health. *BMC Med.* **2018**, *16*, 123. [CrossRef]
225. Yang, L.; Wong, L.Y.; Grivel, M.M.; Hasin, D.S. Stigma and substance use disorders. *Curr. Opin. Psychiatry* **2017**, *30*, 378. [CrossRef] [PubMed]
226. Schulte, E.M.; Avena, N.M.; Gearhardt, A.N. Which foods may be addictive? The roles of processing, fat content, and glycemic load. *PLoS ONE* **2015**, *10*, e0117959. [CrossRef] [PubMed]
227. Ayaz, A.; Nergiz-Unal, R.; Dedebayraktar, D.; Akyol, A.; Pekcan, A.G.; Besler, H.T.; Buyuktuncer, Z. How does food addiction influence dietary intake profile? *PLoS ONE* **2018**, *13*, e0195541. [CrossRef] [PubMed]
228. Hall, K.D.; Ayuketah, A.; Brychta, R.; Cai, H.; Cassimatis, T.; Chen, K.Y.; Chung, S.T.; Costa, E.; Courville, A.; Darcey, V.; et al. Ultra-Processed Diets Cause Excess Calorie Intake and Weight Gain: An Inpatient Randomized Controlled Trial of Ad Libitum Food Intake. *Cell Metab.* **2019**, *30*, 67–77. [CrossRef] [PubMed]
229. Juul, F.; Martinez-Steele, E.; Parekh, N.; Monteiro, C.A.; Chang, V.W. Ultra-processed food consumption and excess weight among US adults. *Br. J. Nutr.* **2018**, *120*, 90–100. [CrossRef]
230. Rico-Campà, A.; Martínez-González, M.A.; Alvarez-Alvarez, I.; de Mendonça, R.; de la Fuente-Arrillaga, C.; Gómez-Donoso, C.; Bes-Rastrollo, M. Association between consumption of ultra-processed foods and all cause mortality: SUN prospective cohort study. *BMJ* **2019**, *365*, l1949. [CrossRef]

231. Ruddock, H.K.; Hardman, C.A. Food Addiction Beliefs Amongst the Lay Public: What Are the Consequences for Eating Behaviour? *Curr. Addict. Rep.* **2017**, *4*, 110–115. [CrossRef]
232. Moran, A.; Musicus, A.; Soo, J.; Gearhardt, A.N.; Gollust, S.E.; Roberto, C.A. Believing that certain foods are addictive is associated with support for obesity-related public policies. *Prev. Med.* **2016**, *90*, 39–46. [CrossRef]
233. Rodgers, R.F.; Sonneville, K. Research for leveraging food policy in universal eating disorder prevention. *Int. J. Eat. Disord.* **2018**, *51*, 503–506. [CrossRef] [PubMed]
234. Mallarino, C.; Gómez, L.F.; González-Zapata, L.; Cadena, Y.; Parra, D.C. Advertising of ultra-processed foods and beverages: Children as a vulnerable population. *Rev. Saúde Pública* **2013**, *47*, 1006–1010. [CrossRef] [PubMed]
235. Freeman, B.; Kelly, B.; Vandevijvere, S.; Baur, L. Young adults: Beloved by food and drink marketers and forgotten by public health? *Health Promot. Int.* **2016**, *31*, 954–961. [CrossRef] [PubMed]
236. Story, M.; French, S. Food Advertising and Marketing Directed at Children and Adolescents in the US. *Int. J. Behav. Nutr. Phys.* **2004**, *1*, 3. [CrossRef] [PubMed]
237. Grier, S.A.; Kumanyika, S.K. The Context for Choice: Health Implications of Targeted Food and Beverage Marketing to African Americans. *Am. J. Public Health* **2008**, *98*, 1616–1629. [CrossRef]
238. Grier, S.; Kumanyika, S.K. Targeting Interventions for Ethnic Minority and Low-Income Populations. *Future Child.* **2006**, *16*, 187–207. [CrossRef]
239. Gearhardt, A.; Roberts, M.; Ashe, M. If Sugar is Addictive ... What Does it Mean for the Law? *J. Law Med. Ethics* **2013**, *41*, 46–49. [CrossRef]
240. Bragg, M.A.; Pageot, Y.K.; Amico, A.; Miller, A.N.; Gasbarre, A.; Rummo, P.E.; Elbel, B. Fast food, beverage, and snack brands on social media in the United States: An examination of marketing techniques utilized in 2000 brand posts. *Pediatr. Obes.* **2019**, *15*, e12606. [CrossRef]
241. Gearhardt, A.N.; Yokum, S.; Harris, J.L.; Epstein, L.H.; Lumeng, J.C. Neural response to fast food commercials in adolescents predicts intake. *Am. J. Clin. Nutr.* **2020**, *111*, 493–502. [CrossRef]
242. Thoits, P.A. Stress and Health: Major Findings and Policy Implications. *J. Health Soc. Behav* **2010**, *51*, S41–S53. [CrossRef]
243. Wiss, D.A. A Biopsychosocial Overview of the Opioid Crisis: Considering Nutrition and Gastrointestinal Health. *Front. Public Health* **2019**, *7*, 193. [CrossRef] [PubMed]

Publisher's Note: MDPI stays neutral with regard to jurisdictional claims in published maps and institutional affiliations.

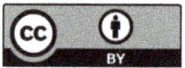

© 2020 by the authors. Licensee MDPI, Basel, Switzerland. This article is an open access article distributed under the terms and conditions of the Creative Commons Attribution (CC BY) license (http://creativecommons.org/licenses/by/4.0/).

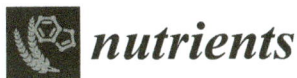

Review

Food Addiction and Tobacco Use Disorder: Common Liability and Shared Mechanisms

Laurie Zawertailo [1,2,*,†], **Sophia Attwells** [2,†], **Wayne K. deRuiter** [2], **Thao Lan Le** [2], **Danielle Dawson** [2] and **Peter Selby** [2,3,4,5]

1. Department of Pharmacology and Toxicology, University of Toronto, 1 King's College Circle, Toronto, ON M5S 1A8, Canada
2. Centre for Addiction and Mental Health, 1025 Queen Street West, Toronto, ON M6J 1H4, Canada; sophia.attwells@camh.ca (S.A.); wayne.deruiter@camh.ca (W.K.d.); thaolan.le@gmail.com (T.L.L.); danielle.dawson@camh.ca (D.D.); peter.selby@camh.ca (P.S.)
3. Department of Family and Community Medicine, University of Toronto, 500 University Ave., Toronto, ON M5G 1V7, Canada
4. Department of Psychiatry, University of Toronto, 250 College St., Toronto, ON M5T 1L8, Canada
5. Dalla Lana School of Public Health, University of Toronto, 155 College St, Toronto, ON M5T 3M7, Canada
* Correspondence: laurie.zawertailo@camh.ca; Tel.: +1-416-535-8201 (ext. 77422)
† These authors contributed equally to this work.

Received: 30 October 2020; Accepted: 10 December 2020; Published: 15 December 2020

Abstract: As food addiction is being more commonly recognized within the scientific community, parallels can be drawn between it and other addictive substance use disorders, including tobacco use disorder. Given that both unhealthy diets and smoking are leading risk factors for disability and death, a greater understanding of how food addiction and tobacco use disorder overlap with one another is necessary. This narrative review aimed to highlight literature that investigated prevalence, biology, psychology, and treatment options of food addiction and tobacco use disorder. Published studies up to August 2020 and written in English were included. Using a biopsychosocial lens, each disorder was assessed together and separately, as there is emerging evidence that the two disorders can develop concurrently or sequentially within individuals. Commonalities include but are not limited to the dopaminergic neurocircuitry, gut microbiota, childhood adversity, and attachment insecurity. In addition, the authors conducted a feasibility study with the purpose of examining the association between food addiction symptoms and tobacco use disorder among individuals seeking tobacco use disorder treatment. To inform future treatment approaches, more research is necessary to identify and understand the overlap between the two disorders.

Keywords: food addiction; nicotine; tobacco use disorder; comorbidity

1. Introduction

Smoking and obesity are the two most prevalent causes of preventable chronic disease morbidity and mortality worldwide [1,2]. Smoking and food addiction are both maladaptive behaviors in which an individual experiences loss of control and compulsive engagement in the behavior despite known harmful consequences. We have reached a pivotal time for understanding food addiction, similar to a time when tobacco use disorder was perceived as habit forming and not addictive. While food addiction does meet several of the American Psychiatric Association's diagnostic criteria outlining substance use disorder [3], more research is necessary to determine if certain foods are addictive and how to prevent and treat this condition.

The concept of food addiction represents a relatively new domain of research [4]. Food addiction refers to an "eating behavior involving the overconsumption of specific foods in an addiction-like manner". While the term "food addiction" was introduced to scientific literature in 1956 [5], research investigating the mechanisms, neurobiology, and genetics of food addiction was not pursued until the early 2000s. Food addiction in relation to certain foods has not been widely accepted or studied. As such, the diagnostic criteria of food addiction are not well established and are not formally recognized by the American Psychiatric Association as either a substance use disorder or a behavioral disorder in the Diagnosis and Statistical Manual of Mental Disorders 5 (DSM 5) [3]. Regardless, the criteria for food addiction have been modeled from substance use disorder criteria outlined in the DSM 5 [6].

In the DSM 5, substance use disorder is defined as a complex condition manifested by compulsive substance use despite harmful consequences. Furthermore, regular substance use may develop dependence and tolerance. The DSM 5 currently lists nine distinct disorders (e.g., tobacco use disorder and alcohol use disorder), but nearly all substances are diagnosed on the basis of the same overarching criteria [3]. Hallmark symptoms of food addiction include loss of control and frequent overconsumption, desire or repeated failed attempts to reduce or stop consumption, increased time spent in activities necessary to obtain and eat food, giving up on important activities such as physical exercise, continued consumption despite physical or psychological problems, and clinically significant impairment or distress [7].

Currently, limited research exists pertaining to food addiction and how it relates to other substance use disorders. Given that both unhealthy diets and smoking are among the leading risk factors for all-cause disability-adjusted life years, total deaths, and years lived with disability [8], a greater understanding of how food addiction and tobacco use disorder overlap with one another is necessary [9]. Furthermore, the role of food addiction in the common but understudied phenomenon of post-cessation weight gain among smokers trying to quit has not been researched. The purpose of this narrative review is to present and summarize the most up-to-date research findings on the prevalence, biology, psychology, and treatment of tobacco use disorder and food addiction as individual disorders, identifying overlap and commonalities that may help inform treatment approaches. It is important to understand each individual disorder in the context of the other since there is emerging evidence that the two disorders can develop concurrently or sequentially within individuals. To provide background on food addiction and tobacco use disorder, this review first discusses the prevalence of these disorders, measurements that assess severity, and theories of food addiction. This review then covers various subtopics such as biology, gut microbiome, psychosocial factors, and treatment options. The studies examined for this review mainly focus on food addiction rather than obesity and eating disorders, as these are two separate and complex conditions.

2. Methods

To locate relevant publications on the relationship between food addiction and tobacco use disorder, the following databases were searched: Ovid Medline, PsycInfo, and Embase. The Medline search strategy included both relevant medical subject headings (MESH) and keywords for the concepts of food addiction and tobacco use disorder/cessation. Food addiction-related terms included "food adj3 addict", "eat adj3 addict", "food adj3 dependence", "food use disorder", "compulsive eating", "Yale Food Addiction Scale", "obes", "diabetes", and "binge eating disorder". Smoking terms included "tobacco use disorder", "tobacco depend", "nicotine", "((nicotine or tobacco or smoking) adj3 (cessation or quit or quitting or quits or give up or giving up or stop or stopping or stopped or stops))", "((nicotine or tobacco or smoking) adj3 withdraw)", and "smoking cessation/or tobacco use cessation". The Medline search strategy was adapted for the controlled vocabulary of the other databases searched. All of the search results were limited to English language publications, but no date or study type limitations were applied. Furthermore, the database search was complemented by a manual review of reference lists from the retrieved articles. Articles related to the purpose of this narrative were retrieved from the database search. Studies examining eating disorders and obesity in the absence of food addiction were not reviewed as this was outside of the scope of this review.

3. Discussion

3.1. Prevalence

3.1.1. Prevalence and Severity Measurement of Tobacco Use Disorder

In 2017, 15% of the Canadian population (about 4.6 million people) were current smokers. Within that population, 11% and 4% reported being daily smokers and occasional smokers, respectively [10]. Daily smokers averaged approximately 14 cigarettes per day, with a higher percentage of smokers being male (17%) than female (13%) [10]. Furthermore, in 2018, nearly 34% of Canadian youth reported trying an electronic cigarette (e-cigarette) at least once in their lifetime [11]. Evidence suggests that e-cigarette use in youth increases the risk of developing tobacco use disorder later in life [12]. Similar statistics are reported in the United States, where approximately 12% of the population (or 40 million people) are daily smokers [13].

The DSM 5 replaced the DSM-IV's categories of nicotine abuse and dependence with tobacco use disorder. Within this context, problematic patterns of tobacco use must cause significant impairment and distress for at least two symptoms within a 1 year period to be considered a disorder. Other common measures of nicotine dependence severity include the Fagerstrom Test for Nicotine Dependence (FTND), Heaviness of Smoking Index (HSI), and time to first cigarette (TTFC). The FTND contains six questions scored 0–3 for a total possible score of 0–10. Higher scores indicate greater the physical dependence on nicotine. Similarly, HSI contains two measures: TTFC of the day and daily consumption of cigarettes. These metrics have been used to predict behavioral and biochemical indices of smoking, including ability to quit and cancer incidence and mortality [14]. Both measures are reliable over time and are important predictors of quitting [15,16].

3.1.2. Prevalence and Severity Measurement of Food Addiction

Food addiction is commonly measured using the Yale Food Addiction Scale (YFAS) [17], a 25-item tool developed in accordance with the substance dependence criteria of the DSM-IV [7,18]. The YFAS applies these criteria to the concept of food addiction for the purpose of identifying individuals who possess a predisposition toward the overconsumption of highly palatable foods within the previous 12 months [7,19]. The YFAS is capable of providing two scoring measures: (i) a cutoff score (yes/no) is achieved when an individual fulfills a minimum of three criteria and satisfies a clinical significant impairment or distress criterion, and (ii) a symptom count (0–7) in which the total number of endorsed criteria, with the exception of clinically significant impairment or distress criteria, is added together [7,18]. The YFAS represents a valid and reliable tool in identifying individuals who meet criteria for food addiction [7,20]; however, a major limitation of the YFAS is the reliance on self-reporting of symptoms. To date, there are no biological measurements to confirm the presence or absence of food addiction. Therefore, in conjunction with the lack of formal recognition by the DSM 5, a clinical diagnosis for food addiction does not exist at this time.

With the release of the DSM 5, criteria for diagnosing substance-related and addiction disorders have changed. Consequently, the 35-item YFAS 2.0 was developed to accurately align the concept of food addiction with the new DSM 5 substance use disorder criteria [21]. Another adaptation, the modified version of the YFAS (mYFAS), is an abbreviated nine-item version of the YFAS. Within the mYFAS, each of the seven DSM-4 substance dependence criteria is represented by one question [18]. The remaining two items of the mYFAS pertain to whether food or eating causes an individual clinically significant impairment or distress [18]. Both YFAS 2.0 and mYFAS have demonstrated marginal to good psychometric properties [20,22].

The observed prevalence rate of food addiction in a meta-analysis of 20 studies from North American and European countries was 19.9% (range: 16.3% to 24.0%) [23]. In a more recent meta-analysis of 36 articles, Burrows et al. (2018) concluded that the prevalence of individuals with mental health symptoms who met the cutoff for food addiction was 16.2% (range: 13.6% to 19.3%) [22]. A sex difference was also observed, where higher prevalence of food addiction appeared among females (12.2%) compared to males (6.4%) [23].

Although many individuals may not meet the threshold for food addiction, it is not uncommon for individuals to report specific symptoms. On average, individuals with mental health symptoms endorse approximately three symptoms for food addiction [22,23]. Of the seven YFAS symptoms for food addiction, "persistent desire or unsuccessful attempts to cut down or control eating" is one of the most frequently endorsed symptoms of food addiction [19,23,24].

3.1.3. Theories of Food Addiction

Several theories link specific high-caloric and palatable foods to food addiction. Similar to addictive substances, these foods exist on a spectrum of addiction [7]. For example, individuals meeting the cutoff for food addiction convey significant problems with highly palatable foods such as chocolate, doughnuts, cookies, cake, candy, white bread, pasta, rice, crackers, French fries, and hamburgers compared to their counterparts without food addiction [25,26]. In addition, more frequent consumption of hamburgers, candy bar, milk chocolate, butter, pizza, and low-calorie beverages was associated with meeting the cutoff for food addiction [26]. Conversely, more frequent consumption of dark chocolate, homemade cookies, white rice, and sugar-sweetened beverages was negatively associated with food addiction [26]. Other theories suggest that food itself is not addictive, but the manner in which the food is consumed is an addictive behavior. Specifically, the repetitive behavior of food restriction and dieting leads to periods of overeating and binging. While controversy surrounds the addictive properties of foods, it is important to consider that tobacco took several decades before it was declared an addictive substance [27]. Addictive substances including alcohol, tobacco, and cannabis have gained acceptance at some point and it was not until these substances were recognized as being addictive that society implemented changes that would provide opportunities for individuals to receive treatment [27].

3.2. Biology

3.2.1. Neurobiological Parallels between Food Addiction and Tobacco Use Disorder

Within the past several decades, neuroimaging has allowed the quantification of specific proteins and neurotransmitter receptors, the investigation of food and tobacco cues and their effects on neural activation, and the investigation of the integrity of gray and white matter, using positron emission tomography (PET), functional magnetic resonance imaging (fMRI), and structural MRI, respectively. Although no specific neuroimaging study has investigated the neural correlates of tobacco use disorder with comorbid food addiction, when investigated separately, the effects of food addiction on the brain often resemble those of tobacco use disorder. Specifically, highly palatable foods, such as those with high fat and sugar content, can activate the dopaminergic (DAergic) reward pathways [7,28–30], and specific conditioned food cues such as its sight, smell, and taste may trigger the desire or craving of eating [31]. This suggests that common neural substrates exist for both food and tobacco use disorder, both of which depend on DAergic pathways.

To date, no PET studies have investigated dopamine (DA) receptor availability in individuals with food addiction. Although obesity and food addiction are distinct disorders, most neurobiological literature surrounding food addiction is derived from obesity studies since the two conditions often co-occur. The first human neuroimaging study to examine striatal DA D2 receptor availability in relation to obesity was Wang et al. 2001 [32]. Measured by [^{11}C]raclopride PET, striatal DA D2 receptor availability was significantly lower in obese individuals compared to healthy controls, and body mass index (BMI) was negatively correlated with D2 receptor availability. Similarly, low levels of DA are often reported in individuals addicted to drugs including cocaine [33], alcohol [34], opiates [35], and nicotine [36], and low DA receptor levels are associated with addictive behaviors irrespective of food or addictive drugs [32]. DA deficiency may perpetuate pathological eating to replenish the mesolimbic DAergic pathway, and feeding has been shown to increase extracellular DA levels in the nucleus accumbens (NAcc) [37], a region thought to contribute to the reinforcing effects of euphoria [38]. It is possible that chronic overconsumption of food leads to increases in DA, resulting in DA D2 receptor downregulation. This produces a feed-forward cyclical pattern where overconsumption of food must then be sustained to replenish DA levels to avoid food cravings and withdrawal symptoms [39].

DA receptor availability in individuals with tobacco use disorder has been extensively investigated with [^{11}C]raclopride PET. For example, a 26% to 37% reduction in binding potential, indicative of greater DA release, was observed in the left ventral caudate, NAcc, and left ventral putamen in cigarette smokers compared to nonsmokers [40]. In contrast, several other PET studies using tobacco cigarettes and alternative methods of nicotine administration, such as nicotine nasal sprays and nicotine gum, found no significant changes in binding potential within smokers [41–44]. More recent nonhuman primate PET studies found [^{11}C]PHNO ([^{11}C]-(+)-propyl-hexahydro-naphtho-oxazin) to be more sensitive to nicotine-induced DA release compared to [^{11}C]raclopride [45]. To date, three studies have utilized [^{11}C]PHNO PET in relation to nicotine administration and smoking-associated cues in humans. Specifically, following cigarette smoking, a 12% to 15% reduction in D2 and D3 receptor binding potential was observed compared to control conditions [46]. These findings are likely influenced by genetics, where, during abstinence, slow metabolizers of nicotine had lower [^{11}C]PHNO-binding potential compared to fast metabolizers within the D2 regions of the striatum [47]. Interestingly, there was no change in [^{11}C]PHNO-binding potential in the striatum of nicotine-dependent individuals following the presentation of tobacco-associated cues [48].

The effects of food cues and craving on neural activity and DA receptor binding have been widely investigated. fMRI studies demonstrated that food cues activate the amygdala, insula, orbitofrontal cortex, and striatum brain regions compared to neutral cues [49,50]. These cues of highly palatable foods activate similar reward neurocircuitry to tobacco use disorder [51]. Furthermore, food cravings are associated with increased bold-oxygen-level-dependent (BOLD) signals in the hippocampus, insula, and caudate [50], regions involved in craving, motivation, and memory [52]. PET studies demonstrated a positive association of food cravings and increased dorsal caudate and putamen regional cerebral blood flow [53], as well as an association of DA ligand binding within the dorsal striatum and feeding [54]. In summary, molecular imaging studies food cues provide supportive evidence of DAergic pathway activation.

Similar to food addiction, fMRI studies have examined the neuronal activation patterns produced by nicotine. For example, dose- and time-dependent BOLD signal increases were observed within the anterior cingulate cortex, dorsolateral prefrontal cortex, and medial prefrontal cortex brain regions in cigarette smokers [55]. This pattern of brain activation is consistent with DAergic pathways innervating the frontal cortex, as well as evidence supporting acute nicotine's role in positively enhancing reaction time, short-term memory, working memory, and attention [56]. Furthermore, smoking-cue fMRI studies demonstrated that nicotine-dependent smokers exhibited more BOLD signal activation than nonsmokers in the prefrontal cortex, ventral striatum, and NAcc brain regions [57,58]. In addition, contextual factors such as cigarette availability can affect neural activity, and variation in tobacco use disorder severity and genotype can modulate cue-induced activity [59].

3.2.2. Neurobiology Unique to Tobacco Use Disorder

Nicotine is the main psychoactive component of tobacco, and it specifically acts as an agonist of nicotinic acetylcholine receptors (nAChRs) in the brain. nAChRs containing the α4 and β2 subunits are critical for mediating nicotine reinforcement, nicotine sensitivity, reward motivation, and DA release [60–65]. nAChRs are located throughout the brain, with highest density within the thalamus, basal ganglia, frontal cortex, cingulate cortex, occipital cortex, and insula [66,67]. Most importantly, nicotine stimulates the release of DA in the mesolimbic area, the corpus striatum, and the frontal cortex [68,69]. These DAergic pathways are critical in nicotine-induced rewarding behaviors [70], as well as in regulating reward, motivation, decision-making, learning, and memory [71].

Several preclinical and clinical studies of tobacco use disorder examined the effects of cigarette smoking and smoking-related behaviors on brain function, specifically β2-nAChR desensitization and subsequent upregulation [72]. Preclinical studies assessing nicotine administration in animals and postmortem human studies of smokers demonstrated β2-nAChR upregulation throughout the striatum, frontal cortex, anterior cingulate cortex, temporal cortex, occipital cortex, and cerebellum [73], suggesting greater levels of β2-nAChR desensitization and inactivation produced by long-term smoking or nicotine administration [74]. Brain imaging studies examining β2-nAChR availability in human smokers mimicked these preclinical finding [74–77]. Dysregulation of these brain regions following drug use is commonly associated with processing of drug cues and loss of inhibitory control, the primary contributing factor to relapse [78–80]. Furthermore, human postmortem studies of smokers with variable lifelong smoking histories and former smokers demonstrated that nAChR upregulation was reversible following abstinence [81]. Taken together, many preclinical and clinical brain imaging studies support the theory that long-term nicotine administration or chronic smoking can lead to nAChR desensitization and upregulation in smokers [82], but this upregulation is reversible following extended periods of smoking abstinence [81,83].

3.2.3. Neurobiology Unique to Food Addiction

With the exception of the DAergic system, the literature on other neurocircuits implicated in food addiction is limited. To date, only a few fMRI studies have been conducted in individuals who met the YFAS cutoff threshold for food addiction. The first study by Gearhardt et al. (2011) found a positive correlation between food addiction scores and neural activation in the anterior cingulate cortex, medial orbitofrontal cortex, and amygdala when participants anticipated highly palatable foods [84]. Furthermore, upon tasteless food cue presentation, a negative correlation was observed between food addiction scores and activation in the caudate, a region implicated in reward motivation [84]. In a more recent fMRI study, Schulte et al. (2019) investigated food-cue effects on neural activity in obese women who either met the YFAS 2.0 threshold cutoff or did not [85]. When presented with highly palatable foods, participants with food addiction exhibited moderate, elevated activation in the superior frontal gyrus. Decreased activations were observed when minimally processed food cues were presented. Interestingly, participants in the control group had opposite responses in this region [85]. Most of the literature on the neurobiology of food addiction is derived from studies examining obesity; however, the findings from Schulte et al. (2019) presented food addiction as a unique phenotype within obesity.

Provided the limited neuroimaging research, it is theorized that dysregulation in the hypothalamus may also contribute to food addiction given its role as the main homeostatic regulation center for feeding behaviors. The hypothalamus integrates different hormonal and neuronal signals to control appetite and energy. This regulation system monitors body adiposity by using hormones such as leptin, insulin, and ghrelin [86]. Ghrelin, the "hunger peptide", stimulates DAergic reward pathways, whereas leptin and insulin inhibit these circuits [49]. Several brain regions, such as the amygdala, hippocampus, insula, orbitofrontal cortex, and striatum, are also involved with the regulation of feeding and appetite [49]. These brain structures are involved in learning about food, allocating attention and effort towards food, conditioning reward with specific food cues in the environment, and integrating homeostatic information such as hunger with availability of food in the environment [49,71]. For a recent review of potential mechanisms for food addiction (in the presence of obesity) using a systems approach, see [87].

3.3. Role of the Gut Microbiome

3.3.1. Parallels in the Role of Gut Microbiome in Both Tobacco Use Disorder and Food Addiction

As discussed in the section above, both food addiction and tobacco use disorder reflect an imbalance in the extended reward system in response to environmental stimuli. Peptides that regulate appetite such as glucagon-like peptide 1 (GLP-1), ghrelin, leptin, peptide YY, and neuromedin U are expressed throughout the brain reward circuitry, providing strong evidence that food addiction and tobacco use disorder share overlapping gut–brain axis mechanisms [88]. Endocrine signals play a significant role in reward regulation and dysregulation, which is a hallmark feature of all addictive disorders. The neuropeptides that have been studied most extensively are ghrelin and GLP-1.

There were only a few studies exploring the mechanism via which the gut microbiome affects the behavioral response to drugs of abuse [89–91]. Nonetheless, there is preliminary clinical and preclinical evidence of bacterial dysbiosis in response to drugs of abuse, which requires further investigation [92–96].

3.3.2. Tobacco Use Disorder and the Gut Microbiome

The effect of smoking on the brain–gut axis and its behavioral implications has been largely unexplored. However, it has been shown that smoking induces specific changes in the microbiome. Furthermore, evidence suggests that smoking cessation induces an increase in microbial diversity [97,98], thereby reversing the negative effects of smoking and tobacco dependence on gut microbiota. A study by Biedermann et al. (2013) examined the association between smoking and gut microbiota in smokers without specific diseases [98] and showed that smoking cessation induced an increase in Firmicutes and Actinobacteria and a decrease in Bacteroidetes and Proteobacteria [98]. However, this study was conducted in only 10 subjects, and most of the participants developed an increased BMI following smoking cessation [98]. Previous studies showed that higher BMI is associated with increased Firmicutes and decreased Bacteroidetes in the gut compared to normal BMI [99,100]. Therefore, changes in gut microbiota following smoking cessation [98] might be associated with cessation-induced weight gain, as well as with smoking itself.

In a more recent large-scale cross-sectional study that included current, former, and never male smokers, smoking status influenced gut microbiota composition. Specifically, current smokers had a higher proportion of Bacteroidetes compared to never and former smokers, as well as lower proportions of Firmicutes and Proteobacteria compared with never smokers [89]. There were no observed differences in the composition of gut microbiota between never and former smokers, suggesting that smoking cessation allows gut microbiota composition to recover to pre-smoking status. The three groups did not differ significantly in terms of BMI or nutrient intake, thereby providing stronger evidence for the reversal of gut microbiota changes to normal upon smoking cessation.

Furthermore, a recent study compared the oral and gut microbiota in current smokers, current e-cigarette users, and healthy controls [101]. Tobacco smoking was associated with significant differences in the bacterial profiles in fecal, buccal, and saliva samples, while the e-cigarette users were no different to healthy controls. In keeping with previous studies, tobacco smokers had higher relative abundance of *Prevotella* and lower relative abundance of *Bacteroides* in their gut microbiota. This is in accordance with existing data demonstrating gut microbiotal changes following smoking cessation [98,102]

3.3.3. Food Addiction and the Gut Microbiome

Eating behavior is regulated by both homeostatic and hedonic mechanisms in the central nervous system (CNS). These mechanisms involve orchestrated signaling from several sources including gut peptides, endocrine signals, and neuronal impulses, as well as signals from the gut microbiota. For example, ghrelin signals hunger and craving, putatively via amplification of DA signaling [103]. On the other hand, satiety is signaled by other intestinal hormones such as glucagon-like peptide 1 (GLP-1) and peptide YY [104]. Insulin also triggers hunger and increases the palatability of sugar. There is evidence that the gut microbiota can regulate insulin sensitivity through various mechanisms [105]. As discussed in the previous section, normal eating behavior is under the control of the extended reward network, which is involved in the processing of all rewarding stimuli including but not limited to food-related behaviors. These processes become maladaptive when the salience of a specific type of reward such as highly palatable food is greater than that of other stimuli and becomes preferred at the expense of other rewards, thereby leading to addiction-type behavior. At this point, the hedonic system becomes more prominent than the homeostatic system in the regulation of food intake. Therefore, eating behavior becomes driven predominantly by activation of the salience network of the brain, whereby food cues activate this network leading to increased attentional bias to the food cues at the expense of other cues. This in turn results in the uncontrolled overconsumption of highly palatable food.

While there is currently no evidence in humans that food addiction is caused by an altered gut microbiome or that it is driven by particular gut microbes or microbial metabolites, there is substantial evidence from rodent models that point to a role of the gut microbiome in food addiction-like behaviors. However, there is overwhelming evidence that a high-sugar, high-fat diet results in changes to the gut microbiome, which further "supports" addictive-like eating behaviors [87].

The few studies that examined the relationship between the gut microbiome and its metabolites with addictive-like eating behaviors have shown that tryptophan metabolites are implicated in modulating brain–gut–microbiome interactions [106]. In a recent study [107], the association between microbial profiles and tryptophan metabolites with food addiction was examined in a sample of human females with high BMI. The study found that there was a difference in the gut microbiome of females with food addiction versus those without, whereby levels of *Bacteroides* and *Akkermansia* were negatively associated with food addiction.

3.4. Psychological

3.4.1. Childhood Adversity

Adverse childhood experiences (ACEs) have been shown to have deleterious effects on adult health [108–110]. To standardize the operationalization of childhood adversity within studies, Felitti et al. (1998) developed the ACE Survey, which quantifies an individual's reports of exposure to abuse, neglect, and household dysfunction before the age of 18 [111]. These questions surveyed ACEs by asking about behaviors rather than subjective experiences of trauma. This survey originally encompassed seven categories including three of abuse and four of household dysfunction. More recent versions of the ACE study capture two additional categories of neglect and parental separation or divorce [112]. Cronholm et al. proposed the expansion of the concept of ACEs to include experiences such as witnessing violence, feeling discrimination, living in an unsafe neighborhood, experiencing bullying, and living in foster care to fully understand the influence of childhood adversity on adult substance use [113].

3.4.2. Overlap in Childhood Adversity of Tobacco Use Disorder and Food Addiction

Childhood adversity influences various physiological and behavioral mechanisms that contribute to adult addictive behaviors. Studies demonstrate that chronic stress in childhood may cause changes in the nervous, endocrine, and immune systems. Alterations in these systems may lead to impairments in cognitive, social, and emotional development that predispose individuals with ACEs to adopt addictive behaviors [114–116]. The original ACE study reported that individuals who experienced four or more categories of adversity were 2.2 times more likely to be a current smoker and 1.6 times more likely to have a BMI ≥ 35 (severe obesity) [111]. This study did not evaluate food addiction. While the focus here is on tobacco use disorder and food addiction, individuals who report ACEs also engage in other addictive behaviors including alcohol abuse and drug use [111]. This suggests that childhood adversity may have significant and varying downstream effects on numerous adult health behaviors. While there is research on the relationships between childhood adversity and food addiction and between childhood adversity and tobacco use disorder, research is needed to better understand the overlap of food addiction and tobacco use disorder.

3.4.3. Childhood Adversity and Tobacco Use Disorder

Using the ACE Survey, Felitti et al. (1998) produced a landmark paper describing the gradient relationships between the number of categories of childhood adversity and the prevalence of current smoking. Specifically, 6.8% of participants who reported no adversity (zero categories) and 16.5% of participants who reported four or more categories of adversity were current smokers. Participants who reported four or more categories of adversity were 2.2 times more likely to smoke than those who reported no adversity (odds ratio (OR) adjusted for age, gender, race, and educational attainment) [111]. Since then, a systematic review and a meta-analysis of 37 studies found that individuals who reported at least four categories of ACEs were more than twice as likely to be current smokers. Furthermore, there was a moderate association between childhood adversity and smoking [113].

3.4.4. Childhood Adversity and Food Addiction

There is limited research into food addiction. One study identified childhood abuse as a risk factor for food addiction. This study of 57,321 adult women examined the association between child abuse (specifically, physical and sexual child abuse) and food addiction (defined as three or more clinically significant symptoms on the mYFAS). In this sample, over 8% of participants reported severe physical abuse in childhood, 5.3% reported severe sexual abuse, and 8% met the criteria for food addiction. Findings indicated that women with food addiction had a higher BMI than women without food addiction. Furthermore, severe physical and severe sexual abuse was associated with about 90% increased risk for food addiction (physical abuse: relative risk (RR) 1.92, 95% confidence interval (CI) 1.76 to 2.09; sexual abuse: RR 1.87, 95% CI 1.69 to 2.05). The RR for combined severe physical abuse and sexual abuse was 2.40 (95% CI 2.16 to 2.67) demonstrating the additive effects of adversity [117]. Childhood adversity has also been linked to disordered eating, including food addiction, obesity, and binge eating, which has overlapping characteristics with food addiction [111,118–122].

3.4.5. Attachment Insecurity

Attachment theory describes how individuals internalize experiences with their caregivers to form mental representations of themselves and others. Individuals with high attachment anxiety tend to have negative self-views, are concerned about rejection, magnify their expressions of distress, and prefer close proximity to and support from a partner [123,124]. Individuals with high attachment avoidance tend to report positive self-views [123], suppress expressions of distress, and prefer emotional distance in relationships [124]. Individuals can be characterized by varying levels of attachment anxiety and avoidance, and both types of insecurity can co-occur [124]. The experience of childhood trauma is associated with both attachment anxiety and attachment avoidance in adulthood [125]. Attachment theory provides another framework to understand tobacco use disorder.

3.4.6. Overlap in Attachment Insecurity of Tobacco Use Disorder and Food Addiction

Attachment insecurity may influence several processes that may in turn contribute to tobacco use disorder and food addiction. While there is research on the relationships between attachment insecurity and food addiction and between attachment insecurity and tobacco use disorder, research is needed to better understand the overlap of food addiction and tobacco use disorder. Attachment insecurity is related to affect regulation [126], i.e., "the process by which individuals influence which emotions they have, when they have them, and how they experience and express these emotions" [127]. Emotional regulation involves efforts to up- and downregulate positive and negative emotions [127]. High levels of attachment insecurity are associated with a deficit in affect regulation [128]. Individuals with high attachment insecurity may feel less capable of disengaging from negative feelings and in turn attempt to calm themselves through food or other substances. Food or other substances (e.g., tobacco, alcohol, or drugs), when consumed in order to reduce feelings of insecurity, have been called "external regulators of affect" [129]. Individuals with high attachment insecurity are more likely to use these "external regulators of affect" instead of utilizing more adaptive emotional regulation strategies. Attachment insecurity has been studied in the context of disordered eating, eating disorders, and obesity, but there is still limited research on food addiction [130–132].

3.4.7. Attachment Insecurity and Tobacco Use Disorder

Insecure attachment patterns, specifically attachment anxiety, are associated with the use of tobacco and other drugs [133–136]. Attachment anxiety was associated with increased use of tobacco to reduce stress in college students [135]. In undergraduate and graduate students, significant differences in attachment patterns in tobacco users and nonusers were observed [122]. In a study of adults, findings suggested that attachment anxiety, but not attachment avoidance, was associated with current smoking [137]. In contrast, a study in adult women found that attachment avoidance was associated with being a current smoker [133]. It is currently unclear whether a particular dimension of attachment insecurity, such as attachment avoidance or attachment anxiety, is associated with tobacco use disorder.

3.4.8. Attachment Insecurity and Food Addiction

Few studies examined the association of attachment insecurity and food addiction. One study of a national nonclinical sample of 1841 respondents in the Czech Republic found that attachment insecurity was associated with increased scores of mYFAS 2.0 [138]. In a study of 195 adult women from an eating disorder treatment center, the prevalence of food addiction was 83.6%, and the most frequently reported food addiction criteria were "clinically significant impairment or distress in relation to food", "craving", and "persistent desire or repeated unsuccessful attempts to cut down". Within this sample, no differences in attachment insecurity were found between those meeting the criteria for food addiction and those who did not fulfill the criteria for food addiction [132]. As such, there may be a similarity between food addiction and eating disorders in terms of attachment patterns. The literature suggests that attachment insecurity is associated with unhealthy eating, including anorexia nervosa, bulimia nervosa, nonclinical levels of disordered eating, and obesity [130,131,139–148].

3.5. Treatment

3.5.1. Treating Tobacco Use Disorder

There is a wide array of smoking cessation interventions that are well-established by evidence from several systematic reviews. Individualized treatments such as nicotine replacement therapy (NRT), varenicline, bupropion, behavioral supports, e-cigarettes, and combination therapies have positive outcomes on cessation rates and sustained abstinence. In addition, community- or government-level efforts such as prohibiting smoking in public spaces, advertising restrictions, and health warning labels contribute to reductions in smoking.

NRT is a common first-line, over-the-counter cessation aid that is available in forms such as the patch, lozenge, inhaler, and gum. NRT has a >6.5% sustained abstinence rate after 6 months, more than double that of placebo [149,150]. Compared to placebo, NRT shows no statistically significant differences in adverse events, except nausea, which has been listed as a common side effect [150]. Using the NRT patch together with another type of NRT (e.g., gum, lozenge, mist, or inhaler), can increase that rate by an additional 15–36% [151]. NRT dose and duration also affect quit rate. Quit success is positively correlated with higher-dose NRT patches (25 mg worn over 16 h or 21 mg worn over 24 h) compared to smaller-dose patches (15 mg over 16 h or 14 mg over 24 h) [151].

Varenicline is well established as achieving the highest quit and sustained abstinence rate of all cessation aids, with minimal risk for adverse effects (see, for example, [149–151]). Varenicline more than doubles the chances of quit compared to placebo [152,153], helping approximately 50% more people to quit and have sustained abstinence than the NRT patch, tablets, spray, lozenge, and inhaler, and 70% more than NRT gum [152]. The antidepressant bupropion has similarly high quit success, making it 52–71% more likely that a person will quit [154]. There have been concerns surrounding varenicline and bupropion's linkage to psychiatric adverse events. A systematic review did not support this for varenicline, where the most frequently reported adverse event was nausea [153]. However, there is high-certainty evidence that unwanted mental health side-effects and adverse events linked to taking bupropion lead to lower medication adherence [154]. Furthermore, highest quit and sustained abstinence rates occur when pharmacotherapies are used in combination with behavioral supports. Behavioral therapy has been shown to increase effectiveness of pharmacotherapies by 83% to 97% across different care settings [155]. One systematic review compared the effects of brief physician advice to quit with offering assistance in the form of behavioral support or medication [156]. Physicians who offered assistance generated more quit attempts than those who gave advice to quit on medical grounds. Furthermore, when assistance was delivered in the form of motivational interviewing, a goal-oriented and patient-centered counseling approach that elicits motivation for change, abstinence rates were statistically significant and demonstrated up to 45% greater odds of smoking abstinence than control groups [157].

In recent years, e-cigarettes have become commonly used smoking cessation aids. While evidence is currently limited, the literature suggests the promise of e-cigarettes being an effective smoking cessation aid [158,159]. There is moderate-certainty evidence [using Grading of Recommendations Assessment, Development and Evaluation (GRADE)] from Cochrane systematic review that e-cigarettes with nicotine are more effective at helping people stop smoking for at least 6 months than NRT (three studies; 1498 participants), nicotine-free e-cigarettes (three studies; 802 participants), and no support or behavioral support alone (four studies; 2312 participants) [158]. Of the adverse events reported for e-cigarettes, throat and/or mouth irritation was the most commonly reported. Moderate-certainty evidence indicates the potential for results to change when more evidence becomes available. More research is needed to determine if e-cigarettes with nicotine are the preferred option for smoking cessation.

In summary, combination therapies that include either pharmacotherapy and behavioral support or a lower-risk nicotine product such as NRT or e-cigarettes with behavioral support increased quit attempts and boosted the level of sustained abstinence after one year. Organizational interventions also played a role in the sale and ease of promoting healthier smoking behaviors.

3.5.2. Treatment Options for Food Addiction

There is currently no well-established treatment model for intervening on food addiction. This is unsurprising given that there is no formal recognition of food addiction as a neurological or behavioral disease within the DSM 5 due to the debate of perceiving food addiction as a (non)substance use disorder or as a behavioral addiction. Furthermore, the heterogeneity of addiction makes it difficult to translate addiction into a working treatment model.

In its contextualization along the spectrum of eating disorders within the scientific literature, there are notable behavioral treatment options. Psychosocial interventions for food addiction include reducing access to processed foods, reducing habit-based eating, removing restrictions on eating healthy foods, and behavioral therapies to improve emotional regulation and to help combat submission to cravings and emotional eating [160]. Furthermore, participation in an integrative and psychological weight management group demonstrated promise in treatment efficacy [161]. Learning about mindful eating, keeping a food diary and keeping track of body weight, creating and maintaining an exercise plan, and planning for social eating are tactics that are taught to enable the maintenance of healthy body weight [161]. A systematic review revealed that additional research is needed to develop and test the efficacy of these types of interventions within the context of food addiction [162].

Noninvasive brain stimulation has been used most frequently for the treatment of addictions such as tobacco use disorder [163]. Transcranial direct current stimulation (tDCS) in particular, is a safe, economical, and accessible means of modifying neural activity [163]. A systematic review highlighted that tDCS significantly improved the symptoms of food addiction by reducing food cravings brought on by visual stimuli [164]. Craving was measured before and after stimulation using visual analogue scales, eye tracking, or the Food Craving Questionnaire—State, and tDCS was found to significantly repress the desire to eat, leading to less food consumption [164]. However, due to underpowered studies and the complexity of addiction, more research is necessary to make any definitive comments about the success of tDCS on food addiction. Tailoring neuromodulating interventions to individuals or subgroups, on the basis of cognitive and neural profiling, might prove to be useful [163]. Since food addiction often presents with comorbidities, current research suggests using evidence-based interventions to address other conditions first [162].

4. Current and Future Research Directions

Evidence demonstrates that individuals can expect to gain an average of 4 to 5 kg of weight after successfully achieving smoking cessation [165,166]. For many tobacco users, this potential increase in weight can be a substantial obstacle when attempting smoking cessation [167,168], thereby leading to continued tobacco use. One possible explanation for post-smoking cessation weight gain is that quitting smoking increases the desire to consume highly palatable, high-calorie foods. Consequently, the authors of this review developed a feasibility study with the purpose of examining the association between food addiction symptoms and smoking behavior among individuals seeking treatment for tobacco use disorder. This feasibility study recruited individuals from the Nicotine Dependence Clinic at the Centre for Addiction and Mental Health (CAMH) who had yet to begin their smoking cessation treatment. Those individuals who provided consent to participate in the study were asked to complete a survey which included the FTND and mYFAS questionnaires.

The sample of this feasibility study included 51 participants seeking treatment for tobacco use disorder. The majority of participants in this convenience sample were male (58.8%). Two-thirds of the sample consumed <20 cigarettes per day (CPD). The prevalence of individuals meeting the cutoff for food addiction was 11.8%. The average symptom count for food addiction was 1.5 ± 1.8 (standard deviation (SD)) symptoms.

Spearman rank correlation coefficients were conducted to examine the association between tobacco use disorder, specifically CPD, and food addiction symptom count, as measured by the mYFAS. No significant association was observed between CPD and food addiction symptom count for the overall sample ($r_s = 0.21$, $p = 0.14$) or by sex (male: $r_s = 0.20$, $p = 0.28$; female: $r_s = 0.24$, $p = 0.31$).

The results of this feasibility study, even though underpowered, represent an important initial step in developing future research. Using a cross-sectional study design, we were unable to observe a significant association between food addiction symptom count and CPD. The findings from another cross-sectional study examining the association between smoking and food addiction found that male smokers report twice as many YFAS symptoms compared to male nonsmokers [169]. However, among females, no relationship was observed between food addiction symptoms and smoking [169]. While this study provides some evidence of an association between smoking and food addiction, more research is needed. Applying a longitudinal study design and examining how changes in smoking behavior relate to changes food addiction symptoms could provide greater insight into the relationship between smoking cessation and weight gain. Furthermore, the feasibility study also revealed that the prevalence of food addiction may be lower among individuals seeking smoking cessation treatment compared to the general population, suggesting, perhaps, that food addiction may have a minor role in post-cessation weight gain. Therefore, examining other concepts such as the role that the gut microbiome may have on smoking cessation weight gain could be promising. However, it is also plausible that achieving smoking cessation could result in the adoption of an addictive behavior involving the overconsumption of highly palatable foods, a process known as addiction transfer [170].

E-cigarettes have been demonstrated to be effective smoking cessation aids [158]. As outlined above, e-cigarette users have gut and oral microbiomes that are more similar to healthy controls than to tobacco smokers [103]. Given that *Bacteriodes*, the bacterium that is most commonly significantly decreased in smokers compared to healthy controls and e-cigarette users, is also implicated in obesity [171], there is the potential that switching smokers to e-cigarettes may decrease their risk of cessation-related weight gain. This hypothesis has not yet been tested, and there is no clear evidence that smokers who switch to e-cigarettes avoid weight gain. As such, these are important research gaps to address.

5. Limitations

This was a narrative review; thus, limitations with respect to the scope of literature covered are present. The authors made every attempt to be systematic in their initial literature search, but they may have missed some important publications. Narrative reviews are also subject to bias, but the authors did their best to mitigate this by using systematic approaches to their literature search.

6. Conclusions

Food addiction and tobacco use disorder share similar but not identical neurological, physiological, and behavioral abnormalities. We attempted to summarize these similarities between the two disorders where there is evidence of their existence. Differences between the two disorders should not lead one to conclude that food addiction is not a "real" disorder. As argued in a recent perspective [172], core features of addiction can differ dramatically depending on which substance is being used, reflecting different underlying neurobiological processes at play. For example, the pattern of consumption and symptoms of withdrawal exhibited in cocaine use disorder completely different to what is seen in tobacco use disorder.

Addiction is a complex disorder that we are only beginning to understand at a system level. The role of the gut–brain axis in brain reward mechanisms related to addiction needs to be further researched. In addition, more attention needs to be paid to the role that early life events have on the risk of developing an addictive disorder. Taking learnings from different types of addictive behaviors such as food addiction, as well as newer "behavioral addictions" such as internet gaming, will help to further our understanding of the underlying mechanisms common to all addictive disorders. This will in turn pave the road toward effective treatment options. Exploring the commonalities between tobacco use disorder and food addiction is a step in this direction.

Author Contributions: L.Z. conceptualized the basis and structure of the review. L.Z., S.A., T.L.L., W.K.d., and D.D. wrote the initial drafts and subsequent drafts of the paper. L.Z., S.A., T.L.L., W.K.d., D.D., and P.S. approved the final version. All authors have read and agreed to the published version of the manuscript.

Funding: L.Z.: T.L.L., W.K.d., D.D., and P.S. are paid employees of the Center for Addiction and Mental Health. S.A. is a postdoctoral fellow. Funding for infrastructure was from the Center for Addiction and Mental Health.

Conflicts of Interest: S.A., T.L.L., and D.D. report no conflicts of interest. L.Z. has received peer-reviewed funding from Canadian Institutes of Health Research, Canadian Cancer Society, Ontario Ministry of Health of Long-term Care, including salary support from Pfizer Inc. (GRAND Award) and the Health Services Research Fund from the Ontario Ministry of Health. W.K.d. reports receiving grants from the Public Health Agency of Canada and Pfizer Inc. W.K.d. is also a shareholder of Abbott Laboratories. P.S. reports receiving grants and/or salary and/or research support from the Center for Addiction and Mental Health, Health Canada, Ontario Ministry of Health and Long-term care, Canadian Institutes of Health Research, Canadian Center on Substance Use and Addiction, Public Health Agency of Canada, Ontario Lung Association, Medical Psychiatry Alliance, Extensions for Community Healthcare Outcomes, Canadian Cancer Society Research Institute, Cancer Care Ontario, Ontario Institute for Cancer Research, Ontario Brain Institute, McLaughlin Center, Academic Health Sciences Center, Workplace Safety and Insurance Board, National Institutes of Health, and the Association of Faculties of Medicine of Canada. P.S. also reports receiving funding and/or honoraria from the following commercial organizations: Pfizer Inc./Canada, Shoppers Drug Mart, Bhasin Consulting Fund Inc., Patient-Centered Outcomes Research Institute, ABBVie, and Bristol-Myers Squibb. Furthermore, P.S. reports receiving consulting fees from Pfizer Inc./Canada, Evidera Inc., Johnson & Johnson Group of Companies, Medcan Clinic, Inflexxion Inc., V-CC Systems Inc., MedPlan Communications, Kataka Medical Communications, Miller Medical Communications, Nvision Insight Group, and Sun Life Financial.

References

1. Abdelaal, M.; Le Roux, C.W.; Docherty, N.G. Morbidity and mortality associated with obesity. *Ann. Transl. Med.* **2017**, *5*, 161. [CrossRef]
2. Jamal, A.; Phillips, E.; Gentzke, A.S.; Homa, D.M.; Babb, S.D.; King, B.A.; Neff, L.J. Current Cigarette Smoking Among Adults — United States, 2016. *MMWR. Morb. Mortal. Wkly. Rep.* **2018**, *67*, 53–59. [CrossRef]
3. American Psychiatric Association. *Diagnostic and Statistical Manual of Mental Disorders*, 5th ed.; American Psychiatric Press: Washington, DC, USA, 2013.
4. Schulte, E.M.; Joyner, M.A.; Potenza, M.N.; Grilo, C.M.; Gearhardt, A.N. Current Considerations Regarding Food Addiction. *Curr. Psychiatry Rep.* **2015**, *17*, 1–8. [CrossRef]
5. Randolph, T.G. The Descriptive Features of Food Addiction. Addictive Eating and Drinking. *Q. J. Stud. Alcohol* **1956**, *17*, 198–224. [CrossRef]
6. Meule, A.; Gearhardt, A.N. Food Addiction in the Light of DSM-5. *Nutrients* **2014**, *6*, 3653–3671. [CrossRef]
7. Gearhardt, A.N.; Corbin, W.R.; Brownell, K.D. Preliminary validation of the Yale Food Addiction Scale. *Appetite* **2009**, *52*, 430–436. [CrossRef]
8. Alam, S.; Lang, J.J.; Drucker, A.M.; Gotay, C.; Kozloff, N.; Mate, K.; Patten, S.; Orpana, H.M.; Afshin, A.; Cahill, L.E. Assessment of the burden of diseases and injuries attributable to risk factors in Canada from 1990 to 2016: An analysis of the Global Burden of Disease Study. *CMAJ Open* **2019**, *7*, E140–E148. [CrossRef] [PubMed]
9. Criscitelli, K.; Avena, N.M. The neurobiological and behavioral overlaps of nicotine and food addiction. *Prev. Med.* **2016**, *92*, 82–89. [CrossRef] [PubMed]
10. Government of Canada. Canadian Tobacco, Alcohol and Drugs Survey (CTADS): Summary of Results for 2017. 2018. Available online: https://www.canada.ca/en/health-canada/services/canadian-tobacco-alcohol-drugs-survey/2017-summary.html (accessed on 4 September 2020).
11. Government of Canada. Summary of Results for the Canadian Student Tobacco, Alcohol and Drugs Survey 2018–2019. Available online: https://www.canada.ca/en/health-canada/services/canadian-student-tobacco-alcohol-drugs-survey/2018-2019-summary.html (accessed on 4 September 2020).
12. Spindle, T.R.; Hiler, M.M.; Cooke, M.E.; Eissenberg, T.; Kendler, K.S.; Dick, D.M. Electronic cigarette use and uptake of cigarette smoking: A longitudinal examination of U.S. college students. *Addict. Behav.* **2017**, *67*, 66–72. [CrossRef] [PubMed]
13. Centers for Disease Control and Prevention. Tobacco-Related Mortality. 2020. Available online: https://www.cdc.gov/tobacco/data_statistics/fact_sheets/health_effects/tobacco_related_mortality/index.htm (accessed on 4 September 2020).
14. Ward, R.C.; Tanner, N.T.; A Silvestri, G.; Gebregziabher, M. Impact of Tobacco Dependence in Risk Prediction Models for Lung Cancer Diagnoses and Deaths. *JNCI Cancer Spectr.* **2019**, *3*, pkz014. [CrossRef]
15. Pomerleau, C.S.; Carton, S.M.; Lutzke, M.L.; Flessland, K.A.; Pomerleau, O.F. Reliability of the fagerstrom tolerance questionnaire and the fagerstrom test for nicotine dependence. *Addict. Behav.* **1994**, *19*, 33–39. [CrossRef]
16. Borland, R.; Yong, H.-H.; O'Connor, R.J.; Hyland, A.; Thompson, M.E. The reliability and predictive validity of the Heaviness of Smoking Index and its two components: Findings from the International Tobacco Control Four Country study. *Nicotine Tob. Res.* **2010**, *12*, S45–S50. [CrossRef]
17. Penzenstadler, L.; Soares, C.; Karila, L.; Khazaal, Y. Systematic Review of Food Addiction as Measured with the Yale Food Addiction Scale: Implications for the Food Addiction Construct. *Curr. Neuropharmacol.* **2019**, *17*, 526–538. [CrossRef] [PubMed]
18. Meule, A.; Gearhardt, A.N. Five years of the Yale Food Addiction Scale: Taking stock and moving forward. *Curr. Addict. Rep.* **2014**, *1*, 193–205. [CrossRef]
19. Mies, G.W.; Treur, J.L.; Larsen, J.K.; Halberstadt, J.; Pasman, J.A.; Vink, J.M. The prevalence of food addiction in a large sample of adolescents and its association with addictive substances. *Appetite* **2017**, *118*, 97–105. [CrossRef] [PubMed]
20. Lemeshow, A.R.; Gearhardt, A.N.; Genkinger, J.M.; Corbin, W.R. Assessing the psychometric properties of two food addiction scales. *Eat. Behav.* **2016**, *23*, 110–114. [CrossRef]
21. Supplemental Material for Development of the Yale Food Addiction Scale Version 2.0. *Psychol. Addict. Behav.* **2016**, *30*, 113–121. [CrossRef]

22. Burrows, T.L.; Kay-Lambkin, F.; Pursey, K.; Skinner, J.; Dayas, C. Food addiction and associations with mental health symptoms: A systematic review with meta-analysis. *J. Hum. Nutr. Diet.* **2018**, *31*, 544–572. [CrossRef]
23. Pursey, K.M.; Stanwell, P.; Gearhardt, A.N.; Collins, C.; Burrows, T. The Prevalence of Food Addiction as Assessed by the Yale Food Addiction Scale: A Systematic Review. *Nutr.* **2014**, *6*, 4552–4590. [CrossRef]
24. Goluza, I.; Borchard, J.P.; Kiarie, E.; Mullan, J.; Pai, N. Exploration of food addiction in people living with schizophrenia. *Asian J. Psychiatry* **2017**, *27*, 81–84. [CrossRef]
25. Ayaz, A.; Nergiz-Unal, R.; Dedebayraktar, D.; Akyol, A.; Pekcan, A.G.; Besler, H.T.; Büyüktuncer, Z. How does food addiction influence dietary intake profile? *PLoS ONE* **2018**, *13*, e0195541. [CrossRef] [PubMed]
26. Lemeshow, A.R.; Rimm, E.B.; Hasin, D.S.; Gearhardt, A.N.; Flint, A.J.; Field, A.E.; Genkinger, J.M. Food and beverage consumption and food addiction among women in the Nurses' Health Studies. *Appetite* **2018**, *121*, 186–197. [CrossRef] [PubMed]
27. Ifland, J.; Preuss, H.; Marcus, M.; Rourke, K.; Taylor, W.; Burau, K.; Jacobs, W.; Kadish, W.; Manso, G. Refined food addiction: A classic substance use disorder. *Med Hypotheses* **2009**, *72*, 518–526. [CrossRef] [PubMed]
28. Bassareo, V.; Di Chiara, G. Differential Influence of Associative and Nonassociative Learning Mechanisms on the Responsiveness of Prefrontal and Accumbal Dopamine Transmission to Food Stimuli in Rats FedAd Libitum. *J. Neurosci.* **1997**, *17*, 851–861. [CrossRef]
29. Hernandez, L.; Hoebel, B.G. Food reward and cocaine increase extracellular dopamine in the nucleus accumbens as measured by microdialysis. *Life Sci.* **1988**, *42*, 1705–1712. [CrossRef]
30. Roitman, M.F.; Stuber, G.D.; Phillips, P.E.M.; Wightman, R.M.; Carelli, R.M. Dopamine Operates as a Subsecond Modulator of Food Seeking. *J. Neurosci.* **2004**, *24*, 1265–1271. [CrossRef]
31. Baik, J.-H. Dopamine signaling in food addiction: Role of dopamine D2 receptors. *BMB Rep.* **2013**, *46*, 519–526. [CrossRef]
32. Wang, G.-J.; Volkow, N.D.; Logan, J.; Pappas, N.R.; Wong, C.T.; Zhu, W.; Netusll, N.; Fowler, J.S. Brain dopamine and obesity. *Lancet* **2001**, *357*, 354–357. [CrossRef]
33. Martinez, D.; Broft, A.; Foltin, R.W.; Slifstein, M.; Hwang, D.-R.; Huang, Y.; Perez, A.; Frankel, W.G.; Cooper, T.; Kleber, H.D.; et al. Cocaine Dependence and D2 Receptor Availability in the Functional Subdivisions of the Striatum: Relationship with Cocaine-Seeking Behavior. *Neuropsychopharmacol.* **2004**, *29*, 1190–1202. [CrossRef]
34. Martinez, D.; Gil, R.; Slifstein, M.; Hwang, D.-R.; Huang, Y.; Perez, A.; Kegeles, L.; Talbot, P.; Evans, S.; Krystal, J.; et al. Alcohol Dependence Is Associated with Blunted Dopamine Transmission in the Ventral Striatum. *Biol. Psychiatry* **2005**, *58*, 779–786. [CrossRef]
35. Martinez, D.; Saccone, P.A.; Liu, F.; Slifstein, M.; Orlowska, D.; Grassetti, A.; Cook, S.H.; Broft, A.; Van Heertum, R.; Comer, S.D. Deficits in Dopamine D2 Receptors and Presynaptic Dopamine in Heroin Dependence: Commonalities and Differences with Other Types of Addiction. *Biol. Psychiatry* **2012**, *71*, 192–198. [CrossRef]
36. Fehr, C.; Yakushev, I.; Hohmann, D.P.N.; Buchholz, H.-G.; Landvogt, M.D.C.; Deckers, H.; Eberhardt, A.; Kläger, M.; Smolka, M.D.M.N.; Scheurich, A.; et al. Association of Low Striatal Dopamine D2Receptor Availability With Nicotine Dependence Similar to That Seen with Other Drugs of Abuse. *Am. J. Psychiatry* **2008**, *165*, 507–514. [CrossRef]
37. Bassareo, V.; Di Chiara, G. Differential responsiveness of dopamine transmission to food-stimuli in nucleus accumbens shell/core compartments. *Neurosci.* **1999**, *89*, 637–641. [CrossRef]
38. Pontieri, F.E.; Tanda, G.; Orzi, F.; Di Chiara, G. Effects of nicotine on the nucleus accumbens and similarity to those of addictive drugs. *Nat. Cell Biol.* **1996**, *382*, 255–257. [CrossRef]
39. Wang, G.J.; Volkow, N.D.; Thanos, P.K.; Fowler, J.S. Similarity between obesity and drug addiction as assessed by neurofunctional imaging: A concept review. *J. Addict. Dis.* **2004**, *23*, 39–53. [CrossRef]
40. Brody, A.L.; Olmstead, R.E.; London, E.D.; Farahi, J.; Meyer, J.H.; Grossman, P.; Lee, G.S.; Huang, J.; Hahn, E.L.; Mandelkern, M.A. Smoking-Induced Ventral Striatum Dopamine Release. *Am. J. Psychiatry* **2004**, *161*, 1211–1218. [CrossRef]
41. Barrett, S.P.; Boileau, I.; Okker, J.; Pihl, R.; Dagher, A. The hedonic response to cigarette smoking is proportional to dopamine release in the human striatum as measured by positron emission tomography and [^{11}C]raclopride. *Synapse* **2004**, *54*, 65–71. [CrossRef]

42. Scott, D.J.; Domino, E.F.; Heitzeg, M.M.; Koeppe, R.A.; Ni, L.; Guthrie, S.; Zubieta, J. Smoking modulation of mu-opioid and dopamine D2 receptor-mediated neurotransmission in humans. *Neuropsychopharmacology* **2007**, *32*, 450–457. [CrossRef]
43. Montgomery, A.J.; Lingford-Hughes, A.R.; Egerton, A.; Nutt, D.; Grasby, P.M. The effect of nicotine on striatal dopamine release in man: A [^{11}C]raclopride PET study. *Synapse* **2007**, *61*, 637–645. [CrossRef]
44. Takahashi, H.; Fujimura, Y.; Hayashi, M.; Takano, H.; Kato, M.; Okubo, Y.; Kanno, I.; Ito, H.; Suhara, T. Enhanced dopamine release by nicotine in cigarette smokers: A double-blind, randomized, placebo-controlled pilot study. *Int. J. Neuropsychopharmacol.* **2007**, *11*, 413–417. [CrossRef]
45. Gallezot, J.-D.; Kloczynski, T.; Weinzimmer, D.; Labaree, D.; Zheng, M.-Q.; Lim, K.; Rabiner, E.A.; Ridler, K.; Pittman, B.; Huang, Y.; et al. Imaging Nicotine- and Amphetamine-Induced Dopamine Release in Rhesus Monkeys with [^{11}C]PHNO vs [^{11}C]raclopride PET. *Neuropsychopharmacology* **2014**, *39*, 866–874. [CrossRef]
46. Le Foll, B.; Guranda, M.; A Wilson, A.; Houle, S.; Rusjan, P.M.; Wing, V.C.; Zawertailo, L.; E Busto, U.; Selby, P.; Brody, A.L.; et al. Elevation of Dopamine Induced by Cigarette Smoking: Novel Insights from a [^{11}C]-(+)-PHNO PET Study in Humans. *Neuropsychopharmacology* **2014**, *39*, 415–424. [CrossRef]
47. Di Ciano, P.; Tyndale, R.F.; Mansouri, E.; Hendershot, C.S.; A Wilson, A.; Lagzdins, D.; Houle, S.; Boileau, I.; Le Foll, B. Influence of Nicotine Metabolism Ratio on [^{11}C]-(+)-PHNO PET Binding in Tobacco Smokers. *Int. J. Neuropsychopharmacol.* **2018**, *21*, 503–512. [CrossRef]
48. Chiuccariello, L.; Boileau, I.; Guranda, M.; Rusjan, P.M.; Wilson, A.A.; Zawertailo, L.; Houle, S.; Busto, U.; Le Foll, B. Presentation of Smoking-Associated Cues Does Not Elicit Dopamine Release after One-Hour Smoking Abstinence: A [^{11}C]-(+)-PHNO PET Study. *PLoS ONE* **2013**, *8*, e60382. [CrossRef]
49. Dagher, A. The neurobiology of appetite: Hunger as addiction. *Int. J. Obes.* **2009**, *33*, S30–S33. [CrossRef]
50. Pelchat, M.L. Food Addiction in Humans. *J. Nutr.* **2009**, *139*, 620–622. [CrossRef]
51. Tang, D.; Fellows, L.K.; Small, D.M.; Dagher, A. Food and drug cues activate similar brain regions: A meta-analysis of functional MRI studies. *Physiol. Behav.* **2012**, *106*, 317–324. [CrossRef]
52. Blumenthal, D.M.; Gold, M.S. Neurobiology of food addiction. *Curr. Opin. Clin. Nutr. Metab. Care* **2010**, *13*, 359–365. [CrossRef]
53. Small, D.M.; Zatorre, R.J.; Dagher, A.; Evans, A.C.; Jones-Gotman, M. Changes in brain activity related to eating chocolate: From pleasure to aversion. *Brain* **2001**, *124*, 1720–1733. [CrossRef]
54. Small, D.M.; Jones-Gotman, M.; Daghera, A. Feeding-induced dopamine release in dorsal striatum correlates with meal pleasantness ratings in healthy human volunteers. *NeuroImage* **2003**, *19*, 1709–1715. [CrossRef]
55. Stein, E.A.; Pankiewicz, J.; Harsch, H.H.; Cho, J.-K.; Fuller, S.A.; Hoffmann, R.G.; Hawkins, M.; Rao, S.M.; Bandettini, P.A.; Bloom, A.S. Nicotine-Induced Limbic Cortical Activation in the Human Brain: A Functional MRI Study. *Am. J. Psychiatry* **1998**, *155*, 1009–1015. [CrossRef]
56. Heishman, S.J.; Kleykamp, B.A.; Singleton, E.G. Meta-analysis of the acute effects of nicotine and smoking on human performance. *Psychopharmacology* **2010**, *210*, 453–469. [CrossRef]
57. Due, D.L.; Huettel, S.A.; Hall, W.G.; Rubin, D.C. Activation in Mesolimbic and Visuospatial Neural Circuits Elicited by Smoking Cues: Evidence from Functional Magnetic Resonance Imaging. *Am. J. Psychiatry* **2002**, *159*, 954–960. [CrossRef]
58. David, S.P.; Munafò, M.R.; Johansen-Berg, H.; Smith, S.; Rogers, R.D.; Matthews, P.M.; Walton, R. Ventral Striatum/Nucleus Accumbens Activation to Smoking-Related Pictorial Cues in Smokers and Nonsmokers: A Functional Magnetic Resonance Imaging Study. *Biol. Psychiatry* **2005**, *58*, 488–494. [CrossRef]
59. Azizian, A.; Monterosso, J.; O'Neill, J.; London, E.D. Magnetic Resonance Imaging Studies of Cigarette Smoking. *Bone Regul. Osteoporos. Ther.* **2009**, *192*, 113–143. [CrossRef]
60. Picciotto, M.R.; Zoli, M.; Rimondini, R.; Léna, C.; Marubio, L.M.; Pich, E.M.; Fuxe, K.; Changeux, J.P. Acetylcholine receptors containing the beta2 subunit are involved in the reinforcing properties of nicotine. *Nature* **1998**, *391*, 173–177. [CrossRef]
61. Epping-Jordan, M.P.; Picciotto, M.R.; Changeux, J.-P.; Pich, E.M. Assessment of nicotinic acetylcholine receptor subunit contributions to nicotine self-administration in mutant mice. *Psychopharmacology* **1999**, *147*, 25–26. [CrossRef]
62. Koranda, J.L.; Cone, J.J.; McGehee, D.S.; Roitman, M.F.; Beeler, J.A.; Zhuang, X. Nicotinic receptors regulate the dynamic range of dopamine release in vivo. *J. Neurophysiol.* **2013**, *111*, 103–111. [CrossRef]

63. Cosgrove, K.P.; Esterlis, I.; McKee, S.; Bois, F.; Alagille, D.; Tamagnan, G.D.; Seibyl, J.P.; Krishnan-Sarin, S.; Staley, J.K. Beta2* nicotinic acetylcholine receptors modulate pain sensitivity in acutely abstinent tobacco smokers. *Nicotine Tob. Res.* **2010**, *12*, 535–539. [CrossRef]
64. Brunzell, D.H.; Boschen, K.E.; Hendrick, E.S.; Beardsley, P.M.; McIntosh, J.M. Alpha-conotoxin MII-sensitive nicotinic acetylcholine receptors in the nucleus accumbens shell regulate progressive ratio responding maintained by nicotine. *Neuropsychopharmacology* **2010**, *35*, 665–673. [CrossRef]
65. Perry, D.C.; Xiao, Y.; Nguyen, H.N.; Musachio, J.L.; Dávila-García, M.I.; Kellar, K.J. Measuring nicotinic receptors with characteristics of alpha4beta2, alpha3beta2 and alpha3beta4 subtypes in rat tissues by autoradiography. *J. Neurochem.* **2002**, *82*, 468–481. [CrossRef] [PubMed]
66. Mamede, M.; Ishizu, K.; Ueda, M.; Mukai, T.; Iida, Y.; Fukuyama, H.; Saga, T.; Saji, H. Quantification of human nicotinic acetylcholine receptors with 123I-5IA SPECT. *J. Nucl. Med.* **2004**, *45*, 1458–1470. [PubMed]
67. Ding, Y.S.; Gatley, S.J.; Fowler, J.S.; Volkow, N.D.; Aggarwal, D.; Logan, J.; Dewey, S.L.; Liang, F.; Carroll, F.I.; Kuhar, M.J. Mapping nicotinic acetylcholine receptors with PET. *Synapse* **1996**, *24*, 403–407. [CrossRef]
68. Brody, A.L. Functional brain imaging of tobacco use and dependence. *J. Psychiatr. Res.* **2006**, *40*, 404–418. [CrossRef]
69. Imperato, A.; Mulas, A.; Di Chiara, G. Nicotine preferentially stimulates dopamine release in the limbic system of freely moving rats. *Eur. J. Pharmacol.* **1986**, *132*, 337–338. [CrossRef]
70. Dani, J.A.; De Biasi, M. Cellular mechanisms of nicotine addiction. *Pharmacol. Biochem. Behav.* **2001**, *70*, 439–446. [CrossRef]
71. Wang, G.J.; Volkow, N.D.; Thanos, P.K.; Fowler, J.S. Imaging of brain dopamine pathways: Implications for understanding obesity. *J. Addict. Med.* **2009**, *3*, 8–18. [CrossRef] [PubMed]
72. Sharma, A.; Brody, A.L. In vivo Brain Imaging of Human Exposure to Nicotine and Tobacco. *Handb. Exp. Pharmacol.* **2009**, 145–171. [CrossRef]
73. Cosgrove, K.P.; Esterlis, I.; Sandiego, C.; Petrulli, R.; Morris, E.D. Imaging Tobacco Smoking with PET and SPECT. *Behav. Neurobiol. Anxiety Treat.* **2015**, *24*, 1–17. [CrossRef]
74. Staley, J.K.; Krishnan-Sarin, S.; Cosgrove, K.P.; Krantzler, E.; Frohlich, E.; Perry, E.; Dubin, J.A.; Estok, K.; Brenner, E.; Baldwin, R.M.; et al. Human Tobacco Smokers in Early Abstinence Have Higher Levels of beta2* Nicotinic Acetylcholine Receptors than Nonsmokers. *J. Neurosci.* **2006**, *26*, 8707–8714. [CrossRef]
75. Rourke, S.B.; Dupont, R.M.; Grant, I.; Lehr, P.P.; Lamoureux, G.; Halpern, S.; Yeung, D.W. Reduction in cortical IMP-SPET tracer uptake with recent cigarette consumption in a young group of healthy males. San Diego HIV Neurobehavioral Research Center. *S. Diego HIV Neurobehav. Res. Cent. Eur. J. Nucl. Med.* **1997**, *24*, 422–427.
76. Yamamoto, Y.; Nishiyama, Y.; Monden, T.; Satoh, K.; Ohkawa, M. A study of the acute effect of smoking on cerebral blood flow using 99mTc-ECD SPET. *Eur. J. Nucl. Med. Mol. Imaging* **2003**, *30*, 612–614. [CrossRef] [PubMed]
77. Brašić, J.R.; Zhou, Y.; Musachio, J.L.; Hilton, J.; Fan, H.; Crabb, A.; Endres, C.J.; Reinhardt, M.J.; Dogan, A.S.; Alexander, M.; et al. Single photon emission computed tomography experience with (S)-5-[^{123}I]iodo-3-(2-azetidinylmethoxy)pyridine in the living human brain of smokers and nonsmokers. *Synapse* **2009**, *63*, 339–358. [CrossRef] [PubMed]
78. Goldstein, R.Z.; Volkow, N.D. Dysfunction of the prefrontal cortex in addiction: Neuroimaging findings and clinical implications. *Nat. Rev. Neurosci.* **2011**, *12*, 652–669. [CrossRef] [PubMed]
79. Goldstein, R.Z.; Tomasi, D.; Rajaram, S.; Cottone, L.A.; Zhang, L.; Maloney, T.; Telang, F.; Alia-Klein, N.; Volkow, N.D. Role of the anterior cingulate and medial orbitofrontal cortex in processing drug cues in cocaine addiction. *Neuroscience* **2007**, *144*, 1153–1159. [CrossRef] [PubMed]
80. Feil, J.; Sheppard, D.; Fitzgerald, P.B.; Yücel, M.; Lubman, D.I.; Bradshaw, J.L. Addiction, compulsive drug seeking, and the role of frontostriatal mechanisms in regulating inhibitory control. *Neurosci. Biobehav. Rev.* **2010**, *35*, 248–275. [CrossRef]
81. Breese, C.R.; Marks, M.J.; Logel, J.; Adams, C.E.; Sullivan, B.; Collins, A.C.; Leonard, S. Effect of smoking history on [3H]nicotine binding in human postmortem brain. *J. Pharmacol. Exp. Ther.* **1997**, *282*, 7–13.
82. Brody, A.L.; Mandelkern, M.A.; London, E.D.; Olmstead, R.E.; Farahi, J.; Scheibal, D.; Jou, J.; Allen, V.; Tiongson, E.; Chefer, S.I.; et al. Cigarette smoking saturates brain alpha 4 beta 2 nicotinic acetylcholine receptors. *Arch. Gen. Psychiatry* **2006**, *63*, 907–915. [CrossRef]

83. Jasinska, A.J.; Zorick, T.; Brody, A.L.; Stein, E.A. Dual role of nicotine in addiction and cognition: A review of neuroimaging studies in humans. *Neuropharmacology* **2014**, *84*, 111–122. [CrossRef]
84. Gearhardt, A.N. Neural Correlates of Food Addiction. *Arch. Gen. Psychiatry* **2011**, *68*, 808–816. [CrossRef]
85. Schulte, E.M.; Yokum, S.; Jahn, A.; Gearhardt, A.N. Food cue reactivity in food addiction: A functional magnetic resonance imaging study. *Physiol. Behav.* **2019**, *208*, 112574. [CrossRef] [PubMed]
86. Morton, G.J.; Cummings, D.E.; Baskin, D.G.; Barsh, G.S.; Schwartz, M.W. Central nervous system control of food intake and body weight. *Nat. Cell Biol.* **2006**, *443*, 289–295. [CrossRef] [PubMed]
87. Gupta, A.; Osadchiy, V.; Mayer, E.A. Brain-gut-microbiome interactions in obesity and food addiction. *Nat. Rev. Gastroenterol. Hepatol.* **2020**, *17*, 655–672. [CrossRef] [PubMed]
88. Morganstern, I.; Barson, J.R.; Leibowitz, S.F. Regulation of drug and palatable food overconsumption by similar peptide systems. *Curr. Drug Abus. Rev.* **2011**, *4*, 163–173. [CrossRef] [PubMed]
89. Lee, S.H.; Yun, Y.; Kim, S.J.; Lee, E.-J.; Chang, Y.; Ryu, S.; Shin, H.; Kim, H.-L.; Kim, H.-N.; Lee, J.H. Association between Cigarette Smoking Status and Composition of Gut Microbiota: Population-Based Cross-Sectional Study. *J. Clin. Med.* **2018**, *7*, 282. [CrossRef] [PubMed]
90. Kiraly, D.D.; Walker, D.M.; Calipari, E.S.; LaBonte, B.; Issler, O.; Pena, C.J.; Ribeiro, E.A.; Russo, S.J.; Nestler, E.J. Alterations of the Host Microbiome Affect Behavioral Responses to Cocaine. *Sci. Rep.* **2016**, *6*, 35455. [CrossRef]
91. Kang, M.; Mischel, R.A.; Bhave, S.; Komla, E.; Cho, A.; Huang, C.; Dewey, W.L.; Akbarali, H.I. The effect of gut microbiome on tolerance to morphine mediated antinociception in mice. *Sci. Rep.* **2017**, *7*, srep42658. [CrossRef]
92. E Volpe, G.; Ward, H.; Mwamburi, M.; Dinh, D.; Bhalchandra, S.; Wanke, C.; Kane, A.V. Associations of Cocaine Use and HIV Infection with the Intestinal Microbiota, Microbial Translocation, and Inflammation. *J. Stud. Alcohol Drugs* **2014**, *75*, 347–357. [CrossRef]
93. Temko, J.E.; Bouhlal, S.; Farokhnia, M.; Lee, M.R.; Cryan, J.F.; Leggio, L. The Microbiota, the Gut and the Brain in Eating and Alcohol Use Disorders: A 'Menage a Trois'? *Alcohol Alcohol.* **2017**, *52*, 403–413. [CrossRef]
94. Wang, F.; Roy, S. Gut Homeostasis, Microbial Dysbiosis, and Opioids. *Toxicol. Pathol.* **2016**, *45*, 150–156. [CrossRef]
95. Hillemacher, T.; Bachmann, O.; Kahl, K.G.; Frieling, H. Alcohol, microbiome, and their effect on psychiatric disorders. *Prog. Neuro Psychopharmacol. Biol. Psychiatry* **2018**, *85*, 105–115. [CrossRef] [PubMed]
96. Hofford, R.S.; Russo, S.J.; Kiraly, D.D. Neuroimmune mechanisms of psychostimulant and opioid use disorders. *Eur. J. Neurosci.* **2019**, *50*, 2562–2573. [CrossRef] [PubMed]
97. Cussotto, S.; Clarke, G.; Dinan, T.G.; Cryan, J.F. Psychotropics and the Microbiome: A Chamber of Secrets ... *Psychopharmacology* **2019**, *236*, 1411–1432. [CrossRef] [PubMed]
98. Biedermann, L.; Zeitz, J.; Mwinyi, J.; Sutter-Minder, E.; Rehman, A.; Ott, S.J.; Steurer-Stey, C.; Frei, A.; Frei, P.; Scharl, M.; et al. Smoking Cessation Induces Profound Changes in the Composition of the Intestinal Microbiota in Humans. *PLoS ONE* **2013**, *8*, e59260. [CrossRef]
99. Kaufmann, S. Faculty Opinions recommendation of Microbial ecology: Human gut microbes associated with obesity. *Fac. Opin. Post Publ. Peer Rev. Biomed. Lit.* **2007**, *444*, 1022–1023. [CrossRef]
100. Koliada, A.; Syzenko, G.; Moseiko, V.; Budovska, L.; Puchkov, K.; Perederiy, V.; Gavalko, Y.; Dorofeyev, A.; Romanenko, M.; Tkach, S.; et al. Association between body mass index and Firmicutes/Bacteroidetes ratio in an adult Ukrainian population. *BMC Microbiol.* **2017**, *17*, 120. [CrossRef]
101. Stewart, C.J.; Auchtung, T.A.; Ajami, N.J.; Velasquez, K.; Smith, D.P.; De La Garza, R., 2nd; Salas, R.; Petrosino, J.F. Effects of tobacco smoke and electronic cigarette vapor exposure on the oral and gut microbiota in humans: A pilot study. *PeerJ* **2018**, *6*, e4693. [CrossRef]
102. Biedermann, L.; Brülisauer, K.; Zeitz, J.; Frei, P.; Scharl, M.; Vavricka, S.R.; Fried, M.; Loessner, M.J.; Rogler, G.; Schuppler, M. Tu1771 Smoking Cessation Alters Intestinal Microbiota: Further Insights from Quantitative Investigations on Human Fecal Samples Using FISH and qPCR. *Gastroenterology* **2014**, *146*, 1496–1501. [CrossRef]
103. Skibicka, K.P.; Dickson, S.L. Ghrelin and food reward: The story of potential underlying substrates. *Peptides* **2011**, *32*, 2265–2273. [CrossRef]
104. Steinert, R.E.; Poller, B.; Castelli, M.C.; Drewe, J.; Beglinger, C. Oral administration of glucagon-like peptide 1 or peptide YY 3-36 affects food intake in healthy male subjects. *Am. J. Clin. Nutr.* **2010**, *92*, 810–817. [CrossRef]

105. Bagarolli, R.A.; Tobar, N.; Oliveira, A.G.; Araújo, T.G.; Carvalho, B.M.; Rocha, G.Z.; Vecina, J.F.; Calisto, K.; Guadagnini, D.; Prada, P.O.; et al. Probiotics modulate gut microbiota and improve insulin sensitivity in DIO mice. *J. Nutr. Biochem.* **2017**, *50*, 16–25. [CrossRef]
106. Osadchiy, V.; Labus, J.S.; Gupta, A.; Jacobs, J.; Ashe-McNalley, C.; Hsiao, E.Y.; Mayer, E.A. Correlation of tryptophan metabolites with connectivity of extended central reward network in healthy subjects. *PLoS ONE* **2018**, *13*, e0201772. [CrossRef] [PubMed]
107. Dong, T.S.; Mayer, E.A.; Osadchiy, V.; Chang, C.; Katzka, W.; Lagishetty, V.; Gonzalez, K.; Kalani, A.; Stains, J.; Jacobs, J.P.; et al. A Distinct Brain-Gut-Microbiome Profile Exists for Females with Obesity and Food Addiction. *Obesity* **2020**, *28*, 1477–1486. [CrossRef] [PubMed]
108. Dong, M.; Giles, W.H.; Felitti, V.J.; Dube, S.R.; Williams, J.E.; Chapman, D.P.; Anda, R.F. Insights into causal pathways for ischemic heart disease: Adverse childhood experiences study. *Circulation* **2004**, *110*, 1761–1766. [CrossRef] [PubMed]
109. Anda, R.F.; Brown, D.W.; Dube, S.R.; Bremner, J.D.; Felitti, V.J.; Giles, W.H. Adverse Childhood Experiences and Chronic Obstructive Pulmonary Disease in Adults. *Am. J. Prev. Med.* **2008**, *34*, 396–403. [CrossRef]
110. Brown, D.W.; Anda, R.F.; Felitti, V.J.; Edwards, V.J.; Malarcher, A.; Croft, J.B.; Giles, W.H. Adverse childhood experiences are associated with the risk of lung cancer: A prospective cohort study. *BMC Public Heal.* **2010**, *10*, 20. [CrossRef]
111. Felitti, V.J.; Anda, R.F.; Nordenberg, D.; Williamson, D.F.; Spitz, A.M.; Edwards, V.; Koss, M.P.; Marks, J.S. REPRINT OF: Relationship of Childhood Abuse and Household Dysfunction to Many of the Leading Causes of Death in Adults: The Adverse Childhood Experiences (ACE) Study. *Am. J. Prev. Med.* **2019**, *56*, 774–786. [CrossRef]
112. Dube, S.R.; Felitti, V.J.; Dong, M.; Chapman, D.P.; Giles, W.H.; Anda, R.F. Childhood Abuse, Neglect, and Household Dysfunction and the Risk of Illicit Drug Use: The Adverse Childhood Experiences Study. *Pediatrics* **2003**, *111*, 564–572. [CrossRef]
113. Cronholm, P.F.; Fokre, C.M.; Wade, R.; Bair-Merritt, M.H.; Davis, M.; Harkins-Schwarz, M.; Pachter, L.M.; Fein, J.A. Adverse Childhood Experiences: Expanding the Concept of Adversity. *Am. J. Prev. Med.* **2015**, *49*, 354–361. [CrossRef]
114. Anda, R.F.; Croft, J.B.; Felitti, V.J.; Nordenberg, D.; Giles, W.H.; Williamson, D.F.; Giovino, G.A. Adverse Childhood Experiences and Smoking During Adolescence and Adulthood. *JAMA* **1999**, *282*, 1652–1658. [CrossRef]
115. Dube, S.R.; Anda, R.F.; Felitti, V.J.; Edwards, V.J.; Croft, J.B. Adverse childhood experiences and personal alcohol abuse as an adult. *Addict. Behav.* **2002**, *27*, 713–725. [CrossRef]
116. Dube, S.R.; Cook, M.L.; Edwards, V.J. Health-Related Outcomes of Adverse Childhood Experiences in Texas, 2002. *Prev. Chronic Dis.* **2010**, *7*, 52.
117. Mason, S.M.; Flint, A.J.; Field, A.E.; Austin, S.B.; Rich-Edwards, J.W. Abuse victimization in childhood or adolescence and risk of food addiction in adult women. *Obesity* **2013**, *21*, E775–E781. [CrossRef] [PubMed]
118. Smolak, L.; Murnen, S.K. A meta-analytic examination of the relationship between child sexual abuse and eating disorders. *Int. J. Eat. Disord.* **2002**, *31*, 136–150. [CrossRef]
119. Kinzl, J.F.; Traweger, C.; Guenther, V.; Biebl, W. Family background and sexual abuse associated with eating disorders. *Am. J. Psychiatry* **1994**, *151*, 1127–1131. [CrossRef]
120. Smyth, J.M.; Heron, K.E.; Wonderlich, S.A.; Crosby, R.D.; Thompson, K.M. The influence of reported trauma and adverse events on eating disturbance in young adults. *Int. J. Eat. Disord.* **2008**, *41*, 195–202. [CrossRef]
121. Johnson, J.G.; Cohen, P.; Kasen, S.; Brook, J.S. Eating Disorders During Adolescence and the Risk for Physical and Mental Disorders During Early Adulthood. *Arch. Gen. Psychiatry* **2002**, *59*, 545–552. [CrossRef]
122. Wise, M.H.; Weierbach, F.; Cao, Y.; Phillips, K. Tobacco Use and Attachment Style in Appalachia. *Issues Ment. Heal. Nurs.* **2017**, *38*, 562–569. [CrossRef]
123. Mikulincer, M. Adult attachment style and affect regulation: Strategic variations in self-appraisals. *J. Pers. Soc. Psychol.* **1998**, *75*, 420–435. [CrossRef]
124. Griffin, D.; Bartholomew, K. Models of the self and other: Fundamental dimensions underlying measures of adult attachment. *J. Personal. Soc. Psychol.* **1994**, *67*, 430–445. [CrossRef]
125. Fowler, J.C.; Allen, J.; Oldham, J.M.; Frueh, B.C. Exposure to interpersonal trauma, attachment insecurity, and depression severity. *J. Affect. Disord.* **2013**, *149*, 313–318. [CrossRef]

126. Mikulincer, M.; Shaver, P.R.; Pereg, D. Attachment Theory and Affect Regulation: The Dynamics, Development, and Cognitive Consequences of Attachment-Related Strategies. *Motiv. Emot.* **2003**, *27*, 77–102. [CrossRef]
127. Gross, J.J. The emerging field of emotion regulation: An integrative review. *Rev. Gen. Psychol.* **1998**, *2*, 271–299. [CrossRef]
128. Kobak, R.R.; Cole, H.E.; Ferenz-Gillies, R.; Fleming, W.S.; Gamble, W. Attachment and Emotion Regulation during Mother-Teen Problem Solving: A Control Theory Analysis. *Child Dev.* **1993**, *64*, 231. [CrossRef] [PubMed]
129. Maunder, R.G.; Hunter, J.J. Attachment and Psychosomatic Medicine: Developmental Contributions to Stress and Disease. *Psychosom. Med.* **2001**, *63*, 556–567. [CrossRef]
130. Faber, A.; Dubé, L.; Knäuper, B. Attachment and eating: A meta-analytic review of the relevance of attachment for unhealthy and healthy eating behaviors in the general population. *Appetite* **2018**, *123*, 410–438. [CrossRef]
131. Shakory, S.; Van Exan, J.; Mills, J.S.; Sockalingam, S.; Keating, L.; Taube-Schiff, M. Binge eating in bariatric surgery candidates: The role of insecure attachment and emotion regulation. *Appetite* **2015**, *91*, 69–75. [CrossRef]
132. Fauconnier, M.; Rousselet, M.; Brunault, P.; Thiabaud, E.; Lambert, S.; Rocher, B.; Challet-Bouju, G.; Grall-Bronnec, M. Food Addiction among Female Patients Seeking Treatment for an Eating Disorder: Prevalence and Associated Factors. *Nutrients* **2020**, *12*, 1897. [CrossRef]
133. Ahrens, K.R.; Ciechanowski, P.; Katon, W. Associations between adult attachment style and health risk behaviors in an adult female primary care population. *J. Psychosom. Res.* **2012**, *72*, 364–370. [CrossRef]
134. Cooper, M.L.; Shaver, P.R.; Collins, N.L. Attachment styles, emotion regulation, and adjustment in adolescence. *J. Pers. Soc. Psychol.* **1998**, *74*, 1380–1397. [CrossRef]
135. Kassel, J.D.; Wardle, M.; Roberts, J.E. Adult attachment security and college student substance use. *Addict. Behav.* **2007**, *32*, 1164–1176. [CrossRef] [PubMed]
136. McNally, A.M.; Palfai, T.P.; Levine, R.V.; Moore, B.M. Attachment dimensions and drinking-related problems among young adults: The mediational role of coping motives. *Addict. Behav.* **2003**, *28*, 1115–1127. [CrossRef]
137. Le, T.L.; Mann, R.E.; Levitan, R.D.; George, T.P.; Maunder, R.G. Sex differences in the relationships between childhood adversity, attachment anxiety and current smoking. *Addict. Res. Theory* **2017**, *25*, 146–153. [CrossRef]
138. Pipová, H.; Kaščáková, N.; Fürstová, J.; Tavel, P. Development of the Modified Yale Food Addiction Scale Version 2.0 summary version in a representative sample of Czech population. *J. Eat. Disord.* **2020**, *8*, 16. [CrossRef] [PubMed]
139. Armstrong, J.G.; Roth, D.M. Attachment and separation difficulties in eating disorders: A preliminary investigation. *Int. J. Eat. Disord.* **1989**, *8*, 141–155. [CrossRef]
140. Broberg, A.G.; Hjalmers, I.; Nevonen, L. Eating disorders, attachment and interpersonal difficulties: A comparison between 18- to 24-year-old patients and normal controls. *Eur. Eat. Disord. Rev.* **2001**, *9*, 381–396. [CrossRef]
141. Chassler, L. Understanding Anorexia Nervosa and Bulimia Nervosa from an Attachment Perspective. *Clin. Soc. Work. J.* **1997**, *25*, 407–423. [CrossRef]
142. Kenny, M.; Hart, K. Relationship between parental attachment and eating disorders in an inpatient and a college sample. *J. Couns. Psychol.* **1992**, *39*, 521–526. [CrossRef]
143. Latzer, Y.; Hochdorf, Z.; Bachar, E.; Canetti, L. Attachment Style and Family Functioning as Discriminating Factors in Eating Disorders. *Contemp. Fam. Ther.* **2002**, *24*, 581–599. [CrossRef]
144. Orzolek-Kronner, C. The Effect of Attachment Theory in the Development of Eating Disorders: Can Symptoms Be Proximity-Seeking? *Child Adolesc. Soc. Work. J.* **2002**, *19*, 421–435. [CrossRef]
145. Ward, A.; Ramsay, R.; Treasure, J. Attachment research in eating disorders. *Br. J. Med Psychol.* **2000**, *73*, 35–51. [CrossRef] [PubMed]
146. Illing, V.; Tasca, G.A.; Balfour, L.; Bissada, H. Attachment Insecurity Predicts Eating Disorder Symptoms and Treatment Outcomes in a Clinical Sample of Women. *J. Nerv. Ment. Dis.* **2010**, *198*, 653–659. [CrossRef] [PubMed]
147. Taube-Schiff, M.; Van Exan, J.; Tanaka, R.; Wnuk, S.; Hawa, R.; Sockalingam, S. Attachment style and emotional eating in bariatric surgery candidates: The mediating role of difficulties in emotion regulation. *Eat. Behav.* **2015**, *18*, 36–40. [CrossRef] [PubMed]

1. Introduction

Psychosis is the hallmark feature of various psychiatric illnesses, including schizophrenia (SCZ), schizoaffective disorder, schizophreniform disorder and bipolar disorder [1]. It is a severely debilitating condition with an estimated worldwide prevalence of approximately 4.6 per 1000 people [2]. The American Psychiatric Association and World Health Organization have conceptualized psychosis as consisting of altered perception and impaired reality testing, including positive symptoms such as hallucinations and delusions [3]. Severe mental illnesses additionally are associated with cognitive deficits and negative symptoms, which can drive functional impairment and illness associated disability [4,5].

Antipsychotic (AP) medications are currently the cornerstone treatment for psychotic disorders [6]. Unfortunately, APs are associated with serious metabolic adverse effects [7], which increase patients' risk of developing metabolic syndrome, type 2 diabetes, and cardiovascular disease (CVD). Notably, CVD is the leading cause of premature mortality in severe mental illness, reducing life expectancy by 11–20 years [8–10]. While clozapine and olanzapine carry the greatest metabolic liability [11], all AP medications cause weight gain in younger patients with limited previous AP exposure [12]. Similarly, these medications have been shown, independently of class or individual agent, to increase risk of type 2 diabetes in patients with SCZ [10].

Weight gain, a common consequence of AP treatment, occurs when there is a positive energy balance, meaning that energy intake exceeds energy expenditure [13]. Beyond the metabolic effect of APs, weight gain in psychotic disorders is also, in part, explained by unfavorable behaviours. For instance, patients with SCZ may have higher intake of calorie dense foods and lower intake of healthy foods than the general population [14]. Other contributing factors include lower levels of physical activity and significantly higher rates of smoking and alcohol consumption [15]. All these behaviours are also associated with lower socioeconomic status and higher unemployment among patients with SCZ [15,16]. Furthermore, epidemiological reviews have suggested that approximately 10% of patients with SCZ suffer from binge eating disorder (BED) or night eating syndromes, which is five times higher than in the general population [17]. Thus, disturbed eating behaviour may also contribute to the significant weight gain and metabolic disturbances experienced by these patients.

Looking beyond social, environmental and behavioural factors, energy homeostasis is controlled by intricate physiological pathways. Patients with SCZ may have subclinical metabolic dysregulations including dyslipidemia [18], hyperglycemia and insulin resistance [19] present at the earliest stages of the illness, which are further exacerbated by AP therapy [20,21]. Furthermore, impaired regulation of appetite related hormones including elevated insulin (linked with insulin resistance) and low leptin and adiponectin (secreted by adipose tissue) levels are also implicated in the pathophysiology of weight gain in psychosis spectrum disorders [18,22]. Ghrelin, which stimulates hunger, does not appear to be altered in AP-naïve or largely unmedicated first episode psychosis (FEP) patients [18]; however, olanzapine use may be associated with decreased ghrelin levels, which is a similar phenomenon to what is observed in obesity [23].

While the physiological homeostatic mechanisms underlying altered eating patterns in this population have been the subject of recent meta-analyses and reviews [18,20], less is known about the psychopathological and neurobiological mechanisms that may be implicated in the non-homeostatic regulation of food intake. Non-homeostatic eating behaviour involves the hedonic and reward aspects of food intake that is separate from the physiological drive stimulated by energy requirement [24]. This aspect of eating behaviour is regulated by the reward system, which includes the mesolimbic dopamine circuit (involving the ventral tegmental area and nucleus accumbens), as well as nuclei in the amygdala and hippocampus that are interconnected to the hypothalamus and brainstem (the latter implicated in homeostatic feeding regulation) [25]. Disruption at any level of these complex neural networks regulating eating behaviour may be implicated in the weight gain and metabolic sequalae associated with SCZ. Moreover, these disruptions are likely to involve aspects intrinsic to

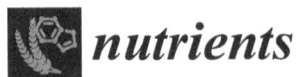

Review

Exploring Patterns of Disturbed Eating in Psychosis: A Scoping Review

Nicolette Stogios [1,2,†], Emily Smith [1,2,†], Roshanak Asgariroozbehani [1,2,†], Laurie Hamel [1], Alexander Gdanski [3], Peter Selby [1,4,5,6], Sanjeev Sockalingam [1,2,6,7], Ariel Graff-Guerrero [1,2,6], Valerie H. Taylor [8], Sri Mahavir Agarwal [1,2,6,‡] and Margaret K. Hahn [1,2,6,*,‡]

1. Centre for Addiction and Mental Health (CAMH), Toronto, ON M6J 1H3, Canada; nicolette.stogios@mail.utoronto.ca (N.S.); emilycc.smith@mail.utoronto.ca (E.S.); roshanak.asgariroozbehani@mail.utoronto.ca (R.A.); laurie.hamel@camh.ca (L.H.); peter.selby@camh.ca (P.S.); sanjeev.sockalingam@camh.ca (S.S.); ariel.graff@camh.ca (A.G.-G.); mahavir.agarwal@camh.ca (S.M.A.)
2. Institute of Medical Science (IMS), University of Toronto, Toronto, ON M5S 1A8, Canada
3. Department of Human Biology, University of Toronto, Toronto, ON M5S 3J6, Canada; alexander.gdanski@mail.utoronto.ca
4. Department of Family and Community Medicine, University of Toronto, Toronto, ON M5G 1V7, Canada
5. Dalla Lana School of Public Health, University of Toronto, Toronto, ON M5T 3M7, Canada
6. Department of Psychiatry, University of Toronto, Toronto, ON M5T 1R8, Canada
7. Bariatric Surgery Program, University Health Network, Toronto, ON M5T 2S8, Canada
8. Department of Psychiatry, University of Calgary, Calgary, AB T2N 1N4, Canada; valerie.taylor3@albertahealthservices.ca
* Correspondence: margaret.hahn@camh.ca; Tel.: +1-(416)-535-8501 (ext. 34368)
† These authors contributed equally to this work.
‡ These authors contributed equally to this work.

Received: 8 November 2020; Accepted: 9 December 2020; Published: 18 December 2020

Abstract: Disturbed eating behaviours have been widely reported in psychotic disorders since the early 19th century. There is also evidence that antipsychotic (AP) treatment may induce binge eating or other related compulsive eating behaviours. It is therefore possible that abnormal eating patterns may contribute to the significant weight gain and other metabolic disturbances observed in patients with psychosis. In this scoping review, we aimed to explore the underlying psychopathological and neurobiological mechanisms of disrupted eating behaviours in psychosis spectrum disorders and the role of APs in this relationship. A systematic search identified 35 studies that met our eligibility criteria and were included in our qualitative synthesis. Synthesizing evidence from self-report questionnaires and food surveys, we found that patients with psychosis exhibit increased appetite and craving for fatty food, as well as increased caloric intake and snacking, which may be associated with increased disinhibition. Limited evidence from neuroimaging studies suggested that AP-naïve first episode patients exhibit similar neural processing of food to healthy controls, while chronic AP exposure may lead to decreased activity in satiety areas and increased activity in areas associated with reward anticipation. Overall, this review supports the notion that AP use can lead to disturbed eating patterns in patients, which may contribute to AP-induced weight gain. However, intrinsic illness-related effects on eating behaviors remain less well elucidated, and many confounding factors as well as variability in study designs limits interpretation of existing literature in this field and precludes firm conclusions from being made.

Keywords: food intake; eating behaviour; diet; overconsumption; binge eating; weight gain; obesity; hedonic pathway; homeostatic pathway

168. Clark, M.M.; Decker, P.A.; Offord, K.P.; A Patten, C.; Vickers, K.S.; Croghan, I.T.; Schaff, H.V.; Hurt, R.D.; Dale, L.C. Weight concerns among male smokers. *Addict. Behav.* **2004**, *29*, 1637–1641. [CrossRef]
169. Owari, Y.; Miyatake, N.; Suzuki, H. Relationship between Food Dependence and Nicotine Dependence in Smokers: A Cross-Sectional Study of Staff and Students at Medical Colleges. *Medicina* **2019**, *55*, 202. [CrossRef]
170. Blum, K.; Bailey, J.; Gonzalez, A.M.; Oscar-Berman, M.; Liu, Y.; Giordano, J.; Braverman, E.; Gold, M. Neuro-genetics of reward deficiency syndrome (RDS) as the root cause of "addiction transfer": A new phenomenon common after bariatric surgery. *J. Genet. Syndr. Gene Ther.* **2011**, S2-001. [CrossRef]
171. Turnbaugh, P.J.; Ley, R.E.; Mahowald, M.A.; Magrini, V.; Mardis, E.R.; Gordon, J.I. An obesity-associated gut microbiome with increased capacity for energy harvest. *Nat. Cell Biol.* **2006**, *444*, 1027–1031. [CrossRef]
172. Fletcher, P.C.; Kenny, P.J. Food addiction: A valid concept? *Neuropsychopharmacology* **2018**, *43*, 2506–2513. [CrossRef]

Publisher's Note: MDPI stays neutral with regard to jurisdictional claims in published maps and institutional affiliations.

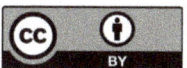

© 2020 by the authors. Licensee MDPI, Basel, Switzerland. This article is an open access article distributed under the terms and conditions of the Creative Commons Attribution (CC BY) license (http://creativecommons.org/licenses/by/4.0/).

148. Wilkinson, L.L.; Rowe, A.C.; Sheldon, C.; Johnson, A.; Brunstrom, J.M. Disinhibited eating mediates differences in attachment insecurity between bariatric surgery candidates/recipients and lean controls. *Int. J. Obes.* **2017**, *41*, 1831–1834. [CrossRef] [PubMed]
149. Wang, D.; Connock, M.; Barton, P.; Fry-Smith, A.; Aveyard, P.; Moore, D. 'Cut down to quit' with nicotine replacement therapies in smoking cessation: A systematic review of effectiveness and economic analysis. *Heal. Technol. Assess.* **2008**, *12*. [CrossRef] [PubMed]
150. Moore, D.; Aveyard, P.; Connock, M.; Wang, D.; Fry-Smith, A.; Barton, P. Effectiveness and safety of nicotine replacement therapy assisted reduction to stop smoking: Systematic review and meta-analysis. *BMJ* **2009**, *338*, b1024. [CrossRef]
151. Lindson, N.; Chepkin, S.C.; Ye, W.; Fanshawe, T.R.; Bullen, C.; Hartmann-Boyce, J. Different doses, durations and modes of delivery of nicotine replacement therapy for smoking cessation. *Cochrane Database Syst. Rev.* **2019**, *4*, CD013308. [CrossRef]
152. Cahill, K.; Stevens, S.; Perera, R.; Lancaster, T. Pharmacological interventions for smoking cessation: An overview and network meta-analysis. *Cochrane Database Syst. Rev.* **2013**, *5*, CD009329. [CrossRef]
153. Cahill, K.; Lindson-Hawley, N.; Thomas, K.H.; Fanshawe, T.R.; Lancaster, T. Nicotine receptor partial agonists for smoking cessation. *Cochrane Database Syst. Rev.* **2016**, *2016*, CD006103. [CrossRef]
154. Howes, S.; Hartmann-Boyce, J.; Livingstone-Banks, J.; Hong, B.; Lindson, N. Antidepressants for smoking cessation. *Cochrane Database Syst. Rev.* **2020**, *4*, CD000031. [CrossRef]
155. Stead, L.F.; Perera, R.; Bullen, C.; Mant, D.; Hartmann-Boyce, J.; Cahill, K.; Lancaster, T. Nicotine replacement therapy for smoking cessation. *Cochrane Database Syst. Rev.* **2012**, *11*, CD000146. [CrossRef] [PubMed]
156. Aveyard, P.; Begh, R.; Parsons, A.; West, R. Brief opportunistic smoking cessation interventions: A systematic review and meta-analysis to compare advice to quit and offer of assistance. *Addiction* **2012**, *107*, 1066–1073. [CrossRef] [PubMed]
157. Heckman, C.J.; Egleston, B.L.; Hofmann, M.T. Efficacy of motivational interviewing for smoking cessation: A systematic review and meta-analysis. *Tob. Control.* **2010**, *19*, 410–416. [CrossRef] [PubMed]
158. Hartmann-Boyce, J.; McRobbie, H.; Lindson, N.; Bullen, C.; Begh, R.; Theodoulou, A.; Notley, C.; A Rigotti, N.; Turner, T.; Butler, A.R.; et al. Electronic cigarettes for smoking cessation. *Cochrane Database Syst. Rev.* **2020**, *10*, CD010216. [CrossRef] [PubMed]
159. Hajek, P.; Phillips-Waller, A.; Przulj, D.; Pesola, F.; Smith, K.M.; Bisal, N.; Li, J.; Parrott, S.; Sasieni, P.; Dawkins, L.; et al. A Randomized Trial of E-Cigarettes versus Nicotine-Replacement Therapy. *N. Engl. J. Med.* **2019**, *380*, 629–637. [CrossRef]
160. Treasure, J.; Leslie, M.; Chami, R.; Fernández-Aranda, F. Are trans diagnostic models of eating disorders fit for purpose? A consideration of the evidence for food addiction. *Eur. Eat. Disord. Rev.* **2018**, *26*, 83–91. [CrossRef]
161. Miller-Matero, L.R.; Brescacin, C.; Clark, S.M.; Troncone, C.L.; Tobin, E.T. Why WAIT? Preliminary evaluation of the weight assistance and intervention techniques (WAIT) group. *Psychol. Heal. Med.* **2019**, *24*, 1029–1037. [CrossRef]
162. Cassin, S.; Sijercic, I.; Montemarano, V. Psychosocial Interventions for Food Addiction: A Systematic Review. *Curr. Addict. Rep.* **2020**, *7*, 9–19. [CrossRef]
163. Luigjes, J.; Segrave, R.; De Joode, N.; Figee, M.; Denys, D. Efficacy of Invasive and Non-Invasive Brain Modulation Interventions for Addiction. *Neuropsychol. Rev.* **2019**, *29*, 116–138. [CrossRef]
164. Sauvaget, A.; Etrojak, B.; Ebulteau, S.; Ejiménez-Murcia, S.; Efernandez-Aranda, F.; Ewolz, I.; Menchón, J.M.; Eachab, S.; Evanelle, J.-M.; Egrall-Bronnec, M. Transcranial direct current stimulation (tDCS) in behavioral and food addiction: A systematic review of efficacy, technical, and methodological issues. *Front. Neurosci.* **2015**, *9*, 349. [CrossRef]
165. Aubin, H.-J.; Farley, A.; Lycett, D.; Lahmek, P.; Aveyard, P. Weight gain in smokers after quitting cigarettes: Meta-analysis. *BMJ* **2012**, *345*, e4439. [CrossRef] [PubMed]
166. Tian, J.; Venn, A.; Otahal, P.; Gall, S. The association between quitting smoking and weight gain: A systematic review and meta-analysis of prospective cohort studies. *Obes. Rev.* **2015**, *16*, 883–901. [CrossRef] [PubMed]
167. Clark, M.M.; Hurt, R.D.; Croghan, I.T.; A Patten, C.; Novotny, P.; Sloan, J.A.; Dakhil, S.R.; Croghan, G.A.; Wos, E.J.; Rowland, K.M.; et al. The prevalence of weight concerns in a smoking abstinence clinical trial. *Addict. Behav.* **2006**, *31*, 1144–1152. [CrossRef] [PubMed]

SCZ, and/or associated with AP treatment [26]. The reward and limbic pathways involved in eating behavior and appetite are depicted in Figure 1 in more detail.

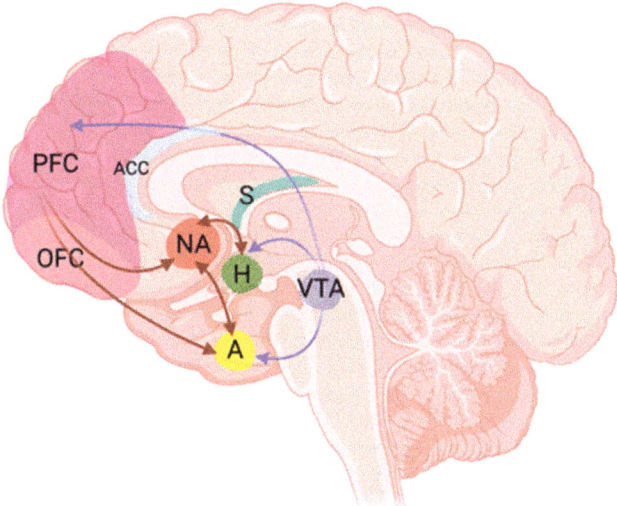

Figure 1. Limbic and reward pathways involved in eating behaviour and appetite. Eating behavior is closely associated with activity of the reward circuitry of the brain, which involves a group of neuronal structures that become activated and release dopamine when exposed to rewarding stimuli like food [27]. The pathway most associated with reward circuitry of the brain is referred to as the mesolimbic dopamine pathway, which starts with production and release of dopamine in the ventral tegmental area (VTA). The mesolimbic dopamine pathway then relays VTA signaling to the nucleus accumbens (NA), an area associated with motivation. The other aspect of the reward system is known as the mesocortical pathway which connects the VTA to the prefrontal cortex (PFC). This region also includes the orbitofrontal cortex (OFC), a key area involved in cognitive processes, such as decision making and memory. The PFC additionally forms connections with sensory and limbic pathways as well. Importantly, the reward pathway is activated, both before and after receipt of a reward suggesting that dopamine increases reward seeking behavior. Thus, any disruption of these pathways could potentially lead to disordered eating behavior. The VTA is also functionally and anatomically connected to the hypothalamus (H), primarily the lateral hypothalamus. The hypothalamus integrates homeostatic signals from various peripheral organs along with reward responses to modulate food intake and energy expenditure according to changes in metabolic state [28]. The arcuate nucleus of the hypothalamus (not shown), where neuropeptide Y (orexigenic) and proopiomelanocortin (anorexigenic) producing neurons reside, is the main area responsible for energy sensing and eating behavior. VTA, ventral tegmental area; NA, nucleus accumbens; H, hypothalamus; PFC, prefrontal cortex; OFC, orbitofrontal cortex; A, amygdala; ACC, anterior cingulate gyrus; S, striatum.

Given the high metabolic comorbidity observed in psychosis spectrum disorders, elucidating the psychopathological and neurobiological mechanisms underlying disrupted eating behaviours is crucial in helping to improve both the physical and psychological well-being of patients. In this scoping review, we aim to provide a comprehensive overview of disordered eating behaviours observed in psychosis spectrum disorders. We synthesize evidence from clinical studies employing self-report questionnaires and surveys to measure changes in food intake, craving and appetite, as well as behavioural neuroimaging studies to further explore the neurobiological mechanisms underlying these disturbances in eating patterns. In an attempt to distinguish illness intrinsic effects from those caused by treatment with APs, we present separately, when possible, results from studies examining

AP-naïve patients (vs. matched healthy controls), and healthy controls (HCs) or AP-naïve patients beginning APs.

2. Methods

Our protocol was developed using the scoping review methodological framework proposed by the Joanna Briggs Institute [29]. The objectives, inclusion criteria and methods for this scoping review were specified in advance and documented in a protocol.

2.1. Search Strategy

An a priori search strategy was developed and tested in consultation with the Education and Liaison Librarian for the Institute of Medical Science at the University of Toronto. Databases searched included Ovid MEDLINE, Ovid EMBASE, Ovid PsychINFO, EBSCO's CINAHL, CENTRAL on Wiley and Scopus. A grey literature search was also performed by mining references from relevant articles and review papers identified in the search, as well as searching SCOPUS for conference proceedings. Vocabulary and syntax were adjusted across databases. There were no language, date or methodology restrictions, with the exception of case studies and opinion pieces, which were excluded from the results. The specific search string for each database can be found in Supplementary Table S1.

2.2. Source of Evidence Screening and Study Selection

Article screening, including automatic duplicate removal, was completed using Covidence [30]. Two authors independently screened and assessed titles and abstracts (NS and AG), while another two independently completed the full-text screening (ES and RA). Conflicts were resolved by discussion and consensus between the authors and in consultation with the senior authors (SMA and MH). At all stages, screening decisions were made according to prespecified inclusion and exclusion criteria which are outlined in Table 1.

Table 1. List of inclusion and exclusion criteria for selected studies.

Inclusion Criteria	Exclusion Criteria

1. Schizophrenia or other Schizophrenia Spectrum Disorders
   a. First episode patients (FEP)
   b. Chronic
   c. AP-naïve
2. Psychosis, psychotic disorders
3. Bipolar disorder
4. Eating disorders
   a. Bulimia nervosa
   b. Binge eating disorder
   c. Night eating syndrome
5. Food addiction
6. Behavioral studies
   a. Neuroimaging
   b. Questionnaires
7. Antipsychotics
   a. First Generation Antipsychotics (FGA)/typical
   b. Second Generation Antipsychotics (SGA)/atypical
	1. Any psychiatric diagnosis not listed in the inclusion criteria (e.g., major depression disorder, anxiety disorders) included as the primary population of interest
	2. Off-label AP use
	3. Opinion pieces, letters
	4. Treatment studies of APs for Anorexia Nervosa
	5. At-risk/subclinical psychosis/psychotic-like experiences included as primary population of interest
	6. Purely physiological studies (i.e., no behavioural/appetite measures)
	7. Pre-clinical studies (mice/rodent, other non-human animals)

2.3. Charting the Data

A data extraction template was created and piloted among study authors (NS, ES, RA) and was refined and finalized based on data extracted from a sample of studies. The information displayed in Table 2 was extracted from each included full-text article.

Table 2. List of information extracted from each full-text article meeting inclusion criteria.

	Extracted Data
1.	Author(s)
2.	Year of publication
3.	Origin/country or ethnicity of participants
4.	Aims/purpose
5.	Type of study
6.	Population and sample size within the source of evidence (if applicable)
7.	Population demographics (Sex/gender, age)
8.	Methodology/methods
9.	Intervention type, comparator and details of these (e.g., duration of the intervention) (if applicable). Duration of the intervention (if applicable)
10.	Outcomes and details of these (e.g., how measured) (if applicable)
11.	Key findings that relate to the scoping review question/s and concepts

2.4. Synthesis and Presentation of Results

Studies were summarized and presented according to their relevant category: (1) Studies describing eating patterns, food preferences and diet composition using dietary recall, food diaries and food frequency questionnaires; (2) studies measuring self-reported appetite, hunger and/or satiety using a mix of validated questionnaires and semi-structured interviews (see Table 3); and (3) studies using neuroimaging methodologies to assess neurobiological changes in relation to aspects of eating or food intake. A narrative summary of each study is reported in its respective subsection, with overlap in other subsections if applicable. Where appropriate, tables were created to concisely summarize characteristics of included studies and relevant findings (see Tables 4–6).

3. Results

3.1. Search Results

Our initial search revealed 3545 results, which was reduced to 2654 after removal of duplicates. Following title and abstract screening, 94 studies were assessed for full-text eligibility. A total of 35 studies that considered dietary composition, food preference and cravings and/or eating patterns in patients with SCZ or HCs exposed to APs were deemed eligible and included in our qualitative synthesis (Figure 2; preferred reporting items for systematic reviews and meta-analyses (PRISMA) flow diagram).

The studies identified in our search used a number of validated methodologies and questionnaires to examine different aspects of eating behavior. The most commonly employed subjective dietary assessments include food diaries, 24-h dietary recall, the Three Factor Eating Questionnaire (TFEQ), the Dutch Eating Behavior Questionnaire (DEBQ), visual analog scales (VAS), the Food Craving Inventory (FCI), the Food Craving Questionnaire (FCQ) and the Food Frequency Questionnaire (FFQ). The TFEQ addresses three aspects of eating behaviour including restriction of food intake, loss of control of food intake and responsivity to internal hunger cues. Previous studies in the general population indicate that increased body weight is positively associated with TFEQ scores [31–33], particularly disinhibition and susceptibility to hunger [34–36]. The DEBQ is a self-report questionnaire designed to assess different factors regulating eating behaviour including desire to restrict food intake, tendency to eat in response to emotions and responsivity to external cues. Overweight and obese individuals generally display greater scores in all DEBQ domains compared to normal weight individuals [37–39], with the most robust relationship found for the emotional eating factor [37,39,40]. General hunger and appetite rating scales (VAS, and Likert scales) are also frequently employed to assess eating behaviour [41], while the FCQ and FCI are used to measure general and specific food cravings, respectively. A more detailed description of these questionnaires can be found in Table 3.

Table 3. Description of self-report questionnaires used to measure subjective appetite and eating behaviour; 'Original Source' indicates the authors who originally developed the questionnaire.

Name	Original Source	Description	Subscales and Other Relevant Information
Three-Factor Eating Questionnaire (TFEQ)	Stunkard and Messick, 1985 [42]	51-item questionnaire measuring three aspects of eating behaviour (cognitive restraint, disinhibition, hunger)	• Cognitive dietary restraint: active attempt to restrict caloric intake and control body weight • Disinhibition: likelihood of overeating when exposed to a favorable environment (e.g., palatable food) or stress • Susceptibility to hunger: susceptibility of individuals to perceive hunger and ingest food as a result; can be triggered by internal and external stimuli • High disinhibition and hunger scores associated with increased weight, obesity [34,35] and overconsumption/binge-eating (DSM-IV/DSM 5 criteria) [43,44])
Dutch Eating Behaviour Questionnaire (DEBQ)	Van Strien et al., 1986 [40]	33-item questionnaire measuring three factors that regulate eating behaviour (restraint, emotion, external factors)	• Restrained eating: the desire or intention to restrict food intake; correlated with TFEQ cognitive restraint • Emotional eating: the tendency to eat in response to negative emotions; associated with overconsumption and obesity; positively correlated with TFEQ disinhibition [35,38,45] • External eating: the tendency to eat in response to environmental triggers and food cues; differs between overweight and normal weight individuals but does not appear to be predictive of weight gain [37,39,45]
Visual Analog Scale (VAS)	Stubbs et al., 2000 (review) [46]	Psychometric tool used to quantify subjective appetite	• The most common method used in appetite research includes a horizontal (100-mm) line anchored by two extremes such as "not at all hungry/as hungry as I've ever felt" • Sensitive to experimental manipulations (e.g., dietary composition, levels of food intake, medication effects) • Best used in conjunction with more objective measures such as calorie intake or physiological changes
Food Craving Questionnaire (FCQ)	Cepeda-Benito et al., 2000 [47]	Questionnaire measuring general food cravings (trait and state version)	• FCQ-Trait (FCQ-T): 9 factors measuring general food cravings and tendencies • FCQ-State (FCQ-S): 5 factors measuring food cravings in response to situational factors • Higher cravings are associated with binge eating and overconsumption • FCQ scores are positively correlated with TFEQ disinhibition and hunger scores

Table 3. *Cont.*

Name	Original Source	Description	Subscales and Other Relevant Information
Food Craving Inventory (FCI)	White et al., 2002 [48]	Questionnaire measuring specific food cravings (carbohydrates, sweets, fats, fast-food fats)	• Considers both intensity and frequency of food cravings, where craving is defined as "an intense desire to consume a particular food (or food type) that is difficult to resist" • Fat craving associated with increased BMI • Positively correlated with TFEQ disinhibition and hunger scores (stronger effect for hunger)
Drug-Related Eating Behavior Questionnaire (DR-EBQ)	Lim et al., 2008 [49]	14-item questionnaire that quantifies changes in appetite, craving and eating behaviour after beginning antipsychotic treatment	• Statements cover feelings of hunger, pre-occupations with food, desire to eat, control of eating and food cravings [50] • For each statement, patients indicate whether the frequency of behaviour/cravings have increased since starting AP therapy using a Likert scale
Questionnaire on Eating and Weight Patterns (QEWP)	Spitzer et al., 1993 [51]	Questionnaire used to evaluate the presence of binge-eating symptomatology and binge-eating related disorders	• Developed using DSM-IV criteria for BED/BN and validated using clinical assessments • Can be used to diagnose BED and BN (purging or non-purging type) • Statements cover social impairment, body image, history of dieting, comorbidities (e.g., depression, alcohol/drug abuse, sexual abuse), compensatory behaviours
Mizes Anorectic Cognitions Questionnaire—Revised (MAC-R)	Mizes et al., 2000 [52]	24-item questionnaire used to assess eating disorder-related cognitions (anorexia nervosa, bulimia nervosa, binge eating disorder)	• Covers three aspects: weight regulation, approval and self-control; statements rated on a 5-point Likert scale (higher scores represent greater dysfunction)

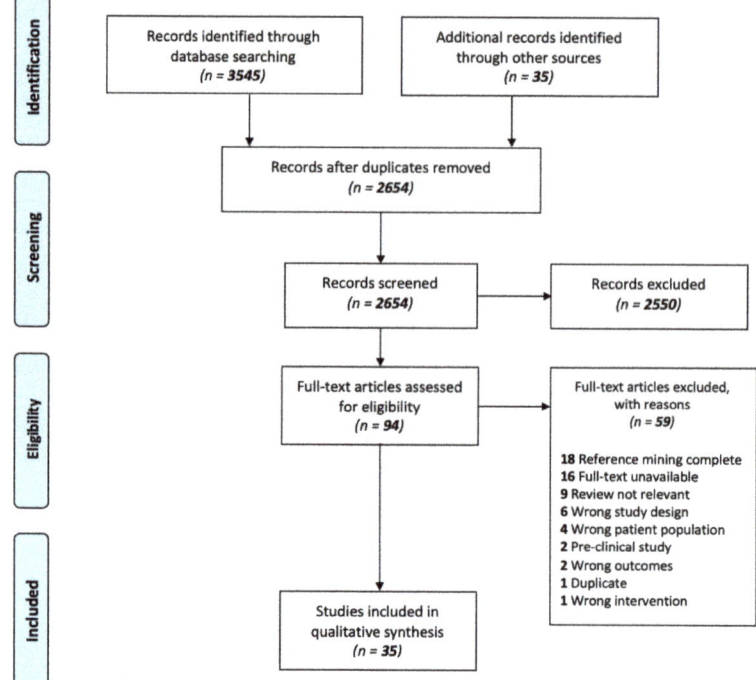

Figure 2. Preferred reporting items for systematic reviews and meta-analyses (PRISMA) flowchart. Literature search and selection process of included studies.

Our search yielded 9 studies that described dietary composition (summarized in Section 1 below); 19 studies that looked at eating patterns and food-related cognitions (summarized in Section 2 below); and 7 studies that used neuroimaging methodologies (summarized in Section 3 below). In order to facilitate elucidation of the specific effects of illness vs. APs, we have divided the results within each of the three methodology-based sections into three subsections based on population type: Patients only, patients (specifying AP-naïve cohorts) vs. controls and HCs exposed to APs.

3.2. Findings from Subjective Food Preference and Dietary Composition Studies

We retrieved nine studies that measured dietary composition and food preference using 24-h dietary recall, food diaries and the Food Frequency Questionnaire (FFQ) [53]. Only two studies indicated that part of the patient population studied were AP-naïve, although no subgroup analyses for these patients were available [54]. Table 4 summarizes the characteristics of included studies in this section, along with main findings.

Table 4. Characteristics of studies reporting on dietary composition.

Study	Design/Aim	Sample (Size, Diagnosis), Mean Age (Years), Mean BMI (kg/m²)	Sex (% F), Race/Ethnicity (%)	Illness Duration/Previous AP Exposure	Assessments	Main Significant Results
Amani 2007 [55]	Cross-sectional (case-control) Dietary preference in patients with SCZ compared to HC	30 SCZ inpatients, 16–76 years Age: 32.3 (M), 32.5 (F) BMI: 22 (M), 26 (F) 30 HCs (matched for age, sex) Age: 35.6 (M), 36.6 (F) BMI: 25.6 (M), 25.4 (F)	SCZ: 37% F HC: 47% F	Illness duration: at least one year; previous AP exposure not stated	Dietary recall (FFQ) Food Guide Pyramid to calculate dietary scores	Females: • Dietary scores ↓ and percent body fat ↑ for patients than HCs. • Consumed ↑ carbonated drinks, but ↓ milk, vegetables and nuts daily than the HCs Males: • Patients ate ↑ hydrogenated fats and full-fat cream, but ↓ red meats, vegetable oils and nuts servings per day than HCs • Male patients ate ↑ vegetables, eggs, cream and chocolate than female patients
Eder 2001 [56]	Longitudinal (8 weeks) Association of olanzapine induced weight gain with an increase in body fat	10 SCZ in patients treated with OLA monotherapy Dose range: 7.5–20 mg/d Age: 30.4 BMI: 22.4 10 HCs (matched for age, sex) Age: 35.2 BMI: 22.1	SCZ: 20% F HC: 20% F	No APs prior to OLA: 5 Previous APs: 5 (flupentixol, fluphenazine, risperidone, or haloperidol)	Semi-standardized structured interview to assess changes in eating behaviour and physical activity	• 70% of patients reported they ingested a significantly greater amount of food than usual during a period of time throughout the study • No change in physical activity
Fountaine 2010 [53]	Randomized, placebo controlled, two treatment crossover study (15 + 15 days, 12-day washout between arms) Comparing food intake and energy expenditure following olanzapine vs. placebo in healthy men	30 male HCs (21 completers) Age: 27 (range: 18–49) BMI: 22.6	All Males	N/A	Food intake monitored and weighed REE, daily activity level	• Mean total food intake in OLA group ↑ 18% (from 3860 kcal to 4230 kcal) relative to PBO • Mean weight change with OLA: 4.1 kg • 43.9% of patients experienced clinically significant weight gain (≥7%) • Early significant weight gain after 2 months of therapy occurred in 23.4% of the patients • ↑REE and respiratory quotient with OLA compared to PBO

185

Table 4. Cont.

Study	Design/Aim	Sample (Size, Diagnosis), Mean Age (Years), Mean BMI (kg/m^2)	Sex (% F), Race/Ethnicity (%)	Illness Duration/Previous AP Exposure	Assessments	Main Significant Results
Gattere 2018 [57]	Cross-sectional Dietary intake in early psychosis	124 early psychotic disorder (PD), 82 (66.1%) FEP patients with <5 years from illness onset Schizophreniform: n = 22 Schizoaffective: n = 12 Psychotic disorder NOS: n = 70 Age: 24.7 BMI: 24.3 36 at-risk mental state (ARMS) Age: 22.2 BMI: 22.2 62 HCs (not matched) Age: 23.5 BMI: 22.2	PD: 34.7% F; 76.6% Caucasian, 9.7% Latino American, 8.1% Arabian, 4.0% Gypsy, 0.8% Black, 0.8% Asian ARMS: 27.8% F; 88.9% Caucasian, 8.3% Latino American, 2.8 Arabian HC: 48.4% F; 95.2% Caucasian, 3.2% Latino America, 1.6% Arabian	PD: Monotherapy: 72 (58.1%) RIS = 31 PAL = 13 OLA = 17 QUE = 1 ARI = 10 Combination: 33 (26.6%) No APs: 19 (15.3%) ARMS: Monotherapy: 7 (19.4%) RIS = 1 OLA = 3 ARI = 3 Combination: 3 (8.3%) No APs: 27 (75%)	24-h dietary recall Food Craving (FCQ-State) IPAQ-short form	• Patients consumed ↑ calories/day and % of calories from saturated fatty acids than HCs • Patients consumed ↓ protein than HCs • Trend towards increased food craving scores (Food Craving Questionnaire; FCQ) with increasing psychopathology (psychotic disorders > at risk mental states > controls) • Both patient groups (PD and ARMS) reported reduced physical activity compared to HCs
Gothelf 2002 [54]	Longitudinal (4 weeks) Food intake and weight gain in adolescent males with SCZ treated with OLA vs. HAL	20 male SCZ inpatients OLA: n = 10 (MD: 14 mg/d) HAL: n = 10 (MD: 6.5 mg/d) Age (both): 17 BMI (OLA only): 24.5	All Males	OLA: mean washout period = 17.6 days Drug naïve = 1 Clomipramine = 1 AP other than OLA = 8	Dietary Evaluation (2-day monitoring of food intake by dietician; food weighed) Daily energy expenditure, REE, physical activity	• BMI ↑ greater for OLA than HAL • ↑ caloric intake (27.7%) in OLA group. • No changes in dietary composition (carbohydrates, fats, or proteins), REE or physical activity levels

Table 4. Cont.

Study	Design/Aim	Sample (Size, Diagnosis), Mean Age (Years), Mean BMI (kg/m²)	Sex (% F), Race/Ethnicity (%)	Illness Duration/Previous AP Exposure	Assessments	Main Significant Results
Nunes 2014 [58]	Cross-sectional (case-control) Evaluating nutritional status, food intake and cardiovascular disease risk in SCZ patients	25 SCZ outpatients Age: 40.5 (range: 18–59) BMI: 29.09 25 HCs (matched for age, sex, BMI) Age: 37.2 BMI: 26.91 Total sample Age: 38.9 BMI: 28.0	SCZ: 40% F HC: 48% F	SGA = 68% FGA = 28% Both = 4%	Dietary recall (FFQ)	• Patients consumed ↑ total calories, calories per kg body weight, protein per kg body weight, and % of carbohydrates and trans fatty acids • Patients consumed ↓ saturated fat, unsaturated fat and omega–6
Strassnig 2003 [59]	Cross-sectional (case-control) Exploring potential causes of weight gain in SCZ patients compared to general population (NHANES III)	146 outpatients with psychosis SCZ, paranoid type: n = 69 Schizoaffective: n = 53 Psychotic disorder NOS: n = 24 Age: 43 BMI: 32.7 Patient data compared to general population (NHANES III)	47% F 54% White, 46% Black	NR	24-h dietary recall	• Patients consumed ↑ total calories, fats and carbohydrates compared to general population (NHANES III). • Relative proportion of each food group (carbohydrates, fat, protein) did not differ between groups.
Stefanska 2017 [60]	Cross-sectional Eating habits and nutritional status in patients with SCZ and affective disorders	60 SCZ, 18–67 years Age: 34.1 (M), 41.3 (F) BMI: 27.6 (M), 27.2 (F) 61 recurrent depressive disorder, 18–67 years Age: 38.0 (M), 46.4 (F) BMI: 26.1 (M), 26.7 (F) 98 HCs (not matched), Age: 33.0 (M), 43.0 (F) (range: 18–69 years) BMI: 27.3 (M), 25.8 (F)	SCZ: 53.3% F Depression: 54.1% F HCs: 61.2% F	AP treatment (FGA or SGA) for at least one year (AP type not specified) Age at onset: 23.3 (M), 30.1 (F) Illness duration (years): 9.5 (M), 10.4 (F)	24-h dietary recall Resting metabolic rate (RMR)	• Patients consumed ↑ fat (with a predominance of saturated fatty acids over polyunsaturated fatty acids), and ↓ protein than HCs • Lower energy intake promoted lower BMI, waist circumference, waist-to-hip ratio and body fat • Female SCZ patients consumed ↑carbohydrates and % of energy from carbohydrates compared to female HCs • Male SCZ patients consumed ↑ fat, particularly saturated fatty acids compared to male HCsb

Table 4. Cont.

Study	Study Description					Main Significant Results
	Design/Aim	Sample (Size, Diagnosis), Mean Age (Years), Mean BMI (kg/m^2)	Sex (% F), Race/Ethnicity (%)	Illness Duration/Previous AP Exposure	Assessments	
Stefanska 2018 [61]	Cross-sectional (case-control) Assessing the nutritional value males consumed by patients with SCZ	85 SCZ outpatients, 18–65 years Age: 37.8 (M), 39.0 (F) BMI: 25.0 (M), 25.1 (F) 70 HCs (not matched) Age: 35.9 (M), 38.2 (F) BMI: 25.9 (M), 24.4 (F)	SCZ: 52.9% F HC: 57.1% F	AP treatment (FGA or SGA) for at least one year (AP type not specified) 1 AP = 39% 2 or 3 APs = 61% Age at onset: 26.7 (M), 273 (F) Illness duration (years): 10.0 (M), 12.3 (F)	24-h dietary recall	• ↑ snacking in patients than HCs • Female SCZ patients consumed ↑ calories and showed an ↑preference for sweets than HCs • Male SCZ patients had ↓ energy intake and content of the majority of assessed nutrients compared to HCs

Note: All main findings reported in this table are statistically significant unless otherwise indicated. SCZ = Schizophrenia, BP = Bipolar Disorder. HC = Healthy controls, FEP: First episode psychosis, AMI = amisulpride, PBO = Placebo, OLA = olanzapine, PAL = Paliperidone, HAL = Haloperidol, RIS = Risperidone, QUE = Quetiapine, ZIP = Ziprasidone, CPZ = Chlorpromazine, FGA = First generation antipsychotics, SGA = Second generation antipsychotic, NR = Not reported, TFEQ = Three-Factor Eating Questionnaire, FCQ = Food Craving Questionnaire, FCI = Food Craving Inventory, VAS = visual analog scale, DR-EBQ = Drug-Related Eating Behaviour Questionnaire, FFQ = Food Frequency Questionnaire, EBA = Eating Behaviour Assessment, DEBQ = Dutch Eating Behaviour Questionnaire, QEWP = Questionnaire on Eating and Weight Patterns, MD = Mean Dose.

3.2.1. Patients vs. Healthy Controls

Seven of the included dietary composition studies compared patients with healthy controls [55–61]; of these studies, only three matched patients to HCs according to key baseline features, such as age, sex and BMI [55,56,58].

Three cross-sectional studies [57–59] revealed that patients consumed significantly more total calories per day than HCs. However, results regarding specific dietary composition (carbohydrates, fat, protein) were less consistent, with the authors reporting either increased protein consumption and decreased saturated fat consumption by patients [58], decreased protein consumption and a trend towards increased saturated fat [57] or no difference between patients and controls [59]. Gattere et al. (2018) noted a trend towards increased scores on the FCQ with increasing psychopathology (psychotic disorders > at risk mental states > controls), suggestive of a relationship between food cravings and disease state, while Nunes et al. (2014) found no significant association between body mass index (BMI) and antipsychotic type (FGA, SGA).

The three remaining case-control studies also noted differences in nutritional patterns between patients and HCs, including increased fat consumption and more frequent snacking in patients [57,62]. Interestingly, these studies also stratified their results by sex, revealing differences in dietary composition and eating behaviour such as snack preference and calorie intake. Details of the differences between males and females are reported in Table 4. Beyond sex effects, Stefanska et al. (2017) also found that in the patient group, lower caloric intake was associated with lower BMI, waist circumference, waist-to-hip ratio and body fat content [60].

The final study included in this section explored eating behaviour differences between HCs and patients with SCZ on OLA treatment. This study revealed that that 70% of the OLA-treated patients reported ingesting a significantly greater amount of food than usual, with no compensatory increase in physical activity levels [56].

3.2.2. Patients Only

Only one dietary composition study explored the effects of APs on food intake and energy expenditure in patients [54]. The study was conducted in males only and compared patients treated with olanzapine to those treated with haloperidol. After four weeks, the olanzapine group experienced a significant increase in BMI and caloric intake, but no difference in dietary composition, energy expenditure or physical activity level. Important to note is that, similar to the aforementioned study by Eder et al. (2001) [56], physical activity levels were low [54], suggesting that olanzapine may lead to weight gain through a combination of increased caloric intake and decreased physical activity.

3.2.3. Healthy Controls Only

Consistent with the patient-only studies discussed above, an HC study conducted by Fountaine et al. revealed that volunteers randomized to receive olanzapine gained more weight and consumed significantly more calories than those randomized to placebo [53]. Interestingly, this weight gain was accompanied by an increase in resting energy expenditure and a trend towards increased physical activity in the olanzapine group, which the authors hypothesize may have occurred to compensate for the increase in caloric intake.

3.3. *Findings from Subjective/Self-Report Questionnaires on Appetite, Satiety and Craving*

In total, there were 19 studies [50,62–79] that examined differences in eating behaviour, subjective appetite and food craving using self-reported questionnaires and interviews. Table 5 presents a detailed summary of these studies. Seven studies specifically considered DSM-IV diagnostic and research criteria for eating disorders (EDs) including binge eating disorder (BED); Section 2.1) [62–68], while the remainder of the studies assessed subjective appetite and/or eating-related cognitions (Section 2.2) [50,69–74,76,77].

Table 5. Characteristics of studies reporting on subjective ratings of appetite, craving and hunger.

Study	Design/Aim	Sample (Size, Diagnosis), Mean Age (Years), Mean BMI (kg/m²)	Sex (% F), Race/Ethnicity	Mean Illness Duration/Previous AP Exposure (n)	Assessments	Main Significant Results
Bromel 1998 [63]	Longitudinal (10 weeks) Effect of CLZ on food craving in patients with SCZ	12 SCZ in patients treated with CLZ (MD: 273 mg/d; range: 81–475 mg/d) SCZ: n = 9 FGA: n = 3 Age: 31 (range: 18–65) BMI: 25.8	50% F	Nine patients treated with psychotropic medication (including APs) prior to starting CLZ (type/duration of previous exposure not specified)	Binge eating/ED symptomatology (DSM-IV) Binary appetite/craving scale	• CLZ treatment ↑ weight, BMI and adiposity • 75% (9/12) of patients reported ↑ appetite/hunger and specific food cravings • 17% (2/12) of patients reported onset of binge eating behaviour • One patient saw remittance and re-occurrence of binge eating after discontinuing and then restarting CLZ
Gebhardt 2007 [64]	Longitudinal (retrospective) Binge-eating symptomatology associated with CLZ and OLA use in patients with psychosis	64 patients being treated for psychotic symptoms with CLZ or OLA SCZ spectrum disorder: 12.3% Mood disorder: 18.5% Substance abuse: 7.7% Personality disorder: 3.1% Other diagnoses: 7.7% Age: 30.7 (range: 13.3–64.6)	47% F	Patients were treated with CLZ or OLA for at least 4 weeks prior to inclusion in study CLZ: n = 33 OLA: n = 31	QEWP (DSM-IV binge-eating) Adverse drug reaction (ADR) scale Appetite (4-point Likert-type scale)	• 69% of patients experienced an increase in appetite after starting CLZ/OLA, with a stronger effect for CLZ • Post-CLZ/OLA weight gain was associated with ↑ appetite • 14% of patients met DSM-IV criteria for BED or bulimia nervosa • ED onset was "definitely" or "probably" linked to CLZ/OLA exposure (Naranjo probability) • Post-CLZ/OLA EDs were more common in patients with a history of EDs
Kluge 2007 [65]	Randomized, double blind, parallel (6 weeks) Effect of CLZ and OLA on food craving and binge eating in patients with SCZ spectrum disorders	30 SCZ (n = 26), Schizoaffective (n = 3), Schizophreniform (n = 1) inpatients, 18–65 years CLZ: n = 15 OLA: n = 15 Age: 36.7 (CLZ), 32.8 (OLA) BMI: 25.4 (CLZ), 24.4 (OLA) Dosing (last 4 weeks of study): mean modal dose = 266.7 mg (CLZ), 21.2 mg (OLA)	CLZ: 53% F OLA: 67% F	Age of illness onset: 30 (CLZ), 28 (OLA)	Binge eating/ED symptomatology (DSM-IV) Binary appetite/craving scale	• CLZ/OLA treatment ↑ body weight and BMI • 97% (29/30) of patients reported ↑ appetite and 90% (27/30) reported ↑ food intake • Patients experienced ↑ binge eating and craving for sweet and fatty foods, with no significant effect of gender

Table 5. Cont.

Study	Design/Aim	Sample (Size, Diagnosis), Mean Age (Years), Mean BMI (kg/m^2)	Sex (% F), Race/Ethnicity	Mean Illness Duration/Previous AP Exposure (n)	Assessments	Main Significant Results
Theisen 2003 [66]	Cross-sectional (BE vs. non-BE) with an exploratory retrospective analysis Comparing binge eating symptomatology in patients with SCZ treated with clozapine and olanzapine	74 SCZ inpatients CLZ: n = 57 OLA: n = 17 Age: 19.8 (range: 15.6–26.6) Two sub-groups based on prevalence of binge eating behaviour Binge eating (BE): n = 37 Non-binge eating (non-BE): n = 37	36% F	Illness duration (years): 2.4 (range = 0.3–7.1)	QEWP (DSM-IV binge-eating)	• 26% (7/27) of females and 11% (5/47) of males met lifetime criteria for full BED or BN • In the BE group, 54% (20/37) of patients reported onset of binge eating episodes during the current CLZ/OLA regime • Patients in the BE group had ↑ current BMI and experienced ↑ weight gain from medication onset to time of study compared to those in the non-BE group
Treuer 2009 [67]	Longitudinal (6 months) Food intake and nutritional factors associated with weight gain in patients with SCZ and BD treated with OLA	622 SCZ or BD outpatients (589 completers) treated with OLA (MD: 11.4 mg/d; mean duration during study: 5.4 months) SCZ: 85% of sample BD: 15% of sample Age: 32.6 years BMI: 23.2	56% F Multinational (China, Romania, Mexico, Taiwan) 61% East Asian, 25% Caucasian, 14% Hispanic	Lifetime AP exposure: 74.5% of sample (duration not specified) Past 6 months: 45.2% of sample	Interview to assess appetite (5-point Likert), frequency of food consumption, subjective energy levels and physical activity	• 44% of patients experienced clinically significant weight gain (≥ 7%) • 49% of patients experienced ↑ appetite relative to baseline and 35% required more food to reach satiety • Weight gain was associated with ↑ frequency and quantity of food intake, ↑ preoccupation with food, and ↓ vigorous physical activity
Khazaal 2006a * [62]	Cross-sectional (case-control) Eating and weight related cognitions in patients with SCZ vs. HCs	40 SGA-treated SCZ outpatients Age: 33.8 40 HCs (matched for BMI) Age: 35.5 Two subgroups (n = 20) for each group: Overweight = BMI > 28 Comparison = BMI < 28	SCZ: 47.5% F HC: 52.5% F	Previous AP exposure (mean duration = 8.3 years): OLA, CLZ, QUE, RIS	Revised version of the Mizes Anorectic cognitive questionnaire (MAC-R)	• Patients had ↑ total MAC-R and weight regulation subscale scores relative to controls • Patients with BMI < 28 had ↑ MAC-R scores on all sub-scales compared to weight-matched controls • Females had ↑ MAC-R scores than men

Table 5. *Cont.*

Study	Design/Aim	Study Description				Main Significant Results
		Sample (Size, Diagnosis), Mean Age (Years), Mean BMI (kg/m²)	Sex (% F), Race/Ethnicity	Mean Illness Duration/Previous AP Exposure (n)	Assessments	
Khazaal 2006b * [68]	Cross-sectional (case-control) Binge eating symptomatology in overweight and obese patients with SCZ vs. HCs	40 SGA-treated SCZ outpatients Age: 33.8 40 HCs (matched for BMI) Age: 35.5 Two subgroups (n = 20) for each group: Overweight = BMI > 28 Comparison = BMI < 28	SCZ: 47.5% F HC: 52.5% F	NR	Binge eating/ED symptomatology (DSM-IV)	• ↑ prevalence of binge-eating symptoms and full BED in SCZ patients with BMI > 28 compared to weight-matched controls
Garriga 2019 [69]	Longitudinal (18 weeks) Effect of CLZ on food craving and consumption in patients with SMI	34 SMI patients SCZ: n = 27 Schizoaffective: n = 5 BD: n = 2 Age: 36.8 (range: 18–65) BMI: 27.3 Dosing: CLZ was initiated with a dose of 12.5–25 mg in the first day of treatment, followed by weekly upward adjustments of 25–50 mg (i.e., standard titration) Two subgroups: Normal weight (NW) = BMI < 25, n = 13 Overweight/obese (OWO) = BMI > 25, n = 21	38% F	Previous AP exposure (mean duration = 8.5 years): SGA = 28 (82.4%) FGA = 3 (8.8%) None = 3 (8.8%)	Food Craving (FCI, Spanish version) Cuestionario de Frecuencia de Consumo de Alimentos (CFCA)	• No significant longitudinal changes in food craving or consumption, however moderating effects of baseline BMI and gender were observed • In the NW group, ↑ cravings for "complex carbohydrates/proteins" and "simple sugar/trans fats" were associated with male gender and recent onset psychosis • NW males had ↑ craving for "fast-food fats" at both time points compared to NW females • In the OWO group, ↑ "fast-food fats" craving at Week 18 was associated with recent onset of psychosis • In both groups, craving scores (FCI) were positively correlated with frequency of consumption (CFCA)

Table 5. Cont.

Study	Design/Aim	Sample (Size, Diagnosis), Mean Age (Years), Mean BMI (kg/m^2)	Sex (% F), Race/Ethnicity	Mean Illness Duration/Previous AP Exposure (n)	Assessments	Main Significant Results
Karagianis 2009 [70]	Randomized, double blind, double dummy study (16 weeks) Effect of OLA on BMI, efficacy scores, weight and subjective appetite in patients with SMI	149 OLA-treated outpatients (115 completers) SCZ: n = 82 BD: n = 41 Schizoaffective: n = 15 Schizophreniform: n = 9 Other related disorder: n = 2 Age: 39 (range: 18-65) BMI: 28.1 Two treatment groups: Orally disintegrating OLA (ODO): n = 84 (MD: 13.87 mg/d) Standard OLA tablets (SOT): n = 65 (MD: 13.23 mg/d)	46% F 52.3% Caucasian, 33.6% Hispanic, 10.1% Black, 2.0% Asian, 1.3% First-nation, 0.7% Other	Previous AP exposure: 5-20 mg/day SOT (duration 4-52 weeks)	Hunger/appetite scale (VAS)	• Patients in both groups experienced ↑ BMI, • Patients in both groups experienced a non-significant trend towards ↓ hunger/appetite
Ryu 2013 [50]	Longitudinal (12 weeks) Effect of SGA treatment on eating behaviour in patients with SCZ	45 SCZ patients treated with SGA monotherapy OLA: n = 13 RIS: n = 24 ARI: n = 8 Age: 32.1 (range: 18-50)	50% F	Treated with current AP for 4-12 weeks (AP-free for 4 weeks prior to starting medication)	Binge eating/ED symptomatology (DSM-IV) Binary appetite/craving scale Food Craving (FCQ) DR-EBQ	• BMI ↑ over time • DR-EBQ total score was positively associated with weight gain and FCQ scores ("pre-occupation with food", "loss of control")
Smith 2012 [71]	Randomized trial (5 months) Effect of OLA and RIS on appetite in patients with chronic SCZ	46 SCZ inpatients OLA: n = 13 (MD: 25.2 mg/d) RIS: n = 17 (MD: 6.1 mg/d) Age: 41.2 (OLA), 42.5 (RIS)	2% F	All patients had been treated with multiple antipsychotics in the past	Hunger/appetite scale (VAS from 0-100) Eating Behavior Assessment (EBA)	• Neither medication had a significant effect on appetite, with a non-significant trend towards ↓ appetite • Both medications resulted in weight gain which was not correlated with changes in appetite (VAS) or eating behaviour (EBA)

Table 5. *Cont.*

Study	Design/Aim	Sample (Size, Diagnosis), Mean Age (Years), Mean BMI (kg/m²)	Sex (% F), Race/Ethnicity	Mean Illness Duration/Previous AP Exposure (n)	Assessments	Main Significant Results
Sentissi 2009 [72]	Cross-sectional (medication type) Effect of SGAs on eating behaviours and motivation in patients with SCZ	153 SCZ in- and outpatients SGA: $n = 93$ FGA: $n = 27$ Untreated: $n = 33$ Age: 33.1 (range: <50) BMI: 25.6 Among the untreated patients, 23 were AP-naïve, and 10 were AP-free for >3 months (mean duration: 7 months; range: 3–29 months)	38.6% F	SGA monotherapy: CLZ = 20 (MD: 374 mg/d) OLA = 23 (MD: 12 mg/d) AMI = 14 (MD: 571.4 mg/d) RIS = 20 (MD: 3.7 mg/d) ARI = 16 (MD: 11.9 mg/d) FGA: mainly HAL ($n = 16$, 59% of sample) or phenothiazines; MD = 289 mg/d (CPZ equivalents) Mean treatment duration (months): 36.2 (range = 3–86) Illness duration: 9.6 years	TFEQ DEBQ	• ↑ BMI was associated with ↑ TFEQ disinhibition (significant) and susceptibility to hunger (nearing significance) • SGA-treated patients displayed ↑ reactivity to external eating cues (DEBQ) compared to FGA-treated, but not untreated patients • Patients with both high restraint and high disinhibition were more likely to be overweight (significant) and to be treated with SGAs (nearing significance)

Table 5. Cont.

Study	Design/Aim	Sample (Size, Diagnosis), Mean Age (Years), Mean BMI (kg/m²)	Sex (% F), Race/Ethnicity	Mean Illness Duration/Previous AP Exposure (n)	Assessments	Main Significant Results
Abbas 2013 [73]	Cross-sectional (case-control) Food craving in OLA- or FGA-treated patients with SCZ vs. HCs	40 SCZ in- and outpatients OLA: n = 20 FGA: n = 20 Age (both): 39.4 (range: 18–65) BMI: 29.5 (OLA), 27.3 (FGA) 20 HCs (un-matched) Age: 40.9 BMI: 25.8	OLA: 45% F FGA: 55% F HC: 55% F	OLA (n = 20) or FGA (n = 20) for at least one month Flupentixol = 6 Zuclopenthixol acetate = 5 CPZ = 3 HAL = 2 Fluphenazine decanoate = 1 Pipotiazine palmitate = 1 Stelazine = 1 Trifluperazine = 1 Mean treatment duration (months): 15.1 (OLA), 19.7 (FGA)	Food Craving (FCI)	• No significant difference in food craving between patients and controls
Blouin 2008 [74]	Cross-sectional (case-control) Adiposity and post-meal challenge eating behaviours in SGA-treated patients with SCZ vs. HCs	18 SCZ outpatients Age: 30.5 (range: 18–65) BMI: 28.8 20 HCs (matched for age and physical activity) Age: 29.5 BMI: 25.0	All Males	Previous AP exposure: FGA or SGA (mean duration = 35.3 months) Current SGA treatment: at least 3 months (mean duration = 24.6 months) OLA = 9 QUE = 3 CLZ = 2 RIS = 2 ZIP = 2	TFEQ Hunger/Appetite Scale (150-mm VAS) Food preference test and spontaneous intake (food weighed) 12 h fast prior to standardized breakfast, followed by an ad libitum buffet-type meal ~3 h later	• Compared to HCs, patients reported ↑ subjective hunger and ↓ satiation following a standardized meal • Compared to HCs, patients displayed ↑ TFEQ scores in all three domains which remained significant after controlling for BMI • Among patients, susceptibility to hunger was positively associated with emotional susceptibility to disinhibition • No significant group differences in spontaneous intake or food preference during ad libitum conditions

195

Table 5. Cont.

Study	Study Description					
	Design/Aim	Sample (Size, Diagnosis, Mean Age (Years), Mean BMI (kg/m^2)	Sex (% F), Race/Ethnicity	Mean Illness Duration/Previous AP Exposure (n)	Assessments	Main Significant Results
Folley 2010 [75]	Cross-sectional (case-control) Relative food preferences and hedonic judgements in SGA-treated patients with SCZ vs. HCs	18 SCZ outpatients treated with SGAs (MD: 93.6 mg/d) Age: 40.5 (range: 21–58) 18 HCs (matched for education and intelligence scores) Age: 38.9 (range: 20–52)	SCZ: 33% F HC: 44% F	Illness duration: 16.4 years	Food preference and food ratings task (Extra scanner task, 5-point Likert scale); participants tested prior to eating lunch	• No significant group differences in response time or food preference during preference task • Both patients and controls were more likely to give positive vs. neutral or negative ratings to food stimuli • In patients, ↓ positive ratings were associated with ↑ anhedonia
Knolle-Veentjer 2008 [76]	Cross-sectional (case-control) Role of eating behaviour in body weight regulation in patients with SCZ vs. HCs	29 SCZ patients Paranoid subtype: n = 27 Disorganized subtype: n = 2 Age: 34 (range: 21–56) BMI: 26.8 23 HCs (matched for age, sex, educational level) Age: 32 (range: 20–58) BMI: 23.9	SCZ: 34.5% F HC: 26.1% F	QUE = 9 (MD: 600 mg/d) RIS = 8 (MD: 5.3 mg/d) OLA = 6 (MD: 15.83 mg/d) AMI = 4 (MD: 700 mg/d) ARI = 1 (MD: 20 mg/d) Flupentixol = 1 (MD: 10 mg/d)	FEV (German version of the TFEQ) Author-developed board game to assess delay of gratification using food reward Behavioral assessment of the dysexecutive syndrome (BADS)	• Patients had ↓ delay of gratification, ↓ executive functioning (BADS), and ↑ BMI compared to controls • In patients, ↑ FEV scores (disinhibition, restraint) were associated with ↓ executive functioning and ↑ BMI • No significant difference in subjective appetite between patients and controls
Schanze 2008 [77]	Cross-sectional Comparing eating behaviours in patients with SCZ and MDD vs. HCs	42 SCZ inpatients Age: 33.6 BMI: 27.28 83 MDD inpatients Age: 40.42 BMI: 26.01 46 HCs (un-matched) Age: 35.7 BMI: 23.51	SCZ: 40.5% F MDD: 47% F HC: 47.8% F	SCZ (last 4 weeks): QUE = 6 RIS = 5 ZIP = 4 OLA = 2 CLZ = 1 SSRI = 1 None = 23 MDD (last 4 weeks): QUE = 1 RIS = 1 SSRI = 15 Mirtazapine = 10 None = 56	TFEQ	• No significant group differences (patients vs. HCs, MDD vs. SCZ) for all TFEQ domains • No significant effect of medication class (antidepressant, antipsychotic, no medication) on TFEQ scores

Table 5. *Cont.*

Study	Study Description					Main Significant Results
	Design/Aim	Sample (Size, Diagnosis), Mean Age (Years), Mean BMI (kg/m²)	Sex (% F), Race/Ethnicity	Mean Illness Duration/Previous AP Exposure (n)	Assessments	
Roerig 2005 [78]	Randomized, double blind, parallel (2 weeks) Effect of OLA and RIS vs. placebo on eating behaviours in HCs	48 HCs, 18–60 years OLA: n = 16 (MD: 8.75 mg/d) RIS: n = 16 (MD: 2.875 mg/d) PLA: n = 16 Age: 33.6 (OLA), 36.2 (RIS), 32.7 (PBO) BMI: 23.6 (OLA), 25.0 (RIS), 24.1 (PBO)	OLA: 87.5% F RIS: 75% F PBO: 68.75% F	N/A	Hunger/appetite scale (100-mm VAS) Feeding laboratory (standardized breakfast, liquid lunch, ad libitum dinner where food was weighed) Resting energy expenditure (REE)	• Participants in both AP groups gained weight, however only the OLA group reached statistical significance • In the OLA group, weight gain was associated with a non-significant ↑ in food intake (kcal/day) and appetite compared to RIS or PBO • None of the groups (OLA, RIS, PBO) showed a significant change in REE
Teff 2015 [79]	Randomized trial (12 days; 9 days of SGA exposure) Effect of acute SGA exposure on hunger and food intake in HCs	30 HCs OLA: n = 10 RIS: n = 10 PBO: n = 10 Age: 26.1 (OLA), 25.9 (ARI), 29.9 (PBO) BMI: 22.1 (OLA), 22.4 (ARI), 21.8 (PBO) reported in [80]	30% F	N/A	Hunger/appetite scale (9-point Likert) Food intake weighed (objective) Activity level (number of steps)	• Neither medication had a significant effect on weight, subjective hunger/fullness or calorie intake compared to PBO • No significant change in physical activity levels in any group

Note: All main findings reported in this table are statistically significant unless otherwise indicated. SCZ = Schizophrenia, BD = Bipolar Disorder, MDD = Major Depressive Disorder, SMI = Severe Mental Illness, HCs = Healthy Controls, FEP = First Episode Psychosis, AMI = amisulpride, OLA = olanzapine, HAL = Haloperidol, RIS = Risperidone, QUE = Quetiapine, ZIP = Ziprasidone, CPZ = Chlorpromazine, PBO = Placebo, FGA = First generation antipsychotics, SGA = Second generation antipsychotic, NR = Not reported, TFEQ = Three-Factor Eating Questionnaire, FCQ = Food Craving Questionnaire, FCI = Food Craving Inventory, VAS = visual analog scale, DR-EBQ = Drug-Related Eating Behaviour Questionnaire, FFQ = Food Frequency Questionnaire, EBA = Eating Behaviour Assessment, DEBQ = Dutch Eating Behaviour Questionnaire, QEWP = Questionnaire on Eating and Weight Patterns, MD = Mean Dose, * = studies from the same cohort (Khazaal 2006a, 2006b).

3.3.1. Binge Eating and Other Eating Disorder-Related Behaviours

Seven studies [62–68] explored the occurrence of binge-eating symptomatology in patients being treated with SGAs. In all cases, binge eating symptomatology was determined based on DSM-IV research criteria for BED unless otherwise specified.

3.3.2. Patients Only

Consistent with the dietary composition studies discussed above, all five patient studies [63–67] found that treatment with clozapine or olanzapine increased appetite, food intake, food craving and/or risk of weight gain in non-FEP patients. Interestingly, the studies further suggest that these changes may be related to AP-mediated induction of binge eating. For example, one study [63] found that 17% of patients reported episodes of binge eating after starting clozapine, with one patient seeing remittance and re-occurrence of binge eating after discontinuing and then restarting treatment. In another study, the authors found that half of all included clozapine- and olanzapine-treated patients screened positively for binge eating behaviour (BE group), with over half reporting *onset* of episodes of binge eating during the current medication regime [66]. A similar retrospective clozapine/olanzapine study [64], found that 14% of patients met DSM-IV diagnostic criteria for an ED, specifically eating disorders not otherwise specified (including BED) or bulimia nervosa. Subsequent comparison of scores from the Questionnaire on Eating and Weight Patterns QEWP [51] and adverse drug reaction (ADR) scale [81] revealed that ED onset was "definitely" or "probably" linked to AP exposure. Prospective studies also appear to support a relationship between clozapine/olanzapine treatment and binge eating, with one showing a significant increase in binge eating episodes from baseline to endpoint [65], and another identifying a positive correlation between olanzapine-induced appetite increases and behaviours similar to DSM-IV BED criteria such as "preoccupation with food" and "eating until uncomfortably full" [67].

3.3.3. Patients vs. Controls

Similar to the findings mentioned above, two case-control studies conducted by Khazaal et al. found evidence of a link between psychosis and disordered eating. In their first study [62], the authors observed altered self-esteem and self-control, greater fear of weight gain, and a greater desire to control weight in patients with SCZ compared to controls as determined by a revised version of the Mizes Anorectic Cognitive Questionnaire (MAC-R). They also found that females had higher MAC-R scores than men, suggestive of sex and/or gender effects. In the second study [68], they found a significantly higher prevalence of DSM-IV binge eating symptoms and BED in overweight/obese patients with SCZ compared to weight-matched controls.

3.4. Subjective Appetite, Hunger and Satiety

Our search identified 12 studies [50,69–74,76,77] that used self-report measures including visual analog scales (VAS), the TFEQ and the DEBQ to measure subjective appetite/hunger and eating-related cognitions.

3.4.1. Patients Only

Conclusions from longitudinal studies regarding the effects of AP medications (particularly SGAs) on appetite were mixed. For example, two studies, one in which patients were randomized to receive olanzapine or risperidone [71], and another where patients were randomized to either disintegrating or standard olanzapine tablets [70] found no significant effect of AP treatment on appetite (Eating Behaviour Assessment and VAS) with a non-significant trend towards decreased appetite. In contrast, two different studies found significant weight-related changes in eating behaviour following AP exposure. In particular, Ryu et al. found that SGA treatment increased weight as well as subjective hunger, appetite and food craving (Drug-Related Eating Behaviour Questionnaire; DR-EBQ) [50].

On the other hand, despite failing to report overall longitudinal changes, Garriga et al. (2019) observed interesting moderating effects of baseline BMI, stage of illness and sex in clozapine-treated patients [69] (see Table 5). The authors also found a significant positive correlation between specific food cravings (FCI) and subsequent consumption (Cuestionario de Frecuencia de Consumo de Alimentos; CFCA), suggesting that psychological desire may translate into behavioural changes.

In the only cross-sectional study identified, Sentissi et al. compared eating behaviour between AP-naïve or AP-free, FGA-treated and SGA-treated patients with SCZ [72]. They found that BMI status was positively associated with TFEQ disinhibition (significant) and hunger (nearing significance) scores. Furthermore, SGA-treated patients showed greater reactivity to external eating cues (DEBQ) than the FGA-treated, but not the untreated patients.

3.4.2. Patients vs. Healthy Controls

All five studies comparing patients and controls were cross-sectional studies. Generally, there were mixed results regarding group differences in appetite/satiety, which highlights a need for longitudinal studies in this area.

In one study, although patients experienced increased hunger (VAS) and decreased satiation compared to HCs following a standardized meal [74], the groups did not differ in spontaneous intake and food preference during a buffet-type meal three hours later. The authors also found that patients had increased TFEQ scores in all three domains (cognitive restraint, disinhibition, susceptibility to hunger), a finding that remained significant after controlling for BMI. A separate study exploring executive functioning (which is known to be impaired in SCZ), found that patients displayed significantly worse delay of gratification and executive functioning than HCs in a task involving food reinforcement [76]. These impairments were associated with increased restrained eating behaviour and disinhibition, as well as increased BMI, suggesting that disease-related dysfunction in the dorsolateral prefrontal cortex (DLPFC) and dorsal anterior cingulate cortex (ACC) (prefrontal-ACC network) may increase susceptibility to overeating, thereby promoting weight gain.

In contrast to the studies discussed above, Schanze et al. (2008) found no group differences between patients with SCZ, patients with major depressive disorder, and HCs in any of the TFEQ domains [77]. Furthermore, they observed no effect of medication class (AP, antidepressant, no medication) on TFEQ scores [77]. Similarly, Abbas et al. (2013) found no significant difference in food craving (FCI) between AP-treated patients with SCZ and HCs [73]. Finally, Folley et al. (2010) found that patients and HCs did not differ in their response time or food preference when asked to choose between two food images [75]. Interestingly, although patients generally gave higher positive ratings to food stimuli than HCs, instances when they gave lower ratings were correlated with increased anhedonia. This led the authors to suggest that while preference judgements appear to be intact in patients, the hedonic value they place on food may be altered.

3.4.3. Controls Only

Our search retrieved two randomized, double-blind, placebo-controlled studies in HCs examining subjective appetite/hunger following short-term SGA exposure. In the first study, Roerig et al. (2005) found that two weeks of either olanzapine or risperidone exposure led to weight gain compared to placebo, although only olanzapine reached statistical significance [78]. The authors also observed a trend towards both greater food intake (kcal/day) and an increase in appetite (measured using a 100 mm VAS) in the olanzapine group relative to the other groups. In contrast, Teff et al. (2015) observed no significant change in weight, subjective hunger/fullness or calorie intake following nine days of SGA exposure [79]. Importantly, in contrast to the aforementioned HC study by Fountaine (2010), neither study reported significant changes in physical activity or energy expenditure in association with AP treatment.

3.5. Findings from Neuroimaging and Brain Structure Studies

Our search yielded seven studies that used neuroimaging methodologies to study food preference and eating behavior in patients with SCZ. The characteristics of these studies and a summary of their main findings can be found in Table 6. Six studies used functional magnetic resonance imaging (fMRI) along with visual analog scales (VAS) and/or eating questionnaires [82–87] and one study used structural MRI to study brain morphology [88]. One study was conducted on AP-naïve ($n = 22$) patients [88], and one was conducted on patients who were AP-naïve ($n = 9$) or had been medication free for at least six weeks ($n = 20$) [86] (Section 3.2).

3.5.1. Patients Only

A study by Stip (2015) and colleagues compared brain activity (fMRI) in response to videos of food in patients with SCZ before and after initiating or switching to olanzapine therapy [84]. The authors found that 16 weeks of olanzapine exposure led to significantly decreased neuronal activation in the salience network (SN), an important network involved in reward processing and reward anticipation. Specific regions affected by olanzapine included the anterior fronto-insular (aFI) cortex, amygdala, thalamus and anterior cingulate cortex (ACC). The decrease in SN activation was associated with a decrease in dietary restraint (TFEQ), leading the authors to suggest that AP-mediated disruptions of the SN may promote changes in eating behaviour.

3.5.2. Patients vs. Healthy Controls

In an earlier publication (conducted in the same cohort as the 2015 study [84], but including a HC comparator), Stip et al. (2012) used static food images and examined subjective appetite (VAS) and TFEQ scores in patients with SCZ before and after starting olanzapine [85]. Using fMRI, they found that 16 weeks of olanzapine treatment led to a significant increase in activation in the supplementary motor area, right fusiform gyrus, insular cortex, amygdala and parahippocampal regions in response to static food images. Comparing these changes in activation to controls, it was found that neural activity in the premotor area, somatosensory cortices and bilaterally in the fusiform gyri of patients with SCZ was normalized, while activity in the insular cortices, amygdala and cerebellum was 'overshot'. Interestingly, this hyperactivation was positively correlated with disinhibition (TFEQ), suggestive of an association between OLA-induced increases in brain activity and dysfunctional processing of food-related stimuli.

An earlier study, using the same patient cohort (but pre-switch to olanzapine) as the two aforementioned studies by Stip and colleagues [84,85], similarly assessed brain activity (fMRI) in response to food cues [83]. Relative to HCs, patients with SCZ showed increased activation in brain regions involved in action planning and regulation of homeostatic signals including the red thalamic nucleus, left parahippocampal gyrus and left middle frontal gyrus. Furthermore, the authors found that activity in the red thalamic nucleus was positively correlated with cognitive restraint (TFEQ Factor 1), while activity in the left middle frontal gyrus was associated with increased disinhibition (TFEQ Factor 2). This led them to suggest that cortical processes may disrupt or override sub-cortical hypothalamic appetite regulation signals in patients with SCZ. Additional correlational analyses controlling for either AP dose (chlorpromazine CPZ equivalents) or disease severity (Positive and Negative Syndrome Scale; PANSS) revealed a significant positive correlation between AP dose and susceptibility to hunger (TFEQ Factor 3) and a significant negative correlation between PANSS score and cognitive restraint. This led to the conclusion that both SCZ and AP medications may contribute to appetite dysregulation in patients, but through different mechanisms.

Table 6. Characteristics of studies with neuroimaging methodologies.

Study	Design/Aim	Sample (Size, Diagnosis), Mean Age (Years), Mean BMI	Sex (% F), Race/Ethnicity	Mean Illness Duration/Previous AP Exposure (n)	Assessments	Main Significant Results
Stip 2015 * [84]	Longitudinal (16 week) study, pre- post with OLA administration	15 SCZ patients not previously exposed to OLA switching to OLA	NR	NR	fMRI (BOLD) during neutral vs. dynamic appetitive stimuli; Hunger/appetite scale (VAS from 0–5); TFEQ	• ↓ Activation of SN (including ACC, aFI, and amygdala) in response to dynamic appetitive stimuli • ↓ ACC and aFI activity were associated with ↑ ghrelin levels and ↓ dietary restraint (TFEQ)
	Examining the salience network in SCZ patients on OLA treatment	Same cohort as 2012 study (authors did not specify switchers vs. AP-naïve, fasted)				
Lungu 2013 * [83]	Cross sectional (case-control)	25 SCZ (20 completers) AP (OLA excluded): n = 21 AP-naïve: n = 3 Age: 34.5 BMI: 26.62	48% F SCZ: 24% F HC: 20% F	RIS = 12 QUE = 6 HAL = 2 CLZ = 1	fMRI (BOLD) during neutral vs. static appetitive stimuli; Hunger/appetite scale (VAS from 0–5); TFEQ	• Common neuronal networks activated in both groups (left insula, primary sensory motor areas, and inferior temporal and parietal cortices) • ↑ Responses to appetitive cues in areas of action planning and homeostatic signals (red thalamic nucleus, left parahippocampus, and left middle frontal gyrus) in SCZ group • PANSS positive symptom scores positively correlated with activity in left middle frontal gyrus (action planning) and TFEQ disinhibition scores • TFEQ restraint scores correlated positively with thalamic activity and negatively with disease severity (PANSS score) • TFEQ hunger scores correlated negatively with parahippocampal activity and positively with AP dose (CPZ equivalents)
	Neuronal correlates of appetite regulation in patients with SCZ vs. HC (3 h since last meal)	11 HCs (10 included) Age: 35.2 BMI: 25.07		Perphenazine = 1 No medication = 3		
Stip 2012 * [85]	Longitudinal intervention (16 weeks) vs. HCs	24 SCZ patients not previously exposed to OLA (15 completers) Switch (no washout): n = 19 AP-naïve: n = 3 Age: 30.04	SCZ: 21% F; 91.66% Caucasians, 8.33% Caribbean	RIS = 12 QUE = 6 HAL = 2 CLZ = 1	fMRI (BOLD) during neutral vs. static appetitive stimuli; Hunger/appetite scale (VAS from 0–5); TFEQ	• OLA treatment ↑ weight gain significantly • OLA treatment ↑ BOLD signal in response to appetitive stimuli in supplementary motor area, right fusiform gyrus, insular cortex, amygdala and parahippocampus • OLA ↑ Neural activity in premotor area, somatosensory cortices and bilaterally in the fusiform gyri of patients to the same levels as HCs • Hyperactivation (vs. HC) in 4 regions (insular cortices, amygdala, and cerebellum) in response to appetitive stimuli • OLA-induced ↑ brain activity in response to appetitive stimuli was negatively correlated with TFEQ (dietary restraint) scores
	Evaluating neural changes associated with appetite in SCZ patients pre, and post OLA treatment vs. HCs (3 h since last meal)	10 HCs Age: 33.9 Same cohort as Lungu 2013	HC: 20% F; 100% Caucasian	Perphenazine = 1 No medication = 3		

Table 6. Cont.

Study	Design/Aim	Sample (Size, Diagnosis), Mean Age (Years), Mean BMI	Sex (% F), Race/Ethnicity	Mean Illness Duration/Previous AP Exposure (n)	Assessments	Main Significant Results
Grimm 2012 [82]	Cross sectional (case-control) Striatal activation during appetitive cues (fasting state)	23 fasted (6h) chronic SCZ in- and outpatients on stable AP medication (MD: 346 mg/d CPZ equivalents) Age: 30.3 23 fasted HCs (matched for age, gender, parental SES, handedness) Age: 28.9	74% F	No change in the medication dose >25% or a switch to a different medication was allowed in the last 4 weeks SGA: n = 22 RIS = 4 OLA = 3 CLZ = 4 AMI = 3 QUE = 3 ARI = 3 ZIP = 1 FGA: n = 1 Flupenthixol = 1 Illness duration: 4.1 years	fMRI (BOLD) during neutral vs. static appetitive stimuli Hunger/appetite scale (VAS)	• ↓ Activation in the dorsal striatal region in patients • Reduced activity remained significant after controlling for AP dose (CPZ equivalents) and body weight • Patients and controls were similar in appetite ratings evoked by presentation of neutral or appetite stimuli
Emsley 2015 [88]	Prospective (13 weeks of AP treatment vs. HC) Morphological changes in brain regions associated with food intake regulation, metabolic parameters (BMI, fasting glucose, lipids) (fasting not specified)	22 AP-naive FEP in- and outpatients randomized to receive RIS or flupenthixol decanoate long-acting injections (n not specified) SCZ: n = 13 Schizophreniform: n = 9 Age: 24.6 (range: 16–45) BMI: 22.1 23 untreated HCs (matched for age, sex, ethnicity, educational status) Age: 27	FEP: 14% F; 64% mixed descent, 36% Black HC: 35% F; 70% mixed descent, 30% Black	No previous AP exposure; mean duration of untreated psychosis: 41 weeks Mean endpoint dose: 31.66 mg 2-weekly (RIS), 13.07 mg 2-weekly (flupenthixol)	Structural MRI changes in prespecified brain regions associated with hedonic and homeostatic body weight regulation	• ↑ Baseline left vDC volumes in patients compared to HCs • Medicated FEP patients had ↓ vDC size (homeostatic), but no difference in prefrontal cortex (hedonic) size • This volume change was also associated with ↑ BMI, dyslipidemia and elevated glucose in patients • ↓ Volumes were not significant following post-hoc testing and were accompanied by ↑ volumes in control group

Table 6. Cont.

Study	Design/Aim	Sample (Size, Diagnosis), Mean Age (Years), Mean BMI	Sex (% F), Race/Ethnicity	Mean Illness Duration/Previous AP Exposure (n)	Assessments	Main Significant Results
Borgan 2019 [86]	Cross-sectional (case-control) Neural responsivity to food cues in unmedicated first episode psychosis (fasting state used)	29 fasted (>12 h), untreated FEP patients SCZ: n = 27 Schizoaffective: n = 2 Age: 26.1 (range: 18–65) BMI: 25.2 28 fasted HCs (matched for age) Age: 26.4 BMI: 24.7	17%, F FEP: 14% F; 12 White, 9 Black African or Black Caribbean, 6 Asian, 2 Mixed HC: 21% F; 10 White, 3 Black African or Black Caribbean, 11 Asian, 4 Mixed	Patients were AP-naïve or free from all psychotropic medication for at least 6 weeks Prior use = 20 AP-naïve = 9 Duration of prior treatment: 4.74 months Illness duration: 21.5 months	fMRI (BOLD signal) during neutral vs. static food cue (low and high calorie) IPAQ Dietary Instrument for Nutrition Education	• ↑BOLD response in HCs vs. patients in the right insula, right anterior, posterior, medial and inferior orbitofrontal gyrus to food cues • Comparing ROIs: ↑ Response to food cues in HCs in nucleus accumbens, but not in insula or hypothalamus • In HCs, BMI was inversely correlated with mean BOLD signal in nucleus accumbens in response to food cues • No group differences in neural responses to food cues between patients and HCs • ↑ Fat consumption in patients than HCs in neural response to food cues
Mathews 2012 [87]	Interventional (pre- post 1-week OLA administration) open-label prospective design Neural activity associated with anticipation and receipt of food rewards after 1 week of OLA (in fasting state)	19 fasted (overnight) HCs Age: 27.5 (range = 18–50) BMI: 25.78 Dosing: 5 mg of OLA on the first night and 10 mg on the subsequent 6 nights	47.4% F 73.7% White, 10.5% African American, 10.5% Hispanic, 5.3% Mixed	N/A	fMRI (BOLD) during appetitive visual stimuli, and in response to receipt of cued food or water control (chocolate milk, tomato juice) Consumption of "liquid breakfast" measured post scan Hunger/appetite scale (5-point Likert) TFEQ	• OLA ↑ Weight (1.1kg) • OLA ↑ activation in regions for anticipatory reward (inferior frontal cortex, striatum, ACC) in response to visual food cues; ↑ activation of reward receipt regions (caudate, putamen); and ↓ activation in regions of inhibitory control of feeding (lateral orbital frontal cortex) • OLA was associated with ↑ consumption of breakfast, and ↑ in disinhibited eating behavior (TFEQ)

Note: All main findings reported in this table are statistically significant unless otherwise indicated. SCZ = Schizophrenia, BP = Bipolar Disorder. HC = Healthy controls, FEP: First episode psychosis, AMI = amisulpride, OLA = olanzapine, HAL = Haloperidol, RIS = Risperidone, QUE = Quetiapine, ZIP = Ziprasidone, CPZ = Chlorpromazine, FGA = First generation antipsychotics, SGA = Second generation antipsychotic, NR = Not reported, TFEQ = Three-Factor Eating Questionnaire, FCQ = Food Craving Questionnaire, FCI = Food Craving Inventory, VAS = visual analog scale, DR-EBQ = Drug-Related Eating Behaviour Questionnaire, FFQ = Food Frequency Questionnaire, EBA = Eating Behaviour Assessment, DEBQ = Dutch Eating Behaviour Questionnaire, QEWP = Questionnaire on Eating and Weight Patterns; BOLD= blood oxygen level dependent response; ACC= anterior cingulate cortex, aFI= Anterior Fronto-insular, vDC= ventral Diencephalon, MD = Mean Dose; * = studies from the same cohort (Lungu 2013, Stip 2012, Stip 2015).

In a similar but independent fMRI study, Grimm et al. (2012) asked chronic patients with SCZ and HCs to rate their appetite levels on a VAS following presentation of neutral or appetitive stimuli [82]. Even after adjusting for body weight and AP dose (CPZ equivalents), patients were found to have significantly weaker activation in the dorsal striatal region (post appetitive stimulus vs. neutral images) compared to controls. In keeping with the findings by Stip et al. 2012 [84], these results led the authors to suggest that SCZ may involve intrinsic disruptions in the SN, leading to altered reward anticipation and eating behavior. However, despite these functional differences (and in contrast to some of the studies already discussed), Grimm et al. found no significant difference in appetite between patients and controls.

3.5.3. First Episode Patients vs. Controls

In a structural MRI study, Emsley and colleagues [88] investigated morphological brain changes after 13 weeks of AP treatment (risperidone or flupentixol injections) in AP-naïve FEP patients with SCZ, in relation to changes in BMI and metabolic indices. Regions of interest included the ventral diencephalon (vDC) and prefrontal cortex (PFC), which respectively represent key homeostatic and hedonic food intake regulatory areas. As there were no differences in MRI or metabolic outcomes between AP treatment groups, patients from both groups were pooled together for analysis. The authors found that compared to HCs, patients experienced a volume reduction in the vDC (a region containing the hypothalamus), which was strongly correlated with BMI and glucose increases and dyslipidemia. In contrast, no changes were observed in the PFC region, leading the authors to suggest that acute AP treatment primarily results in disruption of homeostatic functions (and not reward pathways). However, following post-hoc testing, these volume reductions were no longer significant and increased volumes in the control group were reported, which the authors attributed to random fluctuations due to small sample size.

In a recent fMRI study, Borgan et al. (2019) investigated neural responsiveness to appetitive stimuli in untreated FEP patients and HCs [86]. Comparing fMRI blood oxygen level dependent (BOLD) signaling response to appetitive stimuli between groups, the authors found that patients consistently exhibited the same regional patterns of neural activity observed in controls, indicative of normal neural responses to food cues. This led them to suggest that neural processing of food may be unaltered in the early stages of the illness and may instead be influenced by AP treatment.

3.6. Healthy Controls Only

We retrieved one neuroimaging study in HCs, which examined the effects of seven days of olanzapine administration on fMRI responses to visual stimuli (appetitive and neutral) as well as to receipt of an actual food reward [87]. Olanzapine treatment resulted in increased appetite as measured by both liquid breakfast intake and TFEQ scores (particularly disinhibition). This was accompanied by increased activation in brain regions involved in the reward pathway in response to both anticipation (inferior frontal cortex, striatum and ACC) and receipt (caudate, putamen) of appetitive stimuli. Interestingly, they also observed a concurrent decrease in activation in the lateral orbitofrontal cortex, which is thought to be involved in satiety.

4. Discussion

We performed a scoping review, which aimed to explore associations between psychosis spectrum disorders, food consumption, and disruptions in appetite and eating behaviors. Our search retrieved 35 studies, which we subsequently organized into three sections based on main theme or methodology: (1) Food composition and dietary preference, (2) patterns of eating behaviour and subjective appetite and (3) neural correlates of appetite and eating behavior. These sections are discussed individually, followed by a discussion of postulated mechanisms, and a more general discussion of limitations and future directions of this field.

4.1. Food Composition and Dietary Preference

The studies identified in our search provide evidence that overconsumption, in the form of both increased frequency and quantity of food consumption, differs between patients and HCs [57–60], which may contribute to the high rates of obesity in patient populations. In keeping with the general population, lower calorie intake among patients is associated with lower BMI, waist circumference, waist-to-hip ratio and body fat content [60]. Furthermore, dietary preference appears to be sex-specific [55,60,61], which could explain the differential propensity for weight gain among male and female SCZ spectrum disorder patients [89].

Disentangling the extent to which observed differences in caloric intake and dietary composition relate to biological factors intrinsic to the illness and/or AP treatment is challenging. While work in AP-naïve FEP populations can be helpful in delineating intrinsic illness related factors, only two of the dietary composition studies we retrieved included AP-naïve individuals [56,57]. However, subgroup analyses comparing HCs and AP-naïve patients were not performed, precluding inferences on dietary alterations that may primarily result from intrinsic illness effects. Unfortunately, it is similarly difficult to delineate the relative effects of APs on diet as studies in HCs indicate either no significant difference [78,79] or a significant increase in caloric intake [53] following SGA exposure.

It is also important to consider socioeconomic, environmental, and lifestyle factors that may precipitate a snowball effect on unhealthy dietary patterns among patients. Patients with psychosis spectrum disorders tend to belong to lower socioeconomic status (SES) groups [15,90]. This in turn relates to their ability to afford or have access to a nutritious diet. Notably, none of the dietary composition studies we reviewed matched patients to HCs in terms of SES, including income and education level. Three cross-sectional studies did, however, report significant differences in socio-demographic variables of patients vs. controls [58,60,61]. As such, it is possible that psychosocial stress related to socioeconomic factors, or symptoms of psychosis, may influence food intake in patients. Chronic stress has also been associated with hyperphagia [91] and preference for palatable foods [92]. Thus, failure to match patients to HCs according to key demographic features such as SES is a potential source of variation and should be considered in future studies.

4.2. Eating Behaviour, Cravings and Subjective Appetite

Synthesis of the studies identified in our search revealed a positive association between BMI/weight and altered appetite, hunger and/or food cravings in patients with psychosis spectrum disorders [50,64,65,69,72], as well as between SGA treatment and binge eating symptomatology [62–66,68]. Similar to what is observed in the ED literature [93,94], two studies also noted a relationship between restrictive eating behaviour (high restraint and high disinhibition scores) and increased consumption and weight gain among patients [72,74]. This may potentially suggest a common mechanism between EDs and the disordered eating patterns seen in psychosis patients.

In addition, APs may increase appetite and response to both internal and external hunger cues (as assessed by the TFEQ), putting patients at higher risk of overeating and subsequent weight gain [54,56,74,83,89]; however, the literature appears quite contradictory [70,71,73,82]. Potential explanations for these discrepancies could be choice of rating scale or questionnaire [95] and experimental conditions (i.e., fasting state, meal challenge and type), which differed widely across studies. As such, it is difficult to determine the relative contribution of illness vs. AP drugs on appetite.

Longitudinal HC studies also provide mixed evidence regarding the effects of APs on appetite and eating behaviors. Some studies indicate increased appetite, body weight and food intake following olanzapine treatment, indicative of a potential causal link [53,87], while other studies indicate SGA exposure does not significantly affect appetite or food intake despite inducing weight gain [78] and metabolic changes such as insulin resistance [79]. The latter point may suggest that central insulin and/or leptin resistance resulting from AP-induced weight gain and increases in adiposity may lead to appetite change, rather than appetite driving weight change [79].

4.3. Neural Correlates of Appetite and Eating Behavior

A variety of neuroimaging strategies have been employed to examine neurobiological mechanisms implicated in food intake patterns in patients, with a majority of the work (six out of seven retrieved studies) focusing on functional changes captured by fMRI in response to appetitive cues. Unfortunately, though, the different behavioural paradigms and brain regions of interest of each study made it difficult to draw any broad conclusions or generalizations. Two studies suggest that APs may contribute to disrupted appetite regulation and eating behaviour by increasing activation in areas involved in action planning and homeostatic signals [85], and regions implicated in cognitive and motivational processing of food [83]. However, these findings appear limited to static appetitive stimuli as dynamic stimuli led to decreased activation of the SN [84]. Interestingly, changes in regional activation correlated with disinhibition (TFEQ) scores across all three studies [83–85]. Similarly, AP treatment in HCs appears to [87] enhance activation in the brain reward circuitry, and decrease activation in the lateral orbital frontal cortex, consistent with loss of inhibitory effects on eating behaviour.

In determining the relative effects of illness vs. AP treatment, one AP-naïve study did not report any neural differences between patients or controls, indicating that food-related neural processing is not intrinsically dysregulated in SCZ [86]. In contrast, a different study found that chronic patients with SCZ on stable AP therapy exhibited significantly reduced activation in striatal regions involved in reward processing, an association that persisted even after controlling for AP dose. This suggests that the neural alterations involved in appetite regulation may be related to factors intrinsic to SCZ, which become more prominent as the illness progresses, and further exacerbated by AP therapy. This is consistent with structural MRI findings, which found that AP treatment reduced the volume of the vDC, but not the PFC in AP-naïve FEP patients [88].

4.4. Postulated Neurobiological Mechanisms Involved in Appetite/Feeding Regulation

While the contributing effects of intrinsic illness related factors vs. those of AP medications remain difficult to separate, existing theoretical frameworks may provide a neurobiological rationale for the differences in eating behaviours and appetite between patients with pychosis spectrum disorders and HCs. The postulated disruptions in hedonic/motivational and homeostatic mechanisms in patients with pyschosis spectrum disorders are summarized in Figure 3.

4.5. Hedonic Reward Mechanisms

The mesolimbic dopamine reward system is instantiated by a network of brain structures innervated by dopaminergic projections from the ventral tegmental area (VTA), including the nucleus accumbens (NAc), hypothalamus, amygdala, and PFC regions [96,97] (see Figure 1). Mesolimbic dopamine has primarily been implicated in the incentive motivational dimension of reward, including reward prediction [98], and the attribution of motivational salience to reward-related cues (associated with the concept of 'wanting' or 'craving') [99].

In turn, increased dopaminergic transmission in the striatum is a core neurobiological feature of SCZ that responds to first line AP treatment [100,101]. The striatum integrates inputs received from the majority of the cortex and projects to the mesolimbic dopamine system and cortical salience networks [102]. Its role has been associated with making inferences about the current state of the environment [103], whereas abnormal dopaminergic reactivity in the striatum may lead to misattribution of salience to external or internal cues relating to food or appetite.

Moreover, reward hypoactivity, which is related to negative symptoms of SCZ [104,105], may result in compensatory responses such as increased food consumption to achieve sufficient rewarding stimulation [82,106]. Furthermore, as function in the dorsal striatum is believed to be modulated by body weight, metabolic dysregulations accumulated throughout the course of the illness and perturbated by AP therapy may also be implicated in reduced striatal activity, similar to what is seen in obese individuals [106].

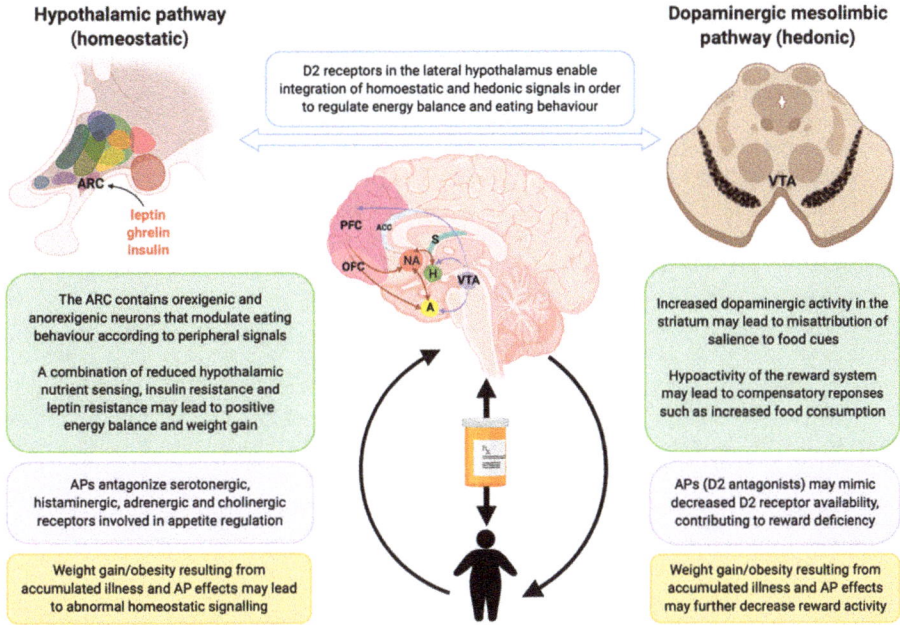

Figure 3. Overview of the homeostatic and hedonic pathways regulating appetite and eating behaviour. Text in green boxes describe the function of each pathway and implications for regulation of eating behaviour; text in purple boxes describes antipsychotic-induced effects; text in yellow boxes describes how weight gain affects pathway function. Abbreviations: VTA, ventral tegmental area; NA, nucleus accumbens; H, hypothalamus; PFC, prefrontal cortex; OFC, orbitofrontal cortex; A, amygdala; ACC, anterior cingulate gyrus; S, striatum; AP, antipsychotic; D2 = dopamine 2.

Additionally, disrupted function in the DLPFC, ACC and mediodorsal nucleus of the thalamus has been associated with impaired executive function in SCZ [107]. Analogous to observations of diminished executive function in the obese population, this may lead to poorer choices in food selection or difficulty in inhibiting responses to cravings. Consistent with this, several studies included in this review suggest that patients with SCZ have increased disinhibition [72,74,83–85], and an increased incidence of binge eating [59,67,68,72,81,108], which may reflect deficits in executive function related to prefrontal-ACC dysfunction [107].

The limited body of literature reporting on AP-naïve FEP patients precludes direct attribution of any dysregulations to inherent illness factors. However, APs share the uniting property of dopamine 2 (D2) receptor antagonism, which may mimic decreased D2 receptor availability, and thus contribute to the reward deficiency/overcompensation phenotype. Indeed, a relationship between reduced D2 receptor function and reward dysfunction has already been observed in obesity [109]. Beyond their effects on the dopamine system, APs also interact with serotonergic, histaminergic, adrenergic, muscarinic and cholinergic receptors, all of which are differentially involved in appetite modulation [84,110]. As such, the role of APs in disturbed eating behaviours is likely complex, involving widespread regions of the brain and signaling networks, with additional interfaces with illness-related disruptions in these pathways.

4.6. Homeostatic Mechanisms

Homeostatic mechanisms of food regulation are thought to be primarily regulated by the hypothalamus, a region anatomically situated to confer accessibility to hormones (leptin, ghrelin, insulin) and nutrients (glucose, fatty acids) in the blood and cerebral spinal fluid (CSF) to relay information about the body's energy stores to the brain [28] (see Figure 3). The topic of impaired hormonal regulation of feeding in SCZ has been the subject of a recent comprehensive review, supporting that early disruptions in these pathways likely progress over the course of illness and are further exacerbated by APs [20]. These homeostatic pathways are also thought to interact with dopamine reward circuits to regulate eating behavior and energy balance [111], potentially mediated by the high concentration of D2 receptors in the lateral hypothalamus [20] Thus, it is possible that the connections between these pathways may be altered in SCZ. For example, Stip et al. (2012) found evidence of increased signaling in the amygdala, a key limbic structure responsible for integrating homeostatic signals with extrinsic influences to modulate eating behavior [85]. However, this field of research is not well developed and is likely further complicated by the interaction between intrinsic aspects of psychosis spectrum disorders, AP treatment and psychological or environmental factors [112,113]. Interestingly, one study included in our review demonstrated volume reductions in the hypothalamus of AP-naïve patients following olanzapine treatment [88]. However, the relevance of changes in hypothalamic size in relation to obesity and metabolic disorders as well as the effects of AP treatment in relation to brain volume changes are controversial [114,115]. Further research combining advanced neuroimaging approaches (functional and structural) with food cues and stimuli relevant to hedonic and non-hedonic aspects of eating and assessments of hormonal activity is needed.

4.7. Strengths, Limitations and Future Directions

A key strength of this scoping review is that the search was broad, allowing for a comprehensive overview of the current state of the literature pertaining to eating behaviours and food consumption in psychosis spectrum disorders. Moreover, to the best of our knowledge, this is the first review to summarize the findings of neuroimaging studies that sought to elucidate the neurobiological mechanisms underlying eating behaviours among psychosis spectrum patients.

Nevertheless, there are some limitations which must be addressed. First, our search revealed high heterogeneity in both study design and questionnaires employed, which made comparing studies difficult and precluded conclusions from being made. Second, the majority of studies used subjective self-report measures of appetite/craving, results of which may be influenced by factors outside of hunger [58]. Additionally, the use of patient recall, as in the case of food diaries or during retrospective interviews, may lead to inaccurate estimations of food intake [57]. This is particularly relevant given that recall is known to be impaired in SCZ [58]. As alluded to by others, future studies that use both subjective and objective measures of appetite (e.g., calorie intake) [71], complemented by neuroimaging approaches [82] are required to move the field forward. Furthermore, only one fMRI study examined the effect of somatosensory (gustatory) stimuli on appetite and eating preferences [87]; the remaining five studies focused solely on visual processing of food-related cues, potentially missing key mediators of altered eating behaviour [116].

Importantly, very few of the studies identified in our search considered AP-naïve FEP patients, with the vast majority involving patients who had previously been exposed to AP therapy. This makes it difficult to determine whether any abnormal eating patterns observed in patients are intrinsic to the illness or secondary to the effects of APs. Additionally, while HC studies are a good way to remove the confounding effect of illness, they preclude identification of any interaction between intrinsic dysfunction in eating and AP effects. Prospective studies in which AP-naïve patients are exposed to APs would be particularly useful in exploring this illness-treatment interaction. Moreover, it should also be considered that studies in chronic patients with SCZ are confounded by cumulative illness associated lifestyle factors and treatments, which may affect both eating patterns and weight gain [7,117]. Further to this point, once obesity and other metabolic comorbidity is established, this may have secondary effects on physiology of feeding regulation [28]. Finally, metabolic consequences of AP treatment are known to be most pronounced in AP-naïve or FEP patients, suggesting that this may represent the critical period to capture early changes in eating behavior and appetite, which drive early weight gain [118]. Unfortunately, at present, the temporal course or trajectory of disordered eating in psychosis cannot be determined as most studies did not report trends over multiple timepoints. This would be a point worth considering when designing future longitudinal studies.

Finally, many of the studies comparing patients with HCs did not match groups on key sociodemographic and physiological (i.e., BMI, gender/sex) factors (see Tables 4–6), constituting a significant confound. To this last point, while sex emerged as an important mediator of appetite and feeding disruptions in some of the studies included in this review, the majority of studies did not account for sex. This is highly relevant given that in the general population, global obesity rates differ for males and females (10% and 18%, respectively [119]), as do TFEQ and DEBQ scores [36,120,121]. Furthermore, in SCZ, females seem to be more at risk for AP-induced metabolic disturbances than males [122,123]. Further investigation is therefore warranted to determine whether sex-related differences in eating behaviors can explain this increased vulnerability.

5. Conclusions

While disruptions in hormones involved in homeostatic mechanisms of appetite control in patients with pychosis spectrum disorders have been the subject of several reviews and meta-analyses, our scoping review highlights the behavioral and neurobiological underpinnings of altered eating behaviour in this population. Our synthesis of evidence from food surveys and self-report questionnaires generally supports the notion that patients with pychosis spectrum disorders exhibit increased appetite and craving for fatty food, increased caloric intake and increased frequency of (over) consumption, which may be associated with increased disinhibition. Early evidence also suggests that disturbed eating behaviours in this population could be mediated by abnormal processing of food-related stimuli within neural systems related to the mesolimbic reward circuit. In addition, it is possible that impaired cognitive restraint and executive functioning intrinsic to psychosis may make patients more susceptible to developing disordered eating patterns in response to weight gain and/or increased appetite and cravings. Future prospective studies with larger samples and AP-naïve populations are needed to improve the evidence base in this field and help dissect the intrinsic and extrinsic illness factors involved in disturbed appetite regulation. This will have important implications for development of pharmacological and behavioral interventions which, by targeting cardiometabolic comorbidities, may have the potential to increase patient life span and improve overall quality of life.

Supplementary Materials: The following are available online at http://www.mdpi.com/2072-6643/12/12/3883/s1, Table S1: Search strategy for Ovid MEDLINE electronic database search.

Author Contributions: Conceptualization, N.S., E.S. and R.A.; methodology, N.S., E.S. and R.A.; screening, N.S., E.S., R.A. and A.G.; data curation, N.S., E.S. and R.A.; investigation, N.S., E.S. and R.A.; writing—original draft preparation, N.S., E.S., R.A., L.H. and A.G.; writing—review and editing, N.S., E.S., R.A., L.H., P.S., S.S., A.G.-G., V.H.T., S.M.A. and M.K.H.; visualization, N.S., E.S. and R.A.; supervision, S.M.A. and M.K.H. All authors have read and agreed to the published version of the manuscript.

Funding: This research received no external funding.

Acknowledgments: All figures were created using BioRender.com. N.S. is supported by the CIHR Canada Graduate Scholarship Master's Program (CGS-M) and the Banting and Best Diabetes Centre (BBDC) Novo-Nordisk Graduate Studentship. E.S. is supported by the CIHR Canada Graduate Scholarship Master's Program (CGS-M) and the Banting and Best Diabetes Centre (BBDC) Novo-Nordisk Graduate Studentship. R.A. is supported by the Banting & Best Diabetes Centre-Novo Nordisk Studentship and the Cleghorn Award. P.S. reports receiving grants and/or salary and/or research support from the Centre for Addiction and Mental Health, Health Canada, Ontario Ministry of Health and Long-term care (MOHLTC), Canadian Institutes of Health Research (CIHR), Canadian Centre on Substance Use and Addiction, Public Health Agency of Canada (PHAC), Ontario Lung Association, Medical Psychiatry Alliance, Extensions for Community Healthcare Outcomes, Canadian Cancer Society Research Institute (CCSRI), Cancer Care Ontario, Ontario Institute for Cancer Research, Ontario Brain Institute, McLaughlin Centre, Academic Health Sciences Centre, Workplace Safety and Insurance Board, National Institutes of Health (NIH), and the Association of Faculties of Medicine of Canada. PS also reports receiving funding and/or honoraria from the following commercial organizations: Pfizer Inc./Canada, Shoppers Drug Mart, Bhasin Consulting Fund Inc., Patient-Centered Outcomes Research Institute, ABBVie, and Bristol-Myers Squibb. Further, PS reports receiving consulting fees from Pfizer Inc./Canada, Evidera Inc., Johnson & Johnson Group of Companies, Medcan Clinic, Inflexxion Inc., V-CC Systems Inc., MedPlan Communications, Kataka Medical

Communications, Miller Medical Communications, Nvision Insight Group, and Sun Life Financial. Through an open tender process Johnson & Johnson, Novartis, and Pfizer Inc. are vendors of record for providing smoking cessation pharmacotherapy, free or discounted, for research studies in which PS is the principal investigator or co-investigator. S.M.A is supported in part by an Academic Scholars Award from the Department of Psychiatry, University of Toronto and has grant support from the Canadian Institutes of Health Research, PSI foundation, Ontario, and the CAMH Discovery Fund. M.K.H. is supported in part by an Academic Scholars Award from the Department of Psychiatry, University of Toronto and has grant support from the Banting and Best Diabetes Center (BBDC) through the New Investigator Award, Canadian Institutes of Health Research (PJT–153262) (CIHR), PSI foundation, Ontario, and holds the Kelly and Michael Meighen Chair in Psychosis Prevention and Cardy Schizophrenia Research Chair. M.K.H. has also received consultant fees from Alkeremes.

Conflicts of Interest: The authors declare no conflict of interest.

References

1. Prentice, P. Psychosis and schizophrenia. *Arch. Dis. Child. Educ. Pract. Ed.* **2013**, *98*, 128–130. [CrossRef]
2. Moreno-Küstner, B.; Martín, C.; Pastor, L. Prevalence of psychotic disorders and its association with methodological issues. A systematic review and meta-analyses. *PLoS ONE* **2018**, *13*, e0195687. [CrossRef] [PubMed]
3. Arciniengas, D.B. Psychosis. *Continuum* **2015**, *21*, 715–736.
4. Bowie, C.R.; Harvey, P.D. Cognition in schizophrenia: Impairments, determinants, and functional importance. *Psychiatr. Clin. N. Am.* **2005**, *28*, 613–633. [CrossRef] [PubMed]
5. Harvey, P.D.; Strassnig, M. Predicting the severity of everyday functional disability in people with schizophrenia: Cognitive deficits, functional capacity, symptoms, and health status. *World Psychiatry* **2012**, *11*, 73–79. [CrossRef]
6. Maric, N.P.; Jovicic, M.J.; Mihaljevic, M.; Miljevic, C. Improving current treatments for schizophrenia. *Drug Dev. Res.* **2016**, *77*, 357–367. [CrossRef]
7. De Hert, M.; Cohen, D.; Bobes, J.; Cetkovich-Bakmas, M.; Leucht, S.; Ndetei, D.M.; Newcomer, J.W.; Uwakwe, R.; Asai, I.; Möller, H.J.; et al. Physical illness in patients with severe mental disorders. II. Barriers to care, monitoring and treatment guidelines, plus recommendations at the system and individual level. *World Psychiatry* **2011**, *10*, 138–151. [CrossRef]
8. Hennekens, C.H.; Hennekens, A.R.; Hollar, D.; Casey, D.E. Schizophrenia and increased risks of cardiovascular disease. *Am. Heart J.* **2005**, *150*, 1115–1121. [CrossRef]
9. Kredentser, M.S.; Martens, P.J.; Chochinov, H.M.; Prior, H.J. Cause and rate of death in people with schizophrenia across the lifespan: A population-based study in Manitoba, Canada. *J. Clin. Psychiatry* **2014**, *75*, 154–161. [CrossRef]
10. Rajkumar, A.P.; Horsdal, H.T.; Wimberley, T.; Cohen, D.; Mors, O.; Borglum, A.D.; Gasse, C. Endogenous and antipsychotic-related risks for diabetes mellitus in young people with schizophrenia: A Danish population-based cohort study. *Am. J. Psychiatry* **2017**, *174*, 686–694. [CrossRef]
11. Musil, R.; Obermeier, M.; Russ, P.; Hamerle, M. Weight gain and antipsychotics: A drug safety review. *Expert Opin. Drug Saf.* **2015**, *14*, 73–96. [CrossRef] [PubMed]
12. Alvarez-Jiménez, M.; González-Blanch, C.; Crespo-Facorro, B.; Hetrick, S.; Rodríguez-Sánchez, J.M.; Pérez-Iglesias, R.; Vázquez-Barquero, J.L. Antipsychotic-induced weight gain in chronic and first-episode psychotic disorders: A systematic critical reappraisal. *CNS Drugs* **2008**, *22*, 547–562. [CrossRef] [PubMed]
13. Hill, J.O.; Wyatt, H.R.; Peters, J.C. The importance of energy balance. *Eur. Endocrinol.* **2013**, *9*, 111–115. [CrossRef] [PubMed]
14. Dipasquale, S.; Pariante, C.M.; Dazzan, P.; Aguglia, E.; McGuire, P.; Mondelli, V. The dietary pattern of patients with schizophrenia: A systematic review. *J. Psychiatr. Res.* **2013**, *47*, 197–207. [CrossRef]
15. Heald, A.; Pendlebury, J.; Anderson, S.; Narayan, V.; Guy, M.; Gibson, M.; Haddad, P.; Livingston, M. Lifestyle factors and the metabolic syndrome in Schizophrenia: A cross-sectional study. *Ann. Gen. Psychiatry* **2017**, *16*, 12. [CrossRef]
16. Suvisaari, J.; Keinänen, J.; Eskelinen, S.; Mantere, O. Diabetes and Schizophrenia. *Curr. Diabetes Rep.* **2016**, *16*, 16. [CrossRef]
17. Kouidrat, Y.; Amad, A.; Lalau, J.D.; Loas, G. Eating disorders in schizophrenia: Implications for research and management. *Schizophr. Res. Treat.* **2014**, *2014*, 791573. [CrossRef]

18. Misiak, B.; Stańczykiewicz, B.; Łaczmański, Ł.; Frydecka, D. Lipid profile disturbances in antipsychotic-naive patients with first-episode non-affective psychosis: A systematic review and meta-analysis. *Schizophr. Res.* **2017**, *190*, 18–27. [CrossRef]
19. Greenhalgh, A.M.; Gonzalez-Blanco, L.; Garcia-Rizo, C.; Fernandez-Egea, E.; Miller, B.; Arroyo, M.B.; Kirkpatrick, B. Meta-analysis of glucose tolerance, insulin, and insulin resistance in antipsychotic-naïve patients with nonaffective psychosis. *Schizophr. Res.* **2017**, *179*, 57–63. [CrossRef]
20. Lis, M.; Stanczykiewicz, B.; Liskiewicz, P.; Misiak, B. Impaired hormonal regulation of appetite in schizophrenia: A narrative review dissecting intrinsic mechanisms and the effects of antipsychotics. *Psychoneuroendocrinology* **2020**, *119*, 104744. [CrossRef] [PubMed]
21. Benarroch, L.; Kowalchuk, C.; Wilson, V.; Teo, C.; Guenette, M.; Chintoh, A.; Nesarajah, Y.; Taylor, V.; Selby, P.; Fletcher, P.; et al. Atypical antipsychotics and effects on feeding: From mice to men. *Psychopharmacology* **2016**, *233*, 2629–2653. [CrossRef] [PubMed]
22. Bartoli, F.; Crocamo, C.; Clerici, M.; Carrà, G. Second-generation antipsychotics and adiponectin levels in schizophrenia: A comparative meta-analysis. *Eur. Neuropsychopharmacol.* **2015**, *25*, 1767–1774. [CrossRef] [PubMed]
23. Goetz, R.L.; Miller, B.J. Meta-analysis of ghrelin alterations in schizophrenia: Effects of olanzapine. *Schizophr. Res.* **2019**, *206*, 21–26. [CrossRef] [PubMed]
24. Matafome, P.; Seiça, R. The role of brain in energy balance. *Adv. Neurobiol.* **2017**, *19*, 33–48. [CrossRef] [PubMed]
25. Yu, Y.H.; Vasselli, J.R.; Zhang, Y.; Mechanick, J.I.; Korner, J.; Peterli, R. Metabolic vs. hedonic obesity: A conceptual distinction and its clinical implications. *Obes. Rev.* **2015**, *16*, 234–247. [CrossRef]
26. Teff, K.L.; Kim, S.F. Atypical antipsychotics and the neural regulation of food intake and peripheral metabolism. *Physiol. Behav.* **2011**, *104*, 590–598. [CrossRef]
27. Adinoff, B. Neurobiologic processes in drug reward and addiction. *Harv. Rev. Psychiatry* **2004**, *12*, 305–320. [CrossRef]
28. Roh, E.; Song, D.K.; Kim, M.S. Emerging role of the brain in the homeostatic regulation of energy and glucose metabolism. *Nat. Publ. Group* **2016**, *48*, 216. [CrossRef]
29. Peters, M.D.; Godfrey, C.M.; Khalil, H.; McInerney, P.; Parker, D.; Soares, C.B. Guidance for conducting systematic scoping reviews. *Int. J. Evid. Based Healthc.* **2015**, *13*, 141–146. [CrossRef]
30. Covidence Systematic Review Software. Available online: www.covidence.org (accessed on 10 June 2020).
31. Lindroos, A.-K.; Lissner, L.; Mathiassen, M.E.; Karlsson, J.; Sullivan, M.; Bengtsson, C.; Sjöström, L. Dietary intake in relation to restrained eating, disinhibition, and hunger in obese and nonobese Swedish women. *Obes. Res.* **1997**, *5*, 175–182. [CrossRef]
32. Westenhoefer, J.; Stunkard, A.J.; Pudel, V. Validation of the flexible and rigid control dimensions of dietary restraint. *Int. J. Eat. Disord.* **1999**, *26*, 53–64. [CrossRef]
33. Provencher, S.W. Automatic quantitation of localized in vivo 1H spectra with LCModel. *NMR Biomed.* **2001**, *14*, 260–264. [CrossRef] [PubMed]
34. Löffler, A.; Luck, T.; Then, F.S.; Sikorski, C.; Kovacs, P.; Böttcher, Y.; Breitfeld, J.; Tönjes, A.; Horstmann, A.; Löffler, M.; et al. Eating behaviour in the general population: An analysis of the factor structure of the German version of the Three-Factor-Eating-Questionnaire (TFEQ) and its association with the body mass index. *PLoS ONE* **2015**, *10*, e0133977. [CrossRef] [PubMed]
35. Bohrer, B.K.; Forbush, K.T.; Hunt, T.K. Are common measures of dietary restraint and disinhibited eating reliable and valid in obese persons? *Appetite* **2015**, *87*, 344–351. [CrossRef]
36. Bryant, E.J.; Rehman, J.; Pepper, L.B.; Walters, E.R. Obesity and eating disturbance: The role of TFEQ restraint and disinhibition. *Curr. Obes. Rep.* **2019**, *8*, 363–372. [CrossRef]
37. Sung, J.; Lee, K.; Song, Y.M. Relationship of eating behavior to long-term weight change and body mass index: The Healthy Twin study. *Eat. Weight Disord. Stud. Anorex. Bulim. Obes.* **2009**, *14*, e98–e105. [CrossRef]
38. Van Strien, T.; Herman, C.P.; Verheijden, M.W. Eating style, overeating, and overweight in a representative Dutch sample. Does external eating play a role? *Appetite* **2009**, *52*, 380–387. [CrossRef]
39. Koenders, P.G.; van Strien, T. Emotional eating, rather than lifestyle behavior, drives weight gain in a prospective study in 1562 employees. *J. Occup. Environ. Med.* **2011**, *53*, 1287–1293. [CrossRef]

40. Van Strien, T.; Frijters, J.E.R.; Bergers, G.P.A.; Defares, P.B. The Dutch Eating Behavior Questionnaire (DEBQ) for assessment of restrained, emotional, and external eating behavior. *Int. J. Eat. Disord.* **1986**, *5*, 295–315. [CrossRef]
41. Gibbons, C.; Hopkins, M.; Beaulieu, K.; Oustric, P.; Blundell, J.E. Issues in measuring and interpreting human appetite (satiety/satiation) and its contribution to obesity. *Curr. Obes. Rep.* **2019**, *8*, 77–87. [CrossRef]
42. Stunkard, A.J.; Messick, S. The three-factor eating questionnaire to measure dietary restraint, disinhibition and hunger. *J. Psychosom. Res.* **1985**, *29*, 71–83. [CrossRef]
43. Vinai, P.; Da Ros, A.; Speciale, M.; Gentile, N.; Tagliabue, A.; Vinai, P.; Bruno, C.; Vinai, L.; Studt, S.; Cardetti, S. Psychopathological characteristics of patients seeking for bariatric surgery, either affected or not by binge eating disorder following the criteria of the DSM IV TR and of the DSM 5. *Eat. Behav.* **2015**, *16*, 1–4. [CrossRef] [PubMed]
44. Bas, M.; Bozan, N.; Cigerim, N. Dieting, dietary restraint, and binge eating disorder among overweight adolescents in Turkey. *Adolescence* **2008**, *43*, 635–648. [PubMed]
45. Van Strien, T.; Peter Herman, C.; Verheijden, M.W. Eating style, overeating and weight gain. A prospective 2-year follow-up study in a representative Dutch sample. *Appetite* **2012**, *59*, 782–789. [CrossRef]
46. Stubbs, R.J.; Hughes, D.A.; Johnstone, A.M.; Rowley, E.; Reid, C.; Elia, M.; Stratton, R.; Delargy, H.; King, N.; Blundell, J.E. The use of visual analogue scales to assess motivation to eat in human subjects: A review of their reliability and validity with an evaluation of new hand-held computerized systems for temporal tracking of appetite ratings. *Br. J. Nutr.* **2000**, *84*, 405–415. [CrossRef] [PubMed]
47. Cepeda-Benito, A.; Gleaves, D.H.; Williams, T.L.; Erath, S.A. The development and validation of the state and trait food-cravings questionnaires. *Behav. Ther.* **2000**, *31*, 151–173. [CrossRef]
48. White, M.A.; Whisenhunt, B.L.; Williamson, D.A.; Greenway, F.L.; Netemeyer, R.G. Development and validation of the food-craving inventory. *Obes. Res.* **2002**, *10*, 107–114. [CrossRef]
49. Lim, M.; Noh, J.; Nam, H.; Kim, J.; Lee, D.; Hong, K. Development and validation of drug-related eating behavior questionnaire in patients receiving antipsychotic medications. *Korean J. Schizophr. Res.* **2008**, *11*, 39–44.
50. Ryu, S.; Nam, H.J.; Oh, S.; Park, T.; Lim, M.; Choi, J.S.; Baek, J.H.; Jang, J.H.; Park, H.Y.; Kim, S.N.; et al. Eating-behavior changes associated with antipsychotic medications in patients with schizophrenia as measured by the Drug-Related Eating Behavior Questionnaire. *J. Clin. Psychopharmacol.* **2013**, *33*, 120–122. [CrossRef]
51. Spitzer, R.L.; Yanovski, S.; Wadden, T.; Wing, R.; Marcus, M.D.; Stunkard, A.; Devlin, M.; Mitchell, J.; Hasin, D.; Horne, R.L. Binge eating disorder: Its further validation in a multisite study. *Int. J. Eat. Disord.* **1993**, *13*, 137–153.
52. Mizes, J.S.; Christiano, B.; Madison, J.; Post, G.; Seime, R.; Varnado, P. Development of the mizes anorectic cognitions questionnaire-revised: Psychometric properties and factor structure in a large sample of eating disorder patients. *Int. J. Eat. Disord.* **2000**, *28*, 415–421. [CrossRef]
53. Fountaine, R.J.; Taylor, A.E.; Mancuso, J.P.; Greenway, F.L.; Byerley, L.O.; Smith, S.R.; Most, M.M.; Fryburg, D.A. Increased food intake and energy expenditure following administration of olanzapine to healthy men. *Obesity* **2010**, *18*, 1646–1651. [CrossRef] [PubMed]
54. Gothelf, D.; Falk, B.; Singer, P.; Kairi, M.; Phillip, M.; Zigel, L.; Poraz, I.; Frishman, S.; Constantini, N.; Zalsman, G.; et al. Weight Gain Associated With Increased Food Intake and Low Habitual Activity Levels in Male Adolescent Schizophrenic Inpatients Treated With Olanzapine. *Am. J. Psychiatry* **2002**, *159*, 1055–1057. [CrossRef] [PubMed]
55. Amani, R. Is dietary pattern of schizophrenia patients different from healthy subjects? *BMC Psychiatry* **2007**, *7*. [CrossRef] [PubMed]
56. Eder, U.; Mangweth, B.; Ebenbichler, C.; Weiss, E.; Hofer, A.; Hummer, M.; Kemmler, G.; Lechleitner, M.; Fleischhacker, W.W. Association of olanzapine-induced weight gain with an increase in body fat. *Am. J. Psychiatry* **2001**, *158*, 1719–1722. [CrossRef] [PubMed]
57. Gattere, G.; Stojanovic-Perez, A.; Monseny, R.; Martorell, L.; Ortega, L.; Montalvo, I.; Sole, M.; Algora, M.J.; Cabezas, A.; Reynolds, R.M.; et al. Gene-environment interaction between the brain-derived neurotrophic factor Val66Met polymorphism, psychosocial stress and dietary intake in early psychosis. *Early Interv. Psychiatry* **2018**, *12*, 811–820. [CrossRef] [PubMed]

58. Nunes, D.; Eskinazi, B.; Camboim Rockett, F.; Delgado, V.B.; Schweigert Perry, I.D. Nutritional status, food intake and cardiovascular disease risk in individuals with schizophrenia in southern Brazil: A case–control study. *Rev. Psiquiatr. Salud Ment.* **2014**, *7*, 72–79. [CrossRef] [PubMed]
59. Strassnig, M.; Singh Brar, J.; Qanguli, R. Nutritional assessment of patients with schizophrenia: A preliminary study. *Schizophr. Bull.* **2003**, *29*, 393–397. [CrossRef]
60. Stefanska, E.; Lech, M.; Wendołowicz, A.; Konarzewska, B.; Waszkiewicz, N.; Ostrowska, L. Eating habits and nutritional status of patients with affective disorders and schizophrenia. *Psychiatr. Pol.* **2017**, *51*, 1107–1120. [CrossRef]
61. Stefańska, E.; Wendołowicz, A.; Lech, M.; Wilczyńska, K.; Konarzewska, B.; Zapolska, J.; Ostrowska, L. The assessment of the nutritional value of meals consumed by patients with recognized schizophrenia. *Rocz. Państwowego Zakładu Hig.* **2018**, *69*, 183–192.
62. Khazaal, Y.; Fresard, E.; Zimmermann, G.; Trombert, N.M.; Pomini, V.; Grasset, F.; Borgeat, F.; Zullino, D. Eating and weight related cognitions in people with Schizophrenia: A case control study. *Clin. Pract. Epidemiol. Ment. Health CP EMH* **2006**, *2*, 29. [CrossRef] [PubMed]
63. Brömel, T.; Blum, W.F.; Ziegler, A.; Schulz, E.; Bender, M.; Fleischhaker, C.; Remschmidt, H.; Krieg, J.C.; Hebebrand, J. Serum leptin levels increase rapidly after initiation of clozapine therapy. *Mol. Psychiatry* **1998**, *3*, 76–80. [CrossRef] [PubMed]
64. Gebhardt, S.; Haberhausen, M.; Krieg, J.C.; Remschmidt, H.; Heinzel-Gutenbrunner, M.; Hebebrand, J.; Theisen, F.M. Clozapine/olanzapine-induced recurrence or deterioration of binge eating-related eating disorders. *J. Neural Transm.* **2007**, *114*, 1091–1095. [CrossRef] [PubMed]
65. Kluge, M.; Schuld, A.; Himmerich, H.; Dalal, M.; Schacht, A.; Wehmeier, P.M.; Hinze-Selch, D.; Kraus, T.; Dittmann, R.W.; Pollmächer, T. Clozapine and olanzapine are associated with food craving and binge eating: Results from a randomized double-blind study. *J. Clin. Psychopharmacol.* **2007**, *27*, 662–666. [CrossRef]
66. Theisen, F.M.; Linden, A.; König, I.R.; Martin, M.; Remschmidt, H.; Hebebrand, J. Spectrum of binge eating symptomatology in patients treated with clozapine and olanzapine. *J. Neural Transm.* **2003**, *110*, 111–121. [CrossRef]
67. Treuer, T.; Hoffmann, V.P.; Chen, A.K.-P.; Irimia, V.; Ocampo, M.; Wang, G.; Singh, P.; Holt, S. Factors associated with weight gain during olanzapine treatment in patients with schizophrenia or bipolar disorder: Results from a six-month prospective, multinational, observational study. *World J. Biol. Psychiatry* **2009**, *10*, 729–740. [CrossRef]
68. Khazaal, Y.; Frésard, E.; Borgeat, F.; Zullino, D. Binge eating symptomatology in overweight and obese patients with schizophrenia: A case control study. *Ann. Gen. Psychiatry* **2006**, *5*, 15. [CrossRef]
69. Garriga, M.; Mallorqui, A.; Serrano, L.; Rios, J.; Salamero, M.; Parellada, E.; Gomez-Ramiro, M.; Oliveira, C.; Amoretti, S.; Vieta, E.; et al. Food craving and consumption evolution in patients starting treatment with clozapine. *Psychopharmacology* **2019**, *236*, 3317–3327. [CrossRef]
70. Karagianis, J.; Grossman, L.; Landry, J.; Reed, V.A.; de Haan, L.; Maguire, G.A.; Hoffmann, V.P.; Milev, R. A randomized controlled trial of the effect of sublingual orally disintegrating olanzapine versus oral olanzapine on body mass index: The PLATYPUS Study. *Schizophr. Res.* **2009**, *113*, 41–48. [CrossRef]
71. Smith, R.C.; Rachakonda, S.; Dwivedi, S.; Davis, J.M. Olanzapine and risperidone effects on appetite and ghrelin in chronic schizophrenic patients. *Psychiatry Res.* **2012**, *199*, 159–163. [CrossRef]
72. Sentissi, O.; Viala, A.; Bourdel, M.C.; Kaminski, F.; Bellisle, F.; Olie, J.P.; Poirier, M.F. Impact of antipsychotic treatments on the motivation to eat: Preliminary results in 153 schizophrenic patients. *Int. Clin. Psychopharmacol.* **2009**, *24*, 257–264. [CrossRef] [PubMed]
73. Abbas, M.J.; Liddle, P.F. Olanzapine and food craving: A case control study. *Hum. Psychopharmacol.* **2013**, *28*, 97–101. [CrossRef] [PubMed]
74. Blouin, M.; Tremblay, A.; Jalbert, M.E.; Venables, H.; Bouchard, R.H.; Roy, M.A.; Alméras, N. Adiposity and eating behaviors in patients under second generation antipsychotics. *Obesity* **2008**, *16*, 1780–1787. [CrossRef] [PubMed]
75. Folley, B.S.; Park, S. Relative food preference and hedonic judgments in schizophrenia. *Psychiatry Res.* **2010**, *175*, 33–37. [CrossRef] [PubMed]
76. Knolle-Veentjer, S.; Huth, V.; Ferstl, R.; Aldenhoff, J.B.; Hinze-Selch, D. Delay of gratification and executive performance in individuals with schizophrenia: Putative role for eating behavior and body weight regulation. *J. Psychiatr. Res.* **2008**, *42*, 98–105. [PubMed]

77. Schanze, A.; Reulbach, U.; Scheuchenzuber, M.; Groschl, M.; Kornhuber, J.; Kraus, T. Ghrelin and eating disturbances in psychiatric disorders. *Neuropsychobiology* **2008**, *57*, 126–130. [CrossRef] [PubMed]
78. Roerig, J.L.; Mitchell, J.E.; de Zwaan, M.; Crosby, R.D.; Gosnell, B.A.; Steffen, K.J.; Wonderlich, S.A. A comparison of the effects of olanzapine and risperidone versus placebo on eating behaviors. *J. Clin. Psychopharmacol.* **2005**, *25*, 413–418.
79. Teff, K.L.; Rickels, K.; Alshehabi, E.; Rickels, M.R. Metabolic impairments precede changes in hunger and food intake following short-term administration of second-generation antipsychotics. *J. Clin. Psychopharmacol.* **2015**, *35*, 579–582. [CrossRef]
80. Teff, K.L.; Rickels, M.R.; Grudziak, J.; Fuller, C.; Nguyen, H.-L.; Rickels, K. Antipsychotic-induced insulin resistance and postprandial hormonal dysregulation independent of weight gain or psychiatric disease. *Diabetes* **2013**, *62*, 3232–3240. [CrossRef]
81. Naranjo, C.A.; Busto, U.; Sellers, E.M.; Sandor, P.; Ruiz, I.; Roberts, E.A.; Janecek, E.; Domecq, C.; Greenblatt, D.J. A method for estimating the probability of adverse drug reactions. *Clin. Pharmacol. Ther.* **1981**, *30*, 239–245. [CrossRef]
82. Grimm, O.; Vollstadt-Klein, S.; Krebs, L.; Zink, M.; Smolka, M.N. Reduced striatal activation during reward anticipation due to appetite-provoking cues in chronic schizophrenia: A fMRI study. *Schizophr. Res.* **2012**, *134*, 151–157. [CrossRef] [PubMed]
83. Lungu, O.; Anselmo, K.; Letourneau, G.; Mendrek, A.; Stip, B.; Lipp, O.; Lalonde, P.; Ait Bentaleb, L.; Stip, E. Neuronal correlates of appetite regulation in patients with schizophrenia: Is there a basis for future appetite dysfunction? *Eur. Psychiatry J. Assoc. Eur. Psychiatr.* **2013**, *28*, 293–301. [CrossRef] [PubMed]
84. Stip, E.; Lungu, O.V. Salience network and olanzapine in schizophrenia: Implications for treatment in anorexia nervosa. *Can. J. Psychiatry Rev. Can. Psychiatr.* **2015**, *60*, S35–S39.
85. Stip, E.; Lungu, O.V.; Anselmo, K.; Letourneau, G.; Mendrek, A.; Stip, B.; Lipp, O.; Lalonde, P.; Bentaleb, L.A. Neural changes associated with appetite information processing in schizophrenic patients after 16 weeks of olanzapine treatment. *Transl. Psychiatry* **2012**, *2*, e128. [CrossRef]
86. Borgan, F.; O'Daly, O.; Hoang, K.; Veronese, M.; Withers, D.; Batterham, R.; Howes, O. Neural responsivity to food cues in patients with unmedicated first-episode psychosis. *JAMA Netw. Open* **2019**, *2*, e186893. [CrossRef]
87. Mathews, J.; Newcomer, J.W.; Mathews, J.R.; Fales, C.L.; Pierce, K.J.; Akers, B.K.; Marcu, I.; Barch, D.M. Neural correlates of weight gain with olanzapine. *Arch. Gen. Psychiatry* **2012**, *69*, 1226–1237. [CrossRef]
88. Emsley, R.; Asmal, L.; Chiliza, B.; du Plessis, S.; Carr, J.; Kidd, M.; Malhotra, A.K.; Vink, M.; Kahn, R.S. Changes in brain regions associated with food-intake regulation, body mass and metabolic profiles during acute antipsychotic treatment in first-episode schizophrenia. *Psychiatry Res.* **2015**, *233*, 186–193. [CrossRef] [PubMed]
89. Gebhardt, S.; Haberhausen, M.; Heinzel-Gutenbrunner, M.; Gebhardt, N.; Remschmidt, H.; Krieg, J.C.; Hebebrand, J.; Theisen, F.M. Antipsychotic-induced body weight gain: Predictors and a systematic categorization of the long-term weight course. *J. Psychiatr. Res.* **2009**, *43*, 620–626. [CrossRef] [PubMed]
90. Vancampfort, D.; Rosenbaum, S.; Schuch, F.B.; Ward, P.B.; Probst, M.; Stubbs, B. Prevalence and predictors of treatment dropout from physical activity interventions in schizophrenia: A meta-analysis. *Gen. Hosp. Psychiatry* **2016**, *39*, 15–23. [CrossRef] [PubMed]
91. Kyrou, I.; Tsigos, C. Chronic stress, visceral obesity and gonadal dysfunction. *Hormones* **2008**, *7*, 287–293. [CrossRef]
92. Dallman, M.F.; Pecoraro, N.; Akana, S.F.; La Fleur, S.E.; Gomez, F.; Houshyar, H.; Bell, M.E.; Bhatnagar, S.; Laugero, K.D.; Manalo, S. Chronic stress and obesity: A new view of "comfort food". *Proc. Natl. Acad. Sci. USA* **2003**, *100*, 11696–11701. [CrossRef] [PubMed]
93. Burger, K.S.; Stice, E. Relation of dietary restraint scores to activation of reward-related brain regions in response to food intake, anticipated intake, and food pictures. *NeuroImage* **2011**, *55*, 233–239. [CrossRef] [PubMed]
94. Spinella, M.; Lyke, J. Executive personality traits and eating behavior. *Int. J. Neurosci.* **2004**, *114*, 83–93. [CrossRef] [PubMed]
95. Case, M.; Treuer, T.; Karagianis, J.; Hoffmann, V.P. The potential role of appetite in predicting weight changes during treatment with olanzapine. *BMC Psychiatry* **2010**, *10*. [CrossRef] [PubMed]

96. Cardinal, R.N.; Parkinson, J.A.; Hall, J.; Everitt, B.J. Emotion and motivation: The role of the amygdala, ventral striatum, and prefrontal cortex. *Neurosci. Biobehav. Rev.* **2002**, *26*, 321–352. [CrossRef]
97. Le Moal, M.; Simon, H. Mesocorticolimbic dopaminergic network: Functional and regulatory roles. *Physiol. Rev.* **1991**, *71*, 155–234. [CrossRef] [PubMed]
98. Schultz, W. Dopamine neurons and their role in reward mechanisms. *Curr. Opin. Neurobiol.* **1997**, *7*, 191–197. [CrossRef]
99. Berridge, K.C. The debate over dopamine's role in reward: The case for incentive salience. *Psychopharmacology* **2007**, *191*, 391–431. [CrossRef]
100. Amato, D.; Vernon, A.C.; Papaleo, F. Dopamine, the antipsychotic molecule: A perspective on mechanisms underlying antipsychotic response variability. *Neurosci. Biobehav. Rev.* **2018**, *85*, 146–159. [CrossRef]
101. Kapur, S. Psychosis as a state of aberrant salience: A framework linking biology, phenomenology, and pharmacology in schizophrenia. *Am. J. Psychiatry* **2003**, *160*, 13–23. [CrossRef]
102. McCutcheon, R.A.; Abi-Dargham, A.; Howes, O.D. Schizophrenia, dopamine and the striatum: From biology to symptoms. *Trends Neurosci.* **2019**, *42*, 205–220. [CrossRef] [PubMed]
103. Nour, M.M.; Dahoun, T.; Schwartenbeck, P.; Adams, R.A.; FitzGerald, T.H.B.; Coello, C.; Wall, M.B.; Dolan, R.J.; Howes, O.D. Dopaminergic basis for signaling belief updates, but not surprise, and the link to paranoia. *Proc. Natl. Acad. Sci. USA* **2018**, *115*, E10167–E10176. [CrossRef] [PubMed]
104. Blanchard, J.J.; Cohen, A.S. The structure of negative symptoms within schizophrenia: Implications for assessment. *Schizophr. Bull.* **2006**, *32*, 238–245. [CrossRef] [PubMed]
105. Strauss, G.P.; Waltz, J.A.; Gold, J.M. A review of reward processing and motivational impairment in schizophrenia. *Schizophr. Bull.* **2014**, *40*, S107–S116. [CrossRef]
106. Stice, E.; Spoor, S.; Bohon, C.; Veldhuizen, M.G.; Small, D.M. Relation of reward from food intake and anticipated food intake to obesity: A functional magnetic resonance imaging study. *J. Abnorm. Psychol.* **2008**, *117*, 924–935. [CrossRef]
107. Minzenberg, M.J.; Laird, A.R.; Thelen, S.; Carter, C.S.; Glahn, D.C. Meta-analysis of 41 functional neuroimaging studies of executive function in schizophrenia. *Arch. Gen. Psychiatry* **2009**, *66*, 811–822. [CrossRef]
108. Khazaal, Y.; Billieux, J.; Fresard, E.; Huguelet, P.; van der Linden, M.; Zullino, D. A Measure of dysfunctional eating-related cognitions in people with psychotic disorders. *Psychiatr. Q.* **2010**, *81*, 49–56. [CrossRef]
109. Benton, D.; Young, H.A. A meta-analysis of the relationship between brain dopamine receptors and obesity: A matter of changes in behavior rather than food addiction? *Int. J. Obes.* **2016**, *40*, S12–S21. [CrossRef]
110. Hahn, M.; Chintoh, A.; Giacca, A.; Xu, L.; Lam, L.; Mann, S.; Fletcher, P.; Guenette, M.; Cohn, T.; Wolever, T.; et al. Atypical antipsychotics and effects of muscarinic, serotonergic, dopaminergic and histaminergic receptor binding on insulin secretion in vivo: An animal model. *Schizophr. Res.* **2011**, *131*, 90–95. [CrossRef]
111. Ahima, R.S.; Antwi, D.A. Brain regulation of appetite and satiety. *NIH Public Access* **2008**, *37*, 811–823. [CrossRef]
112. Agarwal, S.M.; Caravaggio, F.; Costa-Dookhan, K.A.; Castellani, L.; Kowalchuk, C.; Asgariroozbehani, R.; Graff-Guerrero, A.; Hahn, M. Brain insulin action in schizophrenia: Something borrowed and something new. *Neuropharmacology* **2020**, *163*, 107633. [CrossRef] [PubMed]
113. MacKenzie, N.E.; Kowalchuk, C.; Agarwal, S.M.; Costa-Dookhan, K.A.; Caravaggio, F.; Gerretsen, P.; Chintoh, A.; Remington, G.J.; Taylor, V.H.; Mueller, D.J.; et al. Antipsychotics, metabolic adverse effects, and cognitive function in schizophrenia. *Front. Psychiatry* **2018**, *9*, 622. [CrossRef] [PubMed]
114. Thomas, B.L.; Claassen, N.; Becker, P.; Viljoen, M. Validity of commonly used heart rate variability markers of autonomic nervous system function. *Neuropsychobiology* **2019**, *78*, 14–26. [CrossRef]
115. Turkheimer, F.E.; Selvaggi, P.; Mehta, M.A.; Veronese, M.; Zelaya, F.; Dazzan, P.; Vernon, A.C. Normalizing the abnormal: Do antipsychotic drugs push the cortex into an unsustainable metabolic envelope? *Schizophr. Bull.* **2020**, *46*, 484–495. [CrossRef] [PubMed]
116. Lemon, C.H. It's all a matter of taste: Gustatory processing and ingestive decisions. *MO Med.* **2010**, *107*, 247–251. [PubMed]
117. Vancampfort, D.; Knapen, J.; Probst, M.; van Winkel, R.; Deckx, S.; Maurissen, K.; Peuskens, J.; de Hert, M. Considering a frame of reference for physical activity research related to the cardiometabolic risk profile in schizophrenia. *Psychiatry Res.* **2010**, *177*, 271–279. [CrossRef] [PubMed]

118. Mitchell, A.J.; Vancampfort, D.; Sweers, K.; van Winkel, R.; Yu, W.; de Hert, M. Prevalence of metabolic syndrome and metabolic abnormalities in schizophrenia and related disorders—A systematic review and meta-analysis. *Schizophr. Bull.* **2013**, *39*, 306–318. [CrossRef]
119. Garawi, F.; Devries, K.; Thorogood, N.; Uauy, R. Global differences between women and men in the prevalence of obesity: Is there an association with gender inequality? *Eur. J. Clin. Nutr.* **2014**, *68*, 1101–1106. [CrossRef]
120. Burton, P.; Smit, H.J.; Lightowler, H.J. The influence of restrained and external eating patterns on overeating. *Appetite* **2007**, *49*, 191–197. [CrossRef]
121. Bellisle, F.; Clément, K.; Le Barzic, M.; Le Gall, A.; Guy-Grand, B.; Basdevant, A. The eating inventory and body adiposity from leanness to massive obesity: A study of 2509 adults. *Obes. Res.* **2004**, *12*, 2023–2030. [CrossRef]
122. Castellani, L.N.; Costa-Dookhan, K.A.; McIntyre, W.B.; Wright, D.C.; Flowers, S.A.; Hahn, M.K.; Ward, K.M. Preclinical and clinical sex differences in antipsychotic-induced metabolic disturbances: A narrative review of adiposity and glucose metabolism. *J. Psychiatry Brain Sci.* **2019**, *4*. [CrossRef]
123. Seeman, M.V. Men and women respond differently to antipsychotic drugs. *Neuropharmacology* **2020**, *163*, 107631. [CrossRef] [PubMed]

Publisher's Note: MDPI stays neutral with regard to jurisdictional claims in published maps and institutional affiliations.

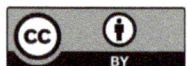

© 2020 by the authors. Licensee MDPI, Basel, Switzerland. This article is an open access article distributed under the terms and conditions of the Creative Commons Attribution (CC BY) license (http://creativecommons.org/licenses/by/4.0/).

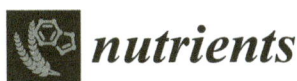 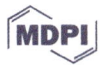

Article

Does Eating Addiction Favor a More Varied Diet or Contribute to Obesity?—The Case of Polish Adults

Marzena Jezewska-Zychowicz, Aleksandra Małachowska * and Marta Plichta

Institute of Human Nutrition Sciences, Warsaw University of Life Sciences (SGGW-WULS), 159C Nowoursynowska Street, 02-787 Warsaw, Poland; marzena_jezewska_zychowicz@sggw.edu.pl (M.J.-Z.); marta_plichta@sggw.edu.pl (M.P.)
* Correspondence: aleksandra_malachowska@sggw.edu.pl; Tel.: +48-(022)-59-37-131

Received: 14 March 2020; Accepted: 29 April 2020; Published: 2 May 2020

Abstract: The rapidly increasing prevalence of overweight and obesity indicates a need to search for their main causes. Addictive-like eating and associated eating patterns might result in overconsumption, leading to weight gain. The aim of the study was to identify the main determinants of food intake variety (FIV) within eating addiction (EA), other lifestyle components, and sociodemographic characteristics. The data for the study were collected from a sample of 898 Polish adults through a cross-sectional survey in 2019. The questionnaire used in the study included Food Intake Variety Questionnaire (FIVeQ), Eating Preoccupation Scale (EPS), and questions regarding lifestyle and sociodemographic factors. High eating addiction was found in more than half of the people with obesity (54.2%). In the study sample, physical activity at leisure time explained FIV in the greatest manner, followed by the EPS factor: eating to provide pleasure and mood improvement. In the group of people with obesity, the score for this EPS factor was the best predictor of FIV, in that a higher score was conducive to a greater variety of food intake. Sociodemographic characteristics differentiated FIV only within groups with normal body weight (age) and with overweight (education). In conclusion, food intake variety (FIV) was associated with physical activity at leisure time, and then with EPS factor "Eating to provide pleasure and mood improvement", whereas sociodemographic characteristics were predictors of FIV only within groups identified by body mass index (BMI). Nevertheless, our observations regarding the eating to provide pleasure and mood improvement factor and its associations with food intake variety indicate a need for further research in this area. Future studies should also use other tools to explicitly explain this correlation.

Keywords: overweight; obesity; food addiction; eating addiction; food intake variety; eating behavior; overeating

1. Introduction

In spite of the growing prevalence of overweight and obesity, determining their main risk factors is still a challenge. Body weight and body mass index (BMI) are greatly influenced by energy intake and its adequacy [1]. However, the link between diet and those anthropometric parameters cannot be solely assessed on the basis of calorie intake, but should also include other elements of dietary patterns (eating frequency, diet quality, food variety, or proportions between different food groups) [2]. Lifestyle-related factors, such as unhealthy dietary patterns but also low physical activity, inadequate sleep hygiene, poor stress management, and tobacco smoking, can majorly alter energy intake and expenditure, and thus induce a positive energy balance [3]. Research shows that lifestyle factors are correlated with each other. Low physical activity is associated with the consumption of unhealthy foods [4,5]. In turn, less stress or negative as well as highly positive effects are associated with engagement in healthy behaviors, especially in physical activity [6]. Physical activity can reduce stress as well as negative emotions and, at the same time, enhance positive emotions. By contrast, human emotional functioning is associated with food, including emotional eating [7]. Physically active emotional eaters may want to eat when under emotional distress; however, they also choose more healthy foods to cope with this distress [8]. These interrelationships between selected lifestyle components, but also within human psychological functioning, implicate the necessity of including such parameters while exploring eating behaviors characteristics.

Some dietary patterns, such as uncontrolled excessive consumption, may resemble addictive behavior, and some foods may have addictive potential [9]. Gearhardt et al. [10] developed the first tool to assess FA, the Yale Food Addiction Scale (YFAS), as well as the follow-up, YFAS 2.0 [11]. These tools enable identification of addictive-like eating behaviors particularly towards highly processed and palatable foods. Elevated YFAS and YFAS 2.0 scores are both positively associated with body mass index (BMI), binge eating symptoms, and weight-cycling [11]. Research suggests that people diagnosed as food addicts consume more calories [12–16], especially derived from processed, energy-dense foods like confectionary, fast-food, and salty snacks, and their diet is higher in fat [12,14,16] than non-food-addicted individuals. Several studies have revealed that food addiction can be correlated with lower consumption of fruit, vegetables, and other core products [13,15].

Overeating might be associated with one of the following eating styles: restrained, emotional, or external. In restrained eating, when someone is following a strict dietary regimen, eating something forbidden may induce an "all-or-nothing" reaction leading to overconsumption [17]. Negative, positive, or neutral emotional states (e.g., sadness, anxiety, joy, boredom) might also increase food intake (emotional eating). Lastly, environmental factors, such as availability of food or presence of others eating, might also affect the consumption in so-called external eating [18]. Studies have found that emotional eating might favor undesirable food behaviors, including higher intake of snacks [19,20], "fast-food" [19], and sweet foods [21,22], whereas external eating may increase total calorie intake [19] as well as predispose to higher consumption of snacks [19,23]. Although dietary restraint can be conducive to lower intake of sweets [19] and total energy intake [19,24,25], it may simultaneously serve as a risk factor for excessive body weight [19,24,25]. The possible explanation of this phenomenon might be related to the possibility that people following strict dietary rules may be more susceptible to external and emotional eating, which can lead to weight gain [26]. Food-related thoughts are believed to be another crucial factor in the etiology of excessive food consumption as they can induce a specific food craving. When the urge to fulfill this craving arises, it can be difficult to resist overeating. Food preoccupation might therefore take the form of obsession [27].

In previous studies, also those using YFAS or YFAS 2.0, dietary assessment did not take into account food intake variety (FIV), which reflects the number of food products consumed by the individual. For many years, FIV was being promoted as a vital component of dietary guidelines. It was believed that a wider range of products will improve intake of macro- and micronutrients and provide adequate nutritional status [28]. Although a systematic review of 26 studies has shown that it is still unclear how total FIV affects body weight and measures of body adiposity [28], this parameter is of special concern to medical scientists and health professionals due to the growing obesity epidemic [29]. Results from the studies assessing the relationship between FIV and diet quality or eating habits remain inconsistent. Some research suggests a negative impact [30,31], whereas several studies have found that FIV might favor healthy eating habits, such as adequate intake of fruit and vegetables [32,33], or predispose to greater diet quality [34,35]. The existing research results suggest that sociodemographic characteristics, such as gender and age, can differentiate assessed variables and their correlations [30,33,34].

We assume that differences in food intake variety (FIV) can be explained by eating addiction assessed using the Eating Preoccupation Scale (EPS). However, we hypothesize that EPS explains the differences in FIV to a lesser extent than some components of lifestyle (i.e., physical activity, following a diet, smoking) but the importance of these factors may vary depending on BMI. Thus, the aim of the study is to assess eating addiction in a group of Polish adults, and to then answer the following questions: (1) Does eating addiction show a relationship with food intake variety? (2) Do such lifestyle components as following a diet, smoking, and physical activity differentiate the food intake variety more than the eating addiction? (3) Do the relationships between the examined variables differ after taking BMI into account?

2. Materials and Methods

2.1. Study Design and Sample Collection

The data were collected from February to March 2019 through a cross-sectional quantitative survey. The study was approved by the Ethics Committee of the Faculty of Human Nutrition and Consumer Science, Warsaw University of Life Sciences, in Poland on the 29 October 2018 (Resolution No. 22/2018). Informed consent to participate in the study was collected from participants.

According to the study design, recruitment and data collection were conducted by a research agency—ARC Market and Opinion. Adults aged 18–65 were recruited from the panel (epanel.pl) of approximately 64,000 adults. After sending an invitation to participate in the study, 2025 people gave their consent to participate in the study. Quota selection using gender, age, place of residence, and education was used to ensure the representativeness of the Polish population. During the recruitment, 78 people stopped filling out the questionnaire during the interview, and 932 people did not qualify due to filling the quota, while eight people were removed from the database at the collection control stage because of errors indicating the lack of credibility of their answers. As a result, the study consisted of 1007 participants. The computer-assisted web interviewing (CAWI) technique was used to collect all data. During the data check, 71 participants were excluded from the sample due to missing data, i.e., body mass and height, which did not allow calculation of the BMI. Then, during the data analysis, one more criterion of exclusion was used, namely being underweight (body mass index (BMI) < 18.5 kg/m^2). Thirty-eight participants were excluded from the analyses due to BMI lower than 18.5 kg/m^2. The total sample consisted of 898 people.

2.2. Food Intake Variety

Food intake variety was assessed using the food consumption frequency method, applying Food Intake Variety Questionnaire (FIVeQ) [36]. Information on the consumption of 63 food product groups over the last 7 days was collected using the FIVeQ questionnaire [36]. Quantity was specified for each product: seven slices for cereal products, seven cups for dairy and beverages with the exception of wine (quantity defined as 1 glass of wine—100 mL) and spirits (one shot of liquor—50 mL), amount sufficient for one slice of bread well covered (approx. 20 g) for cold cuts and sausages, 10 cubes for chocolate, and two tablespoons for the rest of the food products (e.g., groats, nuts, fish, and butter). The participant declared the consumption of such quantity of each product within the last 7 days (Yes/No). Food intake variety is expressed in the food intake variety index (FIVeI). FIVeI was calculated as the number of product groups eaten weekly (maximum 60 products/week) after excluding 3 groups of alcoholic beverages (beer, wine, vodka, and other strong alcohols). According to the methodology and assessment criteria developed by the authors of the questionnaire [35], the following four groups of people with a varied food intake (FIV) were distinguished:

Inadequate FIV (<20 food products weekly)
Sufficient FIV (20–29 food products weekly)
Good FIV (30–39 food products weekly)
Very good FIV (≥40 food products weekly)

2.3. Eating Addiction

Eating Preoccupation Scale (EPS) was used to assess eating addiction [37]. EPS consists of 18 statements, to which the respondent answers on a scale of 1—hardly/never; 2—rarely; 3—sometimes; 4—often; up to 5—almost/always (Table 1). This scale allows measuring an overall score of eating addiction and three EPS factors, which include focusing on eating activities; eating to provide pleasure and mood improvement; and compulsion to eat and loss of control over food. The overall score (range from 18 to 90 points), which was the sum of all ratings, allows evaluating a person's behavioral characteristics for eating addiction (EA) included in EPS. A score above 48 points indicates a high EA, 40–48 points an average EA, and below 40 points a low EA [37].

Table 1. The Eating Preoccupation Scale (EPS).

Statements from the Eating Preoccupation Scale (EPS)	Mean Score ± Standard Deviation *
EPS factor: Focusing on eating activities	
2. I think about eating and about my body weight	3.0 ± 1.2
6. I believe that my relationship with food is terrible	2.3 ± 1.1
8. I feel embarrassed about the amount of food I eat	2.2 ± 1.1
9. I plan ahead for situations when I will be able to eat alone	1.9 ± 1.0
10. I am worried about being unable to control the amount of food consumed	2.3 ± 1.1
16. I have a low self-esteem because of my uncontrolled eating	2.1 ± 1.1
EPS factor: Eating to provide pleasure and mood improvement	
1. Eating is a very important part of my life	3.4 ± 1.1
11. Eating greatly enhances my mood	3.2 ± 1.0
12. Eating is a great pleasure of mine	3.6 ± 1.0
13. I make myself "food feasts" for no clear reason	2.2 ± 1.1
17. I feel great satisfaction after an abundant meal	2.8 ± 1.1
18. I am willing to sacrifice other pleasures for eating	2.3 ± 1.0
EPS factor: Compulsion to eat and loss of control over food	
3. I eat vast amounts of high-calorie foods in a short period of time	2.6 ± 1.0
4. I snack throughout the day	2.9 ± 1.0
5. I eat even when I am not feeling hunger	2.4 ± 1.0
7. I eat more than I had planned	2.7 ± 1.0
14. I wake up to eat at night	1.8 ± 1.0
15. I clear up my plate even when I am not feeling hungry anymore	2.9 ± 1.2

* 5-point scale: 1—hardly/never; 2—rarely, 3—sometimes, 4—often, 5—almost/always.

The internal compliance of the questionnaire was assessed using Cronbach's coefficient, which was 0.89. Internal stability, measured using a correlation coefficient in studies conducted after 6 weeks on a group of 30 women, was 0.72. Validity of the Eating Preoccupation Scale was tested by assessing the correlation of its results with the results of the Eating Related Behaviors Questionnaire [37], which measures the tendency toward habitual and emotional overeating, but also following dietary restrictions.

2.4. Physical Activity and Other Lifestyle Factors

Self-reported physical activity was recorded in the questionnaire on a 3-point scale: 1—"low", 2—"moderate", and 3—"high" [38]. The description of the scale was presented separately for physical activity during leisure and work/school time. For leisure time, "low" was described as "sedentary lifestyle, watching TV, reading the press, books, light housework, taking a walk for 1–2 h a week"; "moderate"—"walks, cycling, gymnastics, gardening or other light physical activity performed for 2–3 h a week ", and "high"—"cycling, running, working on a plot or garden, and other sports activities requiring physical effort, taking up more than 3 h a week". "Low" activity at work/school time was described as "over 70% of the time in a sitting position", "moderate" as "approximately 50% of the time in a sitting position and about 50% of time moving", and "high" as "about 70% of the time in motion or doing physical work associated with a lot of effort" [38].

Two questions were used to assess smoking: *"Do you smoke cigarettes?"* (Yes/No) and *"If you smoke, how many cigarettes a day do you smoke?"* (I smoke occasionally; up to 10 a day, 10–20 a day, more than 20 a day). In addition, respondents answered the question *"Have you followed a special diet in the last 3 months?"* (Yes/No).

2.5. Sociodemographic Characteristics

The questionnaire collected information about sociodemographic characteristics of the study sample, i.e., gender, age, education, and place of residence. Body mass index (BMI) was calculated using self-reported body weight and height and categorized according to International Obesity Task Force (IOTF) standards [39]. During the data analysis, three categories of respondents were identified, i.e., people with normal weight (BMI between 18.5 and 24.99 kg/m^2), overweight (BMI between 25.0 and 29.99 kg/m^2), and obesity (BMI $\geq$ 30 kg/m^2).

2.6. Statistical Analysis

Descriptive statistics were performed. The chi-square test and the one-way analysis of variance ANOVA test were used to compare variables, and $p < 0.05$ was considered significant.

The classification tree was used to determine independent variables explaining differences in food intake variety. This method was used because it allows computing both numerical and categorical data. Moreover, it offers clear graphic data presentation and is easy to interpret [40]. Separate classification trees were made in the study sample, and then in a group of people with normal body weight, overweight, and obesity. The method CHAID (chi-squared automatic interaction detector) was used to build the tree. The first node (node 0) is always the distribution of the dependent variable (FIV). The next nodes can include sociodemographic variables (gender, age, education, place of residence), variables describing eating addiction (eating addiction—overall score, three factors of eating addiction: focusing on eating activities, eating to provide pleasure and mood improvement, compulsion to eat and loss of control over food) and lifestyle variables (following a diet, smoking, physical activity during leisure time, and work/school time).

Statistical analysis was conducted using IBM SPSS Statistics for Windows, version 24.0 (IBM Corp, Armonk, NY, USA).

3. Results

3.1. Characteristics of the Study Sample

The sample consisted of 898 participants (433 women and 465 men) aged 18 to 65 years. Some details concerning sociodemographic characteristics of the study sample are displayed in Table 1.

More men than women were overweight or obese. Among people with normal weight the majority were people of the age of 18–34, while among overweight and people with obesity respondents aged 45–65 were the most numerous in this group. The average age of people with overweight and obesity did not differ, but was significantly higher compared to people with normal body weight. Education and place of residence did not differentiate groups identified according to BMI (Table 2).

3.2. Food Intake Variety and Other Lifestyle Factors

About 60% of the study sample displayed good or very good food intake variety (36.8% and 23.7%, respectively). FIV did not differ in BMI groups (Table 3).

Slightly more than 10% of participants declared following a diet. Almost two-thirds of the study participants (64.0%) declared they did not smoke. In the study sample, there were less heavy smokers (10 or more cigarettes a day) than light smokers (16.6% and 19.4%, respectively). About two-fifths of the study sample (38.3%) described their physical activity at work/school as low, and the same numbers of people evaluated their leisure activities in the same way. More than one-half of people with BMI $\geq$ 30 kg/m^2 (57.6%) declared low physical activity in leisure time. More people with overweight than ones with normal body weight indicated low activity in leisure time (37.7% and 32.8%, respectively) (Table 3).

3.3. Eating Addiction

Over two-fifths of study sample (42.1%) displayed a high eating addiction (EA) on the EPS. The mean value of the overall score from the EPS was 46.4 points, which indicates the average EA. Only differences in the overall score of EPS between people with normal weight and people with obesity were shown. The mean value of the overall score in the obese group exceeded 48 points and, therefore, meant a high EA. Low EA was displayed by 33.7% of people with normal body weight and by almost three times less of those with obesity (13.1%). However, a high EA was found in more than half of the people with obesity (54.2%) and in more than one-third of people with normal body weight (37.7%). Compulsive eating and loss of control of food consumption characterized eating behaviors of people with obesity to a higher extent compared to people with normal body weight. There were differences in the mean score for the "Focusing on eating activities" factor in the BMI groups. The larger the BMI, the more people were focused on eating behaviors were (Table 4).

3.4. Relationship between Food Intake Variety and Eating Addiction

Food intake variety (FIV) has shown differences only due to EPS factor "Eating to provide pleasure and mood improvement" (Figure 1). In the group of people with high or moderate physical activity at leisure time and at work/school time, a higher score for the EPS factor "Eating to provide pleasure and mood improvement" (above 18 points) favored an increase in FIV (nodes 7 and 8). Almost two-fifths of people with a score above 18 had very good FIV. Similarly, in the group of people with low physical activity at leisure time (nodes 5 and 6), a higher score for this EPS factor (above 16 points) was conducive to a greater variety of food intake (Figure 1).

In the group of people with obesity, the score of EPS factor "Eating to provide pleasure and mood improvement" was the most powerful predictor for FIV (nodes 1 and 2). A higher score for this EPS factor (above 16 points) was conducive to a greater variety of food intake. Almost three times more people with a score above 16 (29.5%) than with a score of 16 and below (10.3%) had a very good FIV (Figure 2).

3.5. Relationship between Food Intake Variety and Lifestyle and Sociodemographic Variables

In the study group, FIV has shown differences due to physical activity at leisure time (nodes 1 and 2) and physical activity at work/school (nodes 3 and 4), —as seen in Figure 1. Higher FIV was demonstrated in people with moderate and high physical activity at leisure time ($p < 0.001$). Over one-quarter of people (27.6%) with moderate or high physical activity and 17.7% of those with low physical activity at leisure time were characterized by very good FIV. Twice as many people with low physical activity in their leisure time were characterized by inadequate FIV compared to other people. Twice as many people with high and moderate physical activity in leisure time and the same physical activity at work/school showed very good FIV (32.5%) compared to people with low physical activity at work/school (15.5%) (nodes 3 and 4) (Figure 1).

In the group of people with overweight (nodes 1 and 2), more people with secondary education than the other categories had good FIV (46.8%, 34.9%, respectively) and very good FIV (29.4%, 22.2%, respectively) (Figure 3).

In people with normal body weight, FIV differed among age groups (nodes 1, 2, and 3). The number of people aged 18–24 was the least when it came to showing very good FIV (8.3%), while most people aged 55–65 (31.8%). More than two-thirds of people aged 18–24 had inadequate FIV (11.1%) or sufficient FIV (56.9%). By contrast, more than three-quarters of people aged 25–54 years were characterized by good (40.9%) or very good FIV (25.5%). In this age group (nodes 4 and 5) more people with moderate or high physical activity in leisure time than others had good (44.4%, 34.3%, respectively) and very good (29.9%, 17.2%, respectively) FIV (Figure 4).

Table 2. Characteristics of the study sample.

Variables		Total (N = 898)		18.5 kg/m² ≤ BMI < 25 kg/m² (N = 424)		25.0 kg/m² ≤ BMI < 30 kg/m² (N = 321)		BMI ≥ 30 kg/m² (N = 153)	
		N	%	N	%	N	%	N	%
Gender *	Female	433	48.2	234	55.2	131	40.8	68	44.4
	Male	465	51.8	190	44.8	190	59.2	85	55.6
Education	Lower than secondary	348	38.8	153	36.1	123	38.3	72	47.1
	Secondary	309	34.4	153	36.1	109	34.0	47	30.7
	Higher	241	26.8	118	27.8	89	27.7	34	22.2
Place of residence	Rural area	329	36.6	159	37.5	113	35.2	57	37.3
	City ≤ 100,000 residents	291	32.4	140	33.0	106	33.0	45	29.4
	City > 100,000 residents	278	31.0	125	29.5	102	31.8	51	33.3
Age *	18–24 years	97	10.8	72	17.0	18	5.6	7	4.6
	25–34 years	205	22.8	117	27.6	62	19.3	26	17.0
	35–44 years	209	23.3	105	24.8	67	20.9	37	24.2
	45–54 years	168	18.7	64	15.1	70	21.8	34	22.2
	55–65 years	219	24.4	66	15.5	104	32.4	49	32.0
Age (years)	Mean; standard deviation	42.0; 13.7		38.0 ᵃ; 13.3		45.6 ᵇ; 13.1		45.5 ᵇ; 12.9	
Height (cm)	Mean; standard deviation	171.4; 9.5		170.8 ᵃ; 9.1		172.4 ᵃ; 9.6		170.8 ᵃ; 9.9	
Weight (kg)	Mean; standard deviation	76.6; 15.8		65.7 ᵃ; 9.2		81.0 ᵇ; 10.2		97.6 ᶜ; 13.8	
BMI (kg/m²)	Mean; standard deviation	26.0; 4.5		22.4 ᵃ; 1.8		27.2 ᵇ; 1.4		33.4 ᶜ; 3.6	

N—number of participants; * Significant at $p < 0.001$ between BMI groups (chi-square test); ᵃ,ᵇ,ᶜ Different letters in each line indicate significant differences at $p < 0.05$ between BMI groups (ANOVA test).

Table 3. Food intake variety and other lifestyle characteristics of the study sample.

Variables		Total Sample (N = 898)		18.5 kg/m² ≤ BMI < 25 kg/m² (N = 424)		25.0 kg/m² ≤ BMI < 30 kg/m² (N = 321)		BMI ≥ 30 kg/m² (N = 153)	
		N	%	N	%	N	%	N	%
Food intake variety—FIV	inadequate	79	8.8	38	9.0	25	7.8	16	10.5
	sufficient	276	30.7	139	32.7	92	28.7	45	29.4
	good	330	36.8	147	34.7	125	38.9	58	37.9
	very good	213	23.7	100	23.6	79	24.6	34	22.2
Following a diet	yes	97	10.9	42	10.0	37	11.6	18	12.0
Number of cigarettes smoked **	no smoking	575	64.0	266	62.7	223	69.5	86	56.2
	less than 10 cigarettes a day	174	19.4	91	21.5	56	17.4	27	17.6
	10 or more cigarettes a day	149	16.6	67	15.8	42	13.1	40	26.2
Physical activity during work/school time	low	329	38.3	137	34.3	123	39.4	69	47.3
	moderate	329	38.3	158	39.5	120	38.5	51	34.9
	high	200	23.4	105	26.2	69	22.1	26	17.8
Physical activity during leisure time ***	low	344	38.8	137	32.8	120	37.7	87	57.6
	moderate	415	46.8	208	49.8	153	48.1	54	35.8
	high	128	14.4	73	17.4	45	14.2	10	6.6
Food intake variety—FIV (number of products)	Mean; standard deviation	32.6; 10.7		32.4 a; 10.6		33.0 a; 10.5		32.6 a; 11.3	

N—number of participants; ** Significant at $p < 0.01$; *** Significant at $p < 0.001$ between BMI groups (chi-square test). a Having the same letter means no significant differences at $p < 0.05$ between groups (ANOVA test).

Table 4. Eating addiction in the study sample.

Variables		Total Sample (N = 898)		18.5 kg/m² ≤ BMI < 25 kg/m² (N = 424)		25.0 kg/m² ≤ BMI < 30 kg/m² (N = 321)		BMI ≥ 30 kg/m² (N = 153)	
		N	%	N	%	N	%	N	%
Eating Preoccupation Scale (EPS)—total score ***	low	237	26.4	143	33.7	74	23.1	20	13.1
	average	283	31.5	121	28.6	112	34.8	50	32.7
	high	378	42.1	160	37.7	135	42.1	83	54.2
Eating Preoccupation Scale (EPS)—total score	Mean; standard deviation	46.4; 11.0		45.2 [a]; 11.6		46.7 [a,b]; 10.6		49.1 [b]; 9.9	
EPS factor: Focus on eating activities	Mean; standard deviation	13.7; 4.8		12.9 [a]; 5.0		13.8 [b]; 4.6		15.5 [c]; 4.1	
EPS factor: Eating to provide pleasure and mood improvement	Mean; standard deviation	17.5; 4.4		17.5 [a]; 4.5		17.6 [a]; 4.2		17.5 [a]; 4.3	
EPS factor: Compulsion to eat and loss of control over food	Mean; standard deviation	15.2; 4.2		14.8 [a]; 4.4		15.3 [a,b]; 4.1		16.1 [b]; 3.9	

N—number of participants; *** Significant at $p < 0.001$ between BMI groups (chi-square test). [a,b,c] Different letters in each line mean significant differences at $p < 0.05$ between groups (ANOVA test).

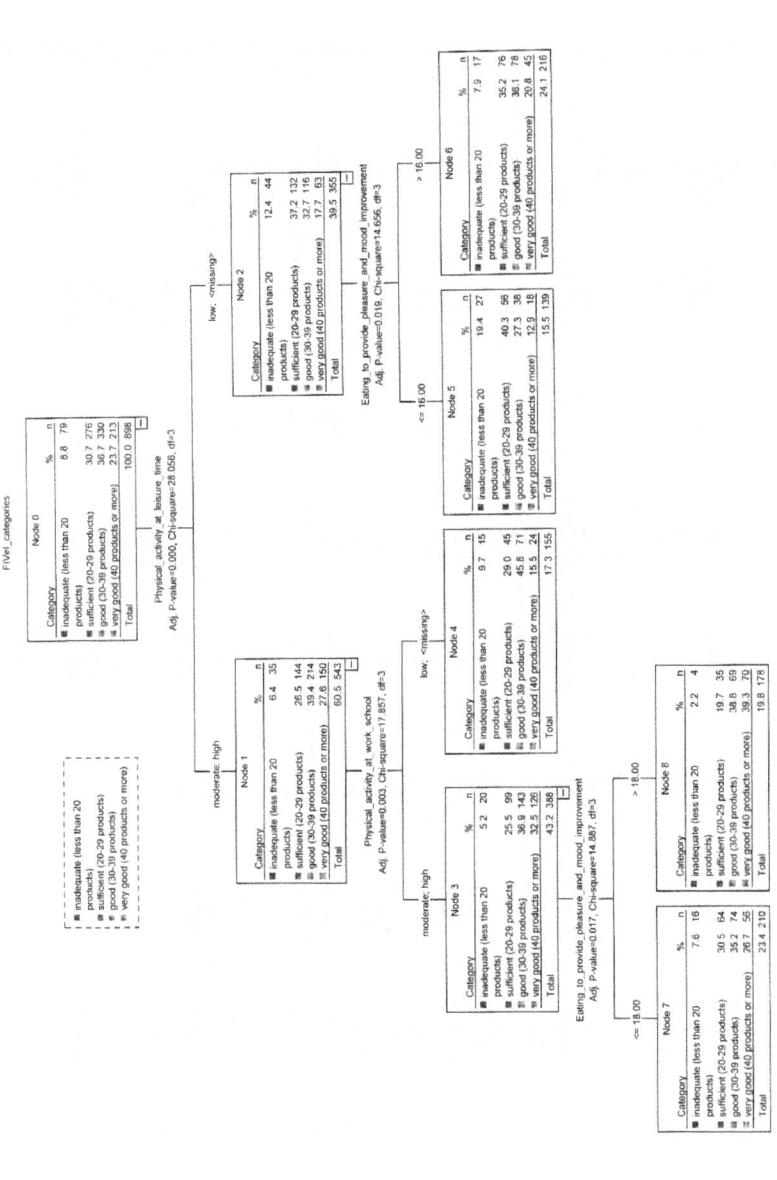

Figure 1. Relationship between food intake variety, eating addiction, selected lifestyles variables and sociodemographic characteristics in the study sample.

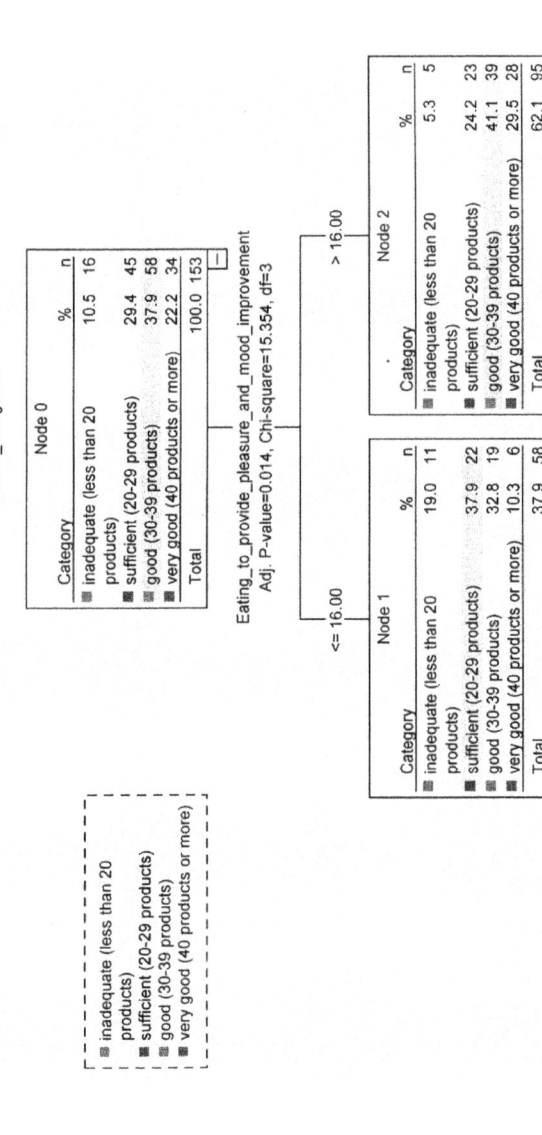

Figure 2. Relationship between food intake variety, eating addiction, selected lifestyles variables and sociodemographic characteristics in the group with obesity.

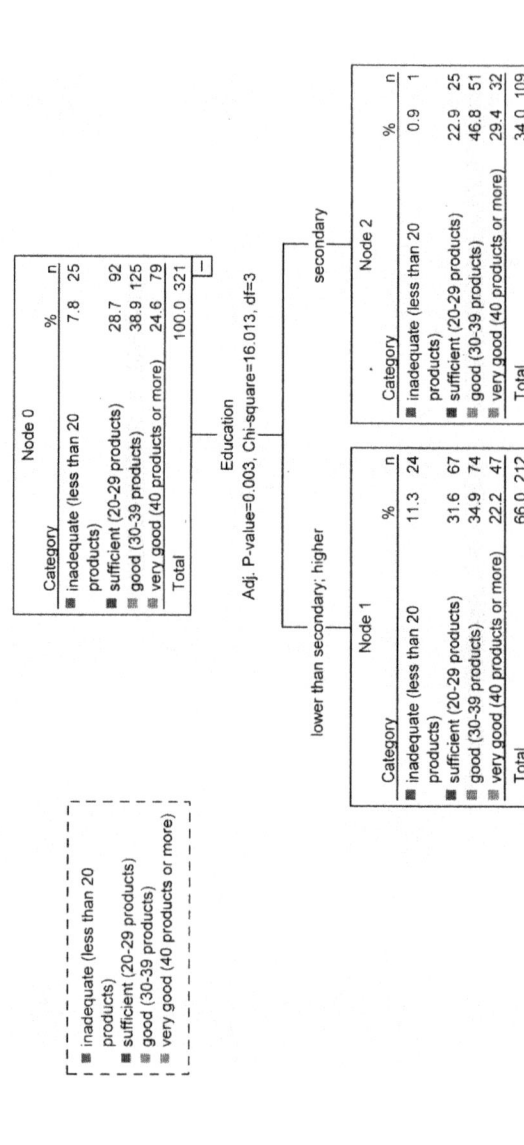

Figure 3. Relationship between food intake variety, eating addiction, selected lifestyles variables and sociodemographic characteristics in the group with overweight.

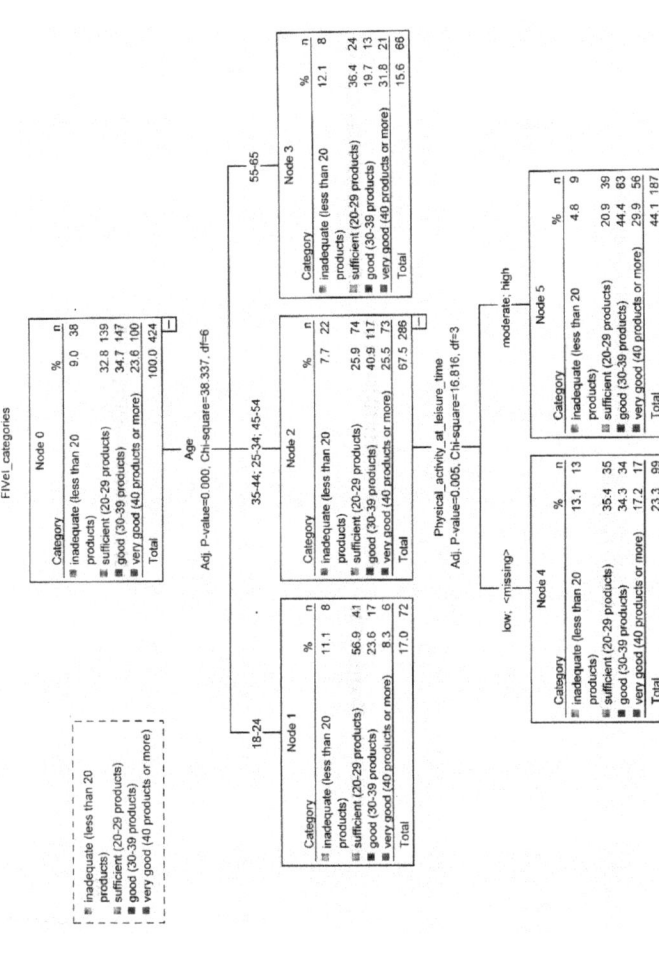

Figure 4. Relationship between food intake variety, eating addiction, selected lifestyles variables, and sociodemographic characteristics in the group with normal body weight.

4. Discussion

The study provided some support for our hypotheses that differences in food intake variety (FIV) can be explained by eating addiction assessed using the Eating Preoccupation Scale (EPS). The results concerning associations between FIV and EPS indicate that only one of the EPS factors, "Eating to provide pleasure and mood improvement", was related to FIV. Moreover, this indicator did not serve as the most important predictor of FIV, as physical activity during leisure time explained this parameter in a greater manner. Other EPS factors and total EPS did not differentiate FIV. In view of the previous research, it can be assumed that "Eating to provide pleasure and mood improvement" as a factor correlated with FIV might favor both overall dietary variety and dietary variety within particular food groups only. Few available studies, which attempted to explain differences in food intake variety, indicate that this parameter might be linked to the amount of food consumed with regard to selected foods [13,41]. People with overeating tendencies usually opt for a wide range of food products, yet it only applies to products considered as palatable. Thus, a wide range of palatable foods might be a factor involved in the development of addictive-like eating behaviors [42]. Other authors also point out that not all foods seem to be equally related to addictive-like eating behaviors. Foods rich in refined carbohydrates and added fat are more likely to be consumed in an addictive manner than low-processed foods [43,44]. High-fat and high-sugar foods were consumed more frequently among individuals who met the criteria of the Yale Food Addiction Scale for food addiction [13]. These foods also appear to trigger behavioral responses that are consistent with addictive-like eating behavior, for example such foods are frequently consumed during binge episodes [45]. Moreover, foods high in fat and sugar are more likely to be intensely craved [41,46,47] and consumed in greater quantities in response to negative affect [48,49]. The results of these studies are consistent with those obtained in our research among people with obesity. Within this group, the EPS factor "Eating to provide pleasure and mood improvement" was the most important factor in explaining FIV. Almost three times more people with a higher score of this EPS factor were characterized by higher FIV in comparison to people scoring lower on this subscale. It might be considered as a cause of overconsumption though longitudinal research is required to determine the direction of causality.

Our hypothesis was also supported, that EPS explains the differences in FIV to a lesser extent than some components of lifestyle (i.e., physical activity, following a diet, smoking) but the importance of these factors may vary depending on BMI. Physical activity at leisure time was the most important predictor of FIV in the study sample, while in the groups distinguished by BMI, differences in FIV predictors were observed. Greater food intake variety (FIV) correlated with moderate or high physical activity during leisure time, which may be the result of higher awareness of healthy lifestyle, healthier food choices, and greater adherence to dietary rules among physically active people [50,51]. Similarly as for the whole study group, the association between food intake variety (FIV) and physical activity in leisure time was supported among individuals with normal body weight aged 25–54, and greater FIV was observed in those more physically active within this age group. According to our best knowledge, an association between FIV and physical activity has not been the subject of previous research. Nevertheless, some studies have shown that physical activity favors healthier food choices among adults [52–54]. However, a few studies have revealed that being physically active might not always determine healthy eating nor prevent unfavorable eating behaviors [55]. On the premise that FIV might be linked to both health benefits and the higher intake of unhealthy foods, our results indicating that greater FIV is observed among physically active people is supported by previous studies.

Higher levels of physical activity observed in individuals presenting eating addiction symptoms might be caused by an attempt to make up for the excessive amount of calories consumed through exercise [56]. Physically active people are able to self-regulate food intake more precisely due to the effect of working out in lowering the reactivity of the brain reward system to food stimuli [57]. Moreover, among individuals in the group of moderate or high physical activity, both in leisure or school/work time, a positive correlation was seen for the result of "Eating to provide pleasure and mood improvement" subscale and FIV, which can be linked to self-contentment associated with satisfaction from living a healthy lifestyle, beneficial for health and wellbeing. A similar correlation was noted in the group with low physical activity in leisure time. It seems that low physical activity can induce food cravings in a manner resembling an addiction mechanism [58]. In those individuals, food can serve as a major source of pleasure, since sedentary behaviors favor food consumption. This association was not seen for the eating addiction total score in our study, and these results are supported by Li et al. [56].

Sociodemographic features as predictors of FIV were noticed only in groups separated due to BMI. Food intake variety in individuals with normal body weight was associated with age, which can be confirmed by previous research. Due to involutional processes along with environmental and psychological factors, older people tend to change their eating habits, which leads to lower calorie as well as macro- and micronutrient intake. Inadequate intake of nutrients increases the risk of malnutrition [59,60]. Greater FIV among older adults in our study, including having the largest number of very good FIV and, at the same time, the largest number of inadequate FIV, indicates that the recommendations on dietary diversity in older people [35,60] are being partly fulfilled. Higher FIV in older people was also noted by Drewnowski et al. [61].

The age was not associated with food intake variety in individuals with overweight and obesity. However, people with overweight with secondary education had greater FIV than the others. The impact of education on FIV in people with overweight may be explained in different ways. Environment, awareness of physical activity, dietary knowledge, and health literacy as well as social roles and cultural norms related to health and nutrition seem to be significant factors affecting this correlation [62]. Among people with lower educational status, a less varied diet might be linked to their living environment with limited access to more diverse and affordable fresh foods, but also to other components of a healthy lifestyle, including safe places for physical activity. On the other hand, alcohol, tobacco, and fast-food might be more accessible, which are conducive to a high-calorie diet combined with sedentary behaviors [63]. By contrast, people with higher education are expected to have more opportunities for being physically active, but also greater access to diverse food products. Educational status might be considerably associated with salary, and thus influence food choices and food variety [64,65]. Moreover, higher educated people should be more predisposed to favoring new or unfamiliar foods [66]. Nonetheless, the above possible explanations and mechanisms involving dietary knowledge and health literacy [67,68] cannot explain the results revealed in our study indicating that among those in the overweight group, people with higher education had lower FIV than individuals with secondary education. Despite having greater nutrition knowledge, more highly educated individuals might conform more to cultural norms, e.g., the thin ideal, which is often perceived as a condition of success [69]. Some authors suggested that body weight dissatisfaction might serve as a driver for unhealthy dieting behaviors [70,71]. It can be assumed that in our study sample, overweight people with higher education could have been particularly susceptible to social norms which, in turn, led to following a strict dietary regimen, thus resulting in lower FIV [70,71].

Strengths and Limitations

The strength of our study is its relatively large sample, representative of the Polish population in terms of the region of residence, gender, education, and age. Although our findings are specific to the Polish population and should not be generalized to populations of other cultural backgrounds, the observations could be of potential use in designing research and interventions. The analysis of relationships between eating addiction and lifestyle elements of great importance for health, i.e., diet (dietary variety and following a diet), and physical activity brought a wider perspective on adequate diet. To the best of our knowledge, this paper is the first to study the association between eating addiction and food intake variety. The use of the hitherto unknown Eating Preoccupation Scale can be considered as both a strength and a weakness. On the one hand, it may be noticed by other researchers and recognized as a tool that deserves further use. On the other hand, the use of this scale is a limitation of our study. The measure of eating addiction used in the present study (EPS) has not been extensively used and there is a need for additional research on its psychometric properties and its association with measures of related constructs such as food addiction, emotional eating, and binge eating. Additionally, this cross-sectional study design does not provide an opportunity to find a causal relationship between food intake variety and other variables. Some limitations are related to the potential biases that may occur when self-reported data are analyzed [72]. People tend to underreport their weight and overreport their body height [73], which may have led to underestimation of individuals with excessive body weight according to the BMI categories in our research. Self-reported indicators of lifestyle can be considered not quite satisfying, however, and using other measurement indicators confirms the results from the analysis of self-reported data [74].

5. Conclusions

The study found that food intake variety (FIV) was associated with physical activity at leisure time, and then with the EPS factor "Eating to provide pleasure and mood improvement", whereas sociodemographic characteristics were predictors of FIV only within groups determined by BMI. In the study sample, physical activity both at leisure and at work/school time proved to be a stronger predictor than the EPS factor related to pleasure and mood. However, the EPS factor "Eating to provide pleasure and mood improvement" was the only predictor of FIV among people with obesity. Sociodemographic characteristics differentiated FIV only within the group with normal body weight (age) and with overweight (education). Based on the findings of this study, it is possible to better understand the relationships between food intake variety and some components of lifestyle, including addictive behaviors. Moreover, additional focus on the groups identified by BMI and the performed analysis will allow the results to be used in dietary practice. However, there is still a need for further research involving the use of tools that can identify the "eating addiction" construct. Symptoms of eating addiction might serve as a marker of disordered eating, while early diagnosis can significantly affect both prevention and treatment of overweight and obesity. Further research attempting to clarify the association between FIV and EA should use also other tools to explicitly explain this correlation.

Author Contributions: M.P. and M.J.-Z. made substantial contributions to the study conception and design; M.P. was involved in the data acquisition; M.J.-Z. analyzed the data; M.J.-Z. and A.M. interpreted the data and wrote the manuscript; M.J.-Z., M.P., and A.M. were involved in critically revising the manuscript, and have given their approval to the manuscript submitted. All authors have read and agreed to the published version of the manuscript.

Funding: This research was funded by Polish Ministry of Science and Higher Education within funds of Faculty of Human Nutrition and Consumer Sciences, Warsaw University of Life Sciences (WULS), for scientific research, grant number 505-10-102500-Q00306-99.

Acknowledgments: We wish to thank all our study participants for their participation.

Conflicts of Interest: The authors declare no conflicts of interest.

References

1. Elmadfa, I.; Meyer, A. Developing Suitable Methods of Nutritional Status Assessment: A Continuous Challenge. *Adv. Nutr.* **2014**, *5*, 590S–598S. [CrossRef] [PubMed]
2. Schulze, M.; Martínez-González, M.; Fung, T.; Lichtenstein, A.; Forouhi, N. Food based dietary patterns and chronic disease prevention. *BMJ* **2018**, *361*, k2396. [CrossRef] [PubMed]
3. Blair, S.N.; Hand, G.A.; Hill, J.O. Energy balance: A crucial issue for exercise and sports medicine. *Br. J. Sports Med.* **2015**, *49*, 970–971. [CrossRef] [PubMed]
4. Hobbs, M.; Pearson, N.; Foster, P.J.; Biddle, S.J. Sedentary behaviour and diet across the lifespan: An updated systematic review. *Br. J. Sports Med.* **2014**, *49*, 1179–1188. [CrossRef]
5. Compernolle, S.; De Cocker, K.; Teixeira, P.J.; Oppert, J.-M.; Roda, C.; Mackenbach, J.D.; Lakerveld, J.; McKee, M.; Glonti, K.; Rutter, H.; et al. The associations between domain-specific sedentary behaviours and dietary habits in European adults: A cross-sectional analysis of the SPOTLIGHT survey. *BMC Public Health* **2016**, *16*, 1057. [CrossRef]

6. Schultchen, D.; Reichenberger, J.; Mittl, T.; Weh, T.R.M.; Smyth, J.M.; Blechert, J.; Pollatos, O. Bidirectional relationship of stress and affect with physical activity and healthy eating. *Br. J. Health Psychol.* **2019**, *24*, 315–333. [CrossRef]
7. Devonport, T.J.; Nicholls, W.; Fullerton, C. A systematic review of the association between emotions and eating behaviour in normal and overweight adult populations. *J. Health Psychol.* **2019**, *24*, 3–24. [CrossRef]
8. Dohle, S.; Hartmann, C.; Keller, C. Physical activity as a moderator of the association between emotional eating and BMI: Evidence from the Swiss Food Panel. *Psychol. Health* **2014**, *29*, 1062–1080. [CrossRef]
9. Gearhardt, A.N.; Corbin, W.R.; Brownell, K.D. Food addiction: An examination of the diagnostic criteria for dependence. *J. Addict. Med.* **2009**, *3*, 1–7. [CrossRef]
10. Gearhardt, A.N.; Corbin, W.R.; Brownell, K.D. Preliminary validation of the Yale Food Addiction Scale. *Appetite* **2009**, *52*, 430–436. [CrossRef]
11. Gearhardt, A.N.; Corbin, W.R.; Brownell, K.D. Development of the Yale Food Addiction Scale Version 2.0. *Psychol Addict. Behav.* **2016**, *30*, 113–121. [CrossRef] [PubMed]
12. Ayaz, A.; Nergiz-Unal, R.; Dedebayraktar, D.; Akyol, A.; Pekcan, A.G.; Besler, H.T.; Buyuktuncer, Z. How does food addiction influence dietary intake profile? *PLoS ONE* **2018**, *13*, e0195541. [CrossRef] [PubMed]
13. Pursey, K.; Collins, C.; Stanwell, P.; Burrows, T. Foods and dietary profiles associated with 'food addiction' in young adults. *Addict. Behav. Rep.* **2015**, *2*, 41–48. [CrossRef] [PubMed]
14. Pedram, P.; Sun, G. Hormonal and dietary characteristics in obese human subjects with and without food addiction. *Nutrients* **2014**, *7*, 223–238. [CrossRef]
15. Burrows, T.; Hides, L.; Brown, R.; Dayas, C.V.; Kay-Lambkin, F. Differences in Dietary Preferences, Personality and Mental Health in Australian Adults with and without Food Addiction. *Nutrients* **2017**, *9*, 285. [CrossRef]
16. Küçükerdönmez, Ö.; Urhan, M.; Altın, M.; Hacıraifoğlu, Ö.; Yıldız, B. Assessment of the relationship between food addiction and nutritional status in schizophrenic patients. *Nutr. Neurosci.* **2019**, *22*, 392–400. [CrossRef]
17. Linardon, J. The relationship between dietary restraint and binge eating: Examining eating-related self-efficacy as a moderator. *Appetite* **2018**, *127*, 126–129. [CrossRef]
18. Denny, K.N.; Loth, K.; Eisenberg, M.E.; Neumark-Sztainer, D. Intuitive eating in young adults. Who is doing it, and how is it related to disordered eating behaviors? *Appetite* **2013**, *60*, 13–19. [CrossRef]
19. Paans, N.; Gibson-Smith, D.; Bot, M.; van Strien, T.; Brouwer, I.; Visser, M.; Penninx, B. Depression and eating styles are independently associated with dietary intake. *Appetite* **2019**, *134*, 103–110. [CrossRef]
20. Camilleri, G.; Méjean, C.; Kesse-Guyot, E.; Andreeva, V.; Bellisle, F.; Hercberg, S.; Péneau, S. The Associations between Emotional Eating and Consumption of Energy-Dense Snack Foods Are Modified by Sex and Depressive Symptomatology. *J. Nutr.* **2014**, *144*, 1264–1273. [CrossRef]
21. Konttinen, H.; Männistö, S.; Sarlio-Lähteenkorva, S.; Silventoinen, K.; Haukkala, A. Emotional eating, depressive symptoms and self-reported food consumption. A population-based study. *Appetite* **2010**, *54*, 473–479. [CrossRef] [PubMed]
22. van Strien, T.; Cebolla, A.; Etchemendy, E.; Gutiérrez-Maldonado, J.; Ferrer-García, M.; Botella, C.; Baños, R. Emotional eating and food intake after sadness and joy. *Appetite* **2013**, *66*, 20–25. [CrossRef] [PubMed]
23. Cleobury, L.; Tapper, K. Reasons for eating 'unhealthy' snacks in overweight and obese males and females. *J. Hum. Nutr. Diet.* **2013**, *27*, 333–341. [CrossRef] [PubMed]
24. Lluch, A.; Herbeth, B.; Méjean, L.; Siest, G. Dietary intakes, eating style and overweight in the Stanislas Family Study. *Int. J. Obes.* **2000**, *24*, 1493–1499. [CrossRef] [PubMed]
25. Klesges, R.C.; Isbell, T.R.; Klesges, L.M. Relationship between dietary restraint, energy intake, physical activity, and body weight: A prospective analysis. *J. Abnorm. Psychol.* **1992**, *101*, 668–674. [CrossRef]
26. van Strien, T.; Konttinen, H.; Ouwens, M.; van de Laar, F.; Winkens, L. Mediation of emotional and external eating between dieting and food intake or BMI gain in women. *Appetite* **2020**, *145*, 104493. [CrossRef]
27. Houben, K.; Jansen, A. When food becomes an obsession: Overweight is related to food-related obsessive-compulsive behavior. *J. Health Psychol.* **2019**, *24*, 1145–1152. [CrossRef]
28. Vadiveloo, M.; Dixon, L.B.; Parekh, N. Associations between dietary variety and measures of body adiposity: A systematic review of epidemiological studies. *Br. J. Nutr.* **2013**, *109*, 1557–1572. [CrossRef]
29. Hruby, A.; Hu, F.B. The Epidemiology of Obesity: A Big Picture. *Pharmacoeconomics* **2015**, *33*, 673–689. [CrossRef]

30. Bezerra, I.N.; Sichieri, R. Household food diversity and nutritional status among adults in Brazil. *Int. J. Behav. Nutr. Phys. Act.* **2011**, *8*, 22. [CrossRef]
31. Zhang, Q.; Chen, X.; Liu, Z.; Varma, D.S.; Wan, R.; Zhao, S. Diet diversity and nutritional status among adults in southwest China. *PLoS ONE* **2017**, *12*, e0172406. [CrossRef] [PubMed]
32. Keim, N.L.; Forester, S.M.; Lyly, M.; Aaron, G.J.; Townsend, M.S. Vegetable variety is a key to improved diet quality in low-income women in California. *J. Acad. Nutr. Diet.* **2014**, *114*, 430–435. [CrossRef] [PubMed]
33. Azadbakht, L.; Esmaillzadeh, A. Dietary diversity score is related to obesity and abdominal adiposity among Iranian female youth. *Public Health Nutr.* **2011**, *14*, 62–69. [CrossRef] [PubMed]
34. Murphy, S.P.; Foote, J.A.; Wilkens, L.R.; Basiotis, P.P.; Carlson, A.; White, K.K.; Yonemori, K.M. Simple measures of dietary variety are associated with improved dietary quality. *J. Am. Diet. Assoc.* **2006**, *106*, 425–429. [CrossRef]
35. Bernstein, M.A.; Tucker, K.L.; Ryan, N.D.; O'Neill, E.F.; Clements, K.M.; Nelson, M.E.; Evans, W.J.; Fiatarone Singh, M.A. Higher dietary variety is associated with better nutritional status in frail elderly people. *J. Am. Diet. Assoc.* **2002**, *102*, 1096–1104. [CrossRef]
36. Niedzwiedzka, E.; Wadolowska, L. Accuracy Analysis of the Food Intake Variety Questionnaire (FIVeQ). Reproducibility Assessment among Older People. *Pakistan J. Nutr.* **2008**, *7*, 426–435. [CrossRef]
37. Ogińska-Bulik, N. *Osobowość Typu D: Teoria i Badania; Type D Personality*; Theory and Research; Wyd.WSHE: Łódź, Poland, 2009.
38. Beliefs and Eating Habits Questionnaire. Behavioral Conditions of Nutrition Team, Committee of Human Nutrition Science. Polish Academy of Science. Warsaw 2014. Available online: http://www.knozc.pan.pl/ (accessed on 15 October 2018).
39. Cole, T.J.; Lobstein, T. Extended international (IOTF) body mass index cut-offs for thinness, overweight and obesity. *Pediatr. Obes.* **2012**, *7*, 284–294. [CrossRef]
40. James, G.; Witten, D.; Hastie, T.; Tibshirani, R. *An Introduction to Statistical Learning*; Springer: New York, NY, USA, 2015; ISBN 978-1-4614-7137-0.
41. Gilhooly, C.H.; Das, S.K.; Golden, J.K.; McCrory, M.A.; Dallal, G.E.; Saltzman, E.; Kramer, F.M.; Robert, S.B. Food cravings and energy regulation: The characteristics of craved foods and their relationship with eating behaviors and weight change during 6 months of dietary energy restriction. *Int. J. Obes.* **2007**, *31*, 1849–1858. [CrossRef]
42. Hebebrand, J.; Albayrak, Ö.; Adan, R.; Antel, J.; Dieguez, C.; de Jong, J.; Leng, G.; Menzies, J.; Mercer, J.G.; Murphy, M.; et al. "Eating addiction", rather than "food addiction", better captures addictive-like eating behavior. *Neurosci. Biobehav. Rev.* **2014**, *47*, 295–306. [CrossRef]
43. Curtis, C.; Davis, C. A qualitative study of binge eating and obesity from an addiction perspective. *Eat. Disord.* **2014**, *22*, 19–32. [CrossRef]
44. Schulte, E.M.; Avena, N.M.; Gearhardt, A.N. Which foods may Be Addictive? The roles of processing, fat content, and glycemic load. *PLoS ONE* **2015**, *10*, e0117959. [CrossRef] [PubMed]
45. Vanderlinden, J.; Dalle Grave, R.; Vandereycken, W.; Noorduin, C. Which factors do provoke binge-eating? An exploratory study in female students. *Eat. Behav.* **2001**, *2*, 79–83. [CrossRef]
46. Ifland, J.R.; Preuss, H.G.; Marcus, M.T.; Rourke, K.M.; Taylor, W.; Theresa Wright, H. Clearing the confusion around processed food addiction. *J. Am. Coll. Nutr.* **2015**, *34*, 240–243. [CrossRef] [PubMed]
47. White, M.A.; Grilo, C.M. Psychometric properties of the Food Craving Inventory among obese patients with binge eating disorder. *Eat. Behav.* **2005**, *6*, 239–245. [CrossRef]
48. Epel, E.; Lapidus, R.; McEwen, B.; Brownell, K. Stress may add bite to appetite in women: A laboratory study of stress-induced cortisol and eating behavior. *Psychoneuroendocrinology* **2001**, *26*, 37–49. [CrossRef]
49. Zellner, D.A.; Loaiza, S.; Gonzalez, Z.; Pita, J.; Morales, J.; Pecora, D.; Wolf, A. Food selection changes under stress. *Physiol. Behav.* **2006**, *87*, 789–793. [CrossRef]
50. Loprinzi, P.; Smit, E.; Mahoney, S. Physical Activity and Dietary Behavior in US Adults and Their Combined Influence on Health. *Mayo Clin. Proc.* **2014**, *89*, 190–198. [CrossRef]
51. Wadolowska, L.; Kowalkowska, J.; Lonnie, M.; Czarnocinska, J.; Jezewska-Zychowicz, M.; Babicz-Zielinska, E. Associations between physical activity patterns and dietary patterns in a representative sample of Polish girls aged 13–21 years: A cross-sectional study (GEBaHealth Project). *BMC Public Health* **2016**, *16*, 698. [CrossRef]

52. Wammes, B.; French, S.; Brug, J. What young Dutch adults say they do to keep from gaining weight: Self-reported prevalence of overeating, compensatory behaviours and specific weight control behaviours. *Public Health Nutr.* **2007**, *10*, 790–798. [CrossRef]
53. Lee, I.; Djoussé, L.; Sesso, H.D.; Wang, L.; Buring, J.E. Physical activity and weight gain prevention. *JAMA* **2010**, *303*, 1173–1179. [CrossRef]
54. Charreire, H.; Kesse-Guyot, E.; Bertrai, S.; Simon, C.; Chaix, B.; Weber, C.; Touvier, M.; Galan, P.; Hercberg, S.; Oppert, J.-M. Associations between dietary patterns, physical activity (leisure-time and occupational) and television viewing in middle-aged French adults. *Br. J. Nutr.* **2011**, *105*, 902–910. [CrossRef] [PubMed]
55. Kesse-Guyot, E.; Bertrais, S.; Peneau, S.; Estaquio, C.; Dauchet, L.; Vergnaud, A.-C.; Czernichow, S.; Galan, P.; Hercberg, S.; Bellisle, F. Dietary patterns and their sociodemographic and behavioural correlates in French middle-aged adults from the SU.VI.MAX cohort. *Eur. J. Clin. Nutr.* **2009**, *63*, 521–528. [CrossRef] [PubMed]
56. Li, J.T.E.; Pursey, K.M.; Duncan, M.J.; Burrows, T. Addictive Eating and Its Relation to Physical Activity and Sleep Behavior. *Nutrients* **2018**, *10*, 1428. [CrossRef]
57. Luo, S.; O'Connor, S.G.; Belcher, B.R.; Page, K.A. Effects of Physical Activity and Sedentary Behavior on Brain Response to High-Calorie Food Cues in Young Adults. *Obesity* **2018**, *26*, 540–546. [CrossRef] [PubMed]
58. Shook, R.; Hand, G.; Drenowatz, C.; Hebert, J.R.; Paluch, A.E.; Blundell, J.E.; Hill, J.O.; Katzmarzyk, P.T.; Church, T.S.; Blair, S.N. Low levels of physical activity are associated with dysregulation of energy intake and fat mass gain over 1 year. *Am. J. Clin. Nutr.* **2015**, *102*, 1332–1338. [CrossRef] [PubMed]
59. Yannakoulia, M.; Mamalaki, E.; Anastasiou, C.; Mourtzi, N.; Lambrinoudaki, I.; Scarmeas, N. Eating habits and behaviors of older people: Where are we now and where should we go? *Maturitas* **2018**, *114*, 14–21. [CrossRef]
60. Tsujim, T.; Yamamoto, K.; Yamasaki, K.; Hayashi, F.; Momoki, C.; Yasui, Y.; Ohfuji, S.; Fukushima, W.; Habu, D. Lower dietary variety is a relevant factor for malnutrition in older Japanese home-care recipients: A cross-sectional study. *BMC Geriatr.* **2019**, *19*, 197. [CrossRef]
61. Drewnowski, A.; Henderson, S.A.; Driscoll, A.; Rolls, B.J. The Dietary Variety Score: Assessing diet quality in healthy young and older adults. *J. Am. Diet. Assoc.* **1997**, *97*, 266–271. [CrossRef]
62. Morozink Boylan, J.; Cundiff, J.M.; Jakubowski, K.P.; Pardini, D.A.; Matthews, K.A. Pathways Linking Childhood SES and Adult Health Behaviors and Psychological Resources in Black and White Men. *Ann. Behav. Med.* **2018**, *52*, 1023–1035. [CrossRef]
63. Adler, N.E.; Stewart, J. Health disparities across the lifespan: Meaning, methods, and mechanisms. *Ann. NY Acad. Sci.* **2010**, *1186*, 5–23. [CrossRef]
64. Pechey, R.; Monsivais, P. Socioeconomic inequalities in the healthiness of food choices: Exploring the contributions of food expenditures. *Prev. Med.* **2016**, *88*, 203–209. [CrossRef] [PubMed]
65. Worsley, A.; Blaschea, R.; Ball, K.; Crawford, D. The relationship between education and food consumption in the 1995 Australian National Nutrition Survey. *Public Health Nutr.* **2004**, *7*, 649–663. [CrossRef] [PubMed]
66. Eertmans, A.; Baeyens, F.; Van den Bergh, O. Food likes and their relative importance in human eating behavior. Review and preliminary suggestions for health promotion. *Health Educ. Res.* **2001**, *16*, 443–456. [CrossRef] [PubMed]
67. Lumbers, M.; Raats, M. Food choices in later life. In *The Psychology of Food Choice*; Frontiers in Nutritional Sciences; Shepherd, R., Raats, M., Eds.; CABI Publishing: Wallingford, UK, 2006; Volume 3, pp. 280–310.
68. Conklin, A.; Forouhi, N.; Suhrcke, M.; Surtees, P.; Wareham, N.; Monsivais, P. Variety More Than Quantity of Fruit And Vegetable Intake Varies By Socioeconomic Status And Financial Hardship. Findings From Older Adults In The EPIC Cohort. *Appetite* **2014**, *83*, 248–255. [CrossRef]
69. Glass, C.; Haas, S.; Reither, E. The Skinny On Success: Body Mass, Gender And Occupational Standing Across The Life Course. *Social Forces* **2010**, *88*, 1777–1806. [CrossRef]
70. Duncan, D.; Wolin, K.; Scharoun-Lee, M.; Ding, E.; Warner, E.; Bennett, G. Does Perception Equal Reality? Weight Misperception in Relation to Weight-Related Attitudes and Behaviors among Overweight and Obese US Adults. *Int. J. Behav. Nutr. Phys. Act.* **2011**, *8*, 20. [CrossRef]
71. Millstein, R.A.; Carlson, S.A.; Fulton, J.E.; Galuska, D.A.; Zhang, J.; Blanck, H.M.; Ainsworth, B.E. Relationships between body size satisfaction and weight control practices among US adults. *Medscape J. Med.* **2008**, *10*, 119.
72. Burton, N.W.; Brown, W.; Dobson, A. Accuracy of body mass index estimated from self-reported height and weight in mid-aged Australian women. *Aust. N. Z. J. Public Health* **2010**, *34*, 620–623. [CrossRef]

73. Visscher, T.L.; Viet, A.L.; Kroesbergen, I.H.; Seidell, J.C. Underreporting of BMI in Adults and Its Effect on Obesity Prevalence Estimations in the Period 1998 to 2001. *Obesity* **2006**, *14*, 2054–2063. [CrossRef]
74. Kurina, L.M.; McClintock, M.K.; Chen, J.-H.; Waite, L.J.; Thisted, R.A.; Lauderdale, D.S. Sleep duration and all-cause mortality: A critical review of measurement and associations. *Ann. Epidemiol.* **2013**, *23*, 361–370. [CrossRef]

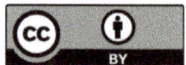

© 2020 by the authors. Licensee MDPI, Basel, Switzerland. This article is an open access article distributed under the terms and conditions of the Creative Commons Attribution (CC BY) license (http://creativecommons.org/licenses/by/4.0/).

MDPI
St. Alban-Anlage 66
4052 Basel
Switzerland
Tel. +41 61 683 77 34
Fax +41 61 302 89 18
www.mdpi.com

Nutrients Editorial Office
E-mail: nutrients@mdpi.com
www.mdpi.com/journal/nutrients

www.ingramcontent.com/pod-product-compliance
Lightning Source LLC
LaVergne TN
LVHW070436100526
838202LV00014B/1606